OXFORD MEDICAL PUBLICATIONS

Hydrocephalus

Dose schedules are being continually revised and new side-effects recognized. Oxford University Press makes no representation, express or implied, that the drug dosages in this book are correct. For these reasons the reader is strongly urged to consult the drug company's printed instructions before administering any of the drugs recommended in this book.

Hydrocephalus

Edited by

PETER H. SCHURR

Consultant Neurosurgeon Emeritus
Guy's Hospital and the Maudsley Hospital
London, UK

and

C. E. POLKEY

Consultant Neurosurgeon
The Maudsley Hospital
London, UK

Oxford   New York   Tokyo
OXFORD UNIVERSITY PRESS
1993

Oxford University Press, Walton Street, Oxford OX2 6DP

Oxford   New York   Toronto
Delhi   Bombay   Calcutta   Madras   Karachi
Kuala Lumpur   Singapore   Hong Kong   Tokyo
Nairobi   Dar es Salaam   Cape Town
Melbourne   Auckland   Madrid

and associated companies in
Berlin   Ibadan

Oxford is a trade mark of Oxford University Press

Published in the United States
by Oxford University Press Inc., New York

A catalogue record for this book is available from the British Library

Library of Congress Cataloging in Publication Data
Hydrocephalus/edited by Peter H. Schurr, C.E. Polkey.
p..   cm.   – – (Oxford medical publications)
Includes bibliography references and index.
1. Hydrocephalus.   I. Schurr, Peter H.   II. Polkey, C.E.   III. Series
[DNLM: 1. Hydrocephalus.   WL 350 H995]
RC331.1193   1993   818.85'8849 – – 0020   92.49516
ISBN 0 19 261863 6

Typeset by EXPO Holdings, Malaysia
Printed by Great Britain by
Bookcraft Ltd. Midsomer Norton, Avon

Preface

The treatment of hydrocephalus has passed beyond the stage of trial and error, and beyond the period in which numerous unsatisfactory techniques were developed and rejected, to a present state of some stability. It is, therefore, appropriate to bring together the experience of a number of well-known workers in this field in order to assess their current practice, their thoughts on the subject, and their knowledge of it.

This book is intended to be a work of reference, covering all aspects of the treatment and diagnosis of this condition in adults as well as children, together with various methods of investigation, and the relevant pathology. Particular attention has been paid, not only to the clinical features, but also to the sociological aspects, including intellectual ability, residual disability, and the quality of life.

It is hoped that the work will provide a source of information for all those involved in the care of patients with hydrocephalus; not only for neurosurgeons, paediatricians, and paediatric neurosurgeons, both established and in training, but also for other workers in the neurosciences, including general neurologists, neuropathologists, neuroradiologists, neurophysiologists, neuropsychologists, physiotherapists, and those concerned with rehabilitation. General practitioners have a special need to be informed of the complications of treatment and the expectations for the future of hydrocephalic patients, since they are being more and more involved in their aftercare.

Nurses and social workers are intimately concerned in the management of the problems which beset these patients and their relatives. It is also essential that they are possessed of up-to-date knowledge in order to give sound advice and comfort to anxious families.

Lastly, there are physicians and surgeons who work in relative isolation in various parts of the world, remote from specialized advice when there are problems. This book is partly written with a view to supplying answers to those questions which are most likely to arise in such circumstances.

The distinguished authors of the various chapters have been most generous in giving of their knowledge, expertise, and above all their time, and we are most grateful to them for this. However, responsibility for the opinions expressed is individual, and their views are not necessarily those of the editors; for this reason we have not sought for absolute uniformity on all points but have outlined the subject matter to be covered in each chapter, so that the book is comprehensive and overlap has been avoided as far as possible.

London   P.H.S.
June 1992   C.E.P.

Contents

Contributors

M.W.B. Bradbury Professor of Physiology, Department of Physiology, King's College London, The Strand, London, WC2R 2LS.

B. Chipchase Psychiatrist, Department of Psychiatry, University of Birmingham, Queen Elizabeth Psychiatric Hospital, Mindelsohn Way, Birmingham, B15 2QZ.

J. Corbett Professor of Developmental Psychiatry, Department of Psychiatry, University of Birmingham, Queen Elizabeth Psychiatric Hospital, Mindelsohn Way, Birmingham, B15 2QZ.

S. Cumella Senior Research Fellow, Department of Psychiatry, University of Birmingham, Queen Elizabeth Psychiatric Hospital, Mindelsohn Way, Birmingham, B15 2QZ.

B.N. Harding Senior Lecturer, Department of Histopathology (Neuropathology), The Hospital for Sick Children, Great Ormond Street, London, WC1N 3HJ.

R. Hemmer Emeritus Professor of Paediatric Neurosurgery, University of Freiburg, Mettackerweg 76, 7800 Freiburg, Germany.

E. Bruce Hendrick Emeritus Professor of Surgery (Neurosurgery), University of Toronto, 63 Legget Avenue, Weston, Ontario, Canada, M9P 1X3.

R.V. Jeffreys Consultant Neurosurgeon, Department of Neurosurgery, Walton Hospital, Rice Lane, Liverpool, L9 1AE.

S. Kida Department of Pathology (Neuropathology), University of Southampton; Level E, Laboratory and Pathology Block, Southampton General Hospital, Tremona Road, Southampton, SO9 4XY.

K.M. Laurence Emeritus Professor of Paediatric Research, University of Wales College of Medicine, Heath Park, Cardiff, CF4 4XN.

B.G.R. Neville Professor of Paediatric Neurology and Developmental Paediatrics, Institute of Child Health, The Wolfson Centre, Mecklenburgh Square, London, WC1N 2AP.

C.E. Polkey Consultant Neurosurgeon, The Neurosurgical Unit, The Maudsley Hospital, Denmark Hill, London, SE5 8AZ.

J. Punt Consultant Neurosurgeon, Department of Neurosurgery, University Hospital, Nottingham, NG7 2UH.

R.O. Robinson   Consultant Paediatric Neurologist, Newcomen Centre, Guy's Hospital, St Thomas Street, London, SE1 9RT.

Peter H. Schurr   Emeritus Consultant Neurosurgeon, Guy's Hospital and the Maudsley Hospital, Neurosurgical Unit of Guy's, Maudsley and King's College Hospital, The Maudsley Hospital, Denmark Hill, London, SE5 8AZ.

D. Simpson   Clinical Professor of Neurosurgery, University of Adelaide, Department of Neurosurgery, Children's Hospital Inc., 72 King William Road, North Adelaide 5006, Australia.

R.O. Weller   Professor of Neuropathology, Department of Pathology (Neuropathology), University of Southampton; Level E, Laboratory and Pathology Block, Southampton General Hospital, Tremona Road, Southampton, SO9 4XY.

1 Causes, incidence, and genetics of hydrocephalus

K.M. Laurence

INTRODUCTION

Hydrocephalus literally means 'water head' or 'water on the brain'. It is best defined as an excessive accumulation of cerebrospinal fluid (CSF) within the brain and cranial cavity.

TYPES OF HYDROCEPHALUS

As the bulk of the CSF is produced by the choroid plexuses, theoretically, hydrocephalus may be brought about by overproduction of the cerebrospinal fluid, defective reabsorption, or obstruction of the CSF pathway. This will result in the dilatation of the whole or part of the ventricular system and, in many instances, part of the extraventricular portion of the CSF pathway as well.

One form of hydrocephalus, '*hydrocephalus ex vacuo*' will be excluded from this chapter (pp. 72–3 and 78–9). Here an increased amount of CSF replaces the brain volume lost through brain destruction or failure to develop, whether this is local, as in schizencephaly and porencephaly, or more general as in hydranencephaly. When the whole brain is small following degeneration as in progressive degeneration of the cerebral cortex of infancy,[1] and senile or presenile dementia, or, occasionally because of failure to develop as in microcephaly, both ventri-cular dilatation and wide extracerebral CSF spaces (especially over the cerebral hemispheres) are usual.

Overproduction of CSF

Overproduction of CSF is now generally conceded to be a phenomenon accompanying choroid plexus papillomata which may be present at birth or develop in early infancy, but most appear in childhood or later in life. The cauliflower-like, friable and vascular tumour, attached to, or replacing a normal choroid plexus,[2] is usually situated in a lateral ventricle but may be found in the third or fourth ventricle. Overproduction of CSF, more than can be reabsorbed, occurs because of the increased bulk of histologically normal, functional choroid plexus tissue and the increased vascularity of the tumour. This causes the whole of the ventricular system and often the basal cisterns to be dilated. Undoubtedly, in many instances, there is an obstructive element as well, probably caused by bleeding from the tumour causing a degree of basal cistern block.

Underabsorption of CSF

Underabsorption of CSF theoretically would be brought about by obstruction of the venous return, as in venous sinus thrombosis. This, however, is not well authenticated and, in nearly every instance where this seems to be the cause of the hydrocephalus, an obstruction of the CSF pathway is found to be the true cause.[3]

Obstruction of the CSF pathway

Obstruction in the CSF pathway is numerically the only significant cause of hydrocephalus and was the main subject of the classical monograph by Dorothy Russell.[4]

The ventricular system dilates proximal to the blockage. When the latter is in the aqueduct of Sylvius both the lateral ventricles dilate. Obstruction of a foramen of Monro will cause just one to be enlarged. When the exit foramina (the foramina of Magendie and of Luschka) are blocked, then the whole of the ventricular system dilates. A basal cistern block causes dilatation of the posterior fossa cistern as well. Blocks may be multiple, especially after inflammatory conditions.

If the hydrocephalus has a developmental aetiology, it may be quite advanced by the time of birth and will be 'congenital' in origin. However, certain prenatal infections, with rubella, cytomegalovirus and herpes simplex virus, or with toxoplasma, may also lead to 'congenital' hydrocephalus. Gliosis of the aqueduct is uncommon. It is likely to be hamartomatous and may be seen as part of the neurofibromatosis complex.[5,6]

DEVELOPMENTAL ABNORMALITIES LEADING TO HYDROCEPHALUS

Distinction has to be made between 'uncomplicated' hydrocephalus, in which the hydrocephalus is the primary condition — usually due to a single anatomical abnormality — and 'complicated' hydrocephalus where it is secondary to another malformation, such as spina bifida (myelocele or myelomeningocele), or part of some malformation complex or syndrome. Hydrocephalus is seen in over 80 per cent of newborn children with myelocele (myelomeningocele) and is usually well established quite early in the second trimester.[7] The only exceptions to this are cases where the spinal lesion is situated in the sacral region. Hydrocephalus often accompanies chromosome disorders such as 13 trisomy and 18 trisomy and triploidy, arhinencephaly, Meckel–Gruber syndrome and Albers–Schönberg syndrome. Ventricular dilatation is occasionally seen complicating quite a number of other malformation syndromes and genetic disorders, such as Apert syndrome, oro–facial–digital syndrome, Hurler syndrome, thanatophoric dysplasia, achondroplasia and osteogenesis imperfecta, and incontinentia pigmentii syndrome, amongst others.[8] In addition, there are increasing reports of apparently rare malformation complexes where hydrocephalus is one of the components.[5,9–14]

The aqueduct of Sylvius, linking the third and fourth ventricles, may be blocked by developmental stenosis where the channel is narrowed and then occluded, or it may be constricted by forking where the single channel splits into two or more smaller branches, some of which may end blindly.[15] The former usually causes the ventricular dilatation in X-linked hydrocephalus, the latter is often found in association with spina bifida.

The Arnold–Chiari malformation which accompanies nearly all cases of myelocele (or myelomeningocele) is one of the causes of the accompanying hydrocephalus. It can be seen as early as the tenth week of gestation, and is a complicated and variable abnormality where the pons and medulla and the cerebellum, together with the fourth ventricle, crowd into a small posterior fossa and upper cervical spinal canal, causing compression of the exit foramina and the subarachnoid space which become fibrosed.[15] In the Dandy–Walker syndrome, the exit foramina fail to develop in the first trimester, giving rise to a large fourth ventricular cyst and cerebellar abnormalities.[16,17]

ACQUIRED CONDITIONS LEADING TO HYDROCEPHALUS

Blood in the CSF may cause blockage of the aqueduct through a blood clot or through denudation of the ependyma followed by a reactive gliosis or blockage of the exit-foramina or basal cisterns, also through a reactive fibrosis. Obvious birth injury is now less common but haemorrhage can occur without very obvious birth trauma or difficulty. Intraventricular haemorrhage caused by periventricular bleeding following hypoxia in very premature or low birthweight infants is, however, more common now because of the increasingly common survival of the very immature.[18] Head injury and haemorrhage in later life may also lead to hydrocephalus.

Intrauterine, neonatal and later intracranial infections of bacterial, protozoal, or viral aetiology also lead to hydrocephalus, usually with aqueduct or basal cistern block. However, in a considerable proportion of cases of hydrocephalus beginning in early infancy with a basal cistern blockage, there is neither any history of birth trauma nor of intracranial infection.

Hydrocephalus may also be caused by congenital tumours or tumours occurring in later infancy or childhood, either through direct obstruction of the CSF pathway by the tumour itself or through haemorrhage from a vascular tumour leading to an inflammatory blockage.

INCIDENCE AND EPIDEMIOLOGY OF HYDROCEPHALUS

Hydrocephalus is a relatively common finding in stillbirth, the newborn period, or early infancy. However, often the condition has been acquired around the time of birth, is secondary to spina bifida, or may be part of a malformation syndrome. In addition, it may be wrongly diagnosed in stillbirths when maceration causes the head to appear relatively large.[17]

'Uncomplicated' congenital hydrocephalus is a less frequent diagnosis in carefully conducted malformation surveys that depend on reliable confirmatory evidence, including post-mortem examination. Prevalences of about 1/1000 births have been reported from eastern USA,[19] Hungary,[20] and Southampton,[21] 0.7/1000 from Belfast,[22] 0.6/1000 from Australia,[23] 0.4/1000 from South Wales,[24] Liverpool,[25] and Sweden.[26] The higher prevalences, 1.5/1000 or more,[27,-29] are probably due to undue reliance on certification, often without confirmatory evidence.

Bearing reporting differences in mind, it is probable that the incidence of 'uncomplicated' congenital hydrocephalus varies little from population to population and has altered little over the years,[30] affecting males about twice as frequently as females.[23] About one third of cases have aqueduct stenosis. Fewer show a block of the fourth ventricular exit-foramina and most of the remainder have a basal cistern block.[17] A considerable proportion of the latter, especially, are probably acquired either in the second half of pregnancy or perinatally, even though there may be no aetiological pointers.

Hydrocephalus complicating spina bifida affects females slightly more frequently than males, and shows considerable geographical variations being most frequent in the British Isles, where South Wales and Ireland have, until recently, had a prevalence of over 4/1000 births. Egypt and northern India also have relatively high prevalence rates.[31] Most of Europe and North America has a prevalence of around 1/1000 births, but there are lower prevalences in Finland, amongst the Jews, the Eastern Asiatics and the Afro-Americans.[31] There has also been a considerable change over time. Not only has the true prevalence dropped very considerably in Britain over the last two decades[32,33] but, in addition, the birth prevalence has dwindled following the introduction of early prenatal diagnosis and selective abortion, so that in South Wales the incidence since 1985 has been only about 0.2/1000 births.[32] (Fig. 1.1).

The occurrence of acquired hydrocephalus varies greatly from population to population and depends largely on the standard of medical care, but no reliable data are available about the incidences in various countries. Improved obstetric services result in less birth trauma and, therefore, less post-haemorrhagic hydrocephalus. However, the survival in recent years of severely premature infants, some of whom develop intraventricular haemorrhage and complicating hydrocephalus, has increased.[18] Neonatal and later meningitis is more effectively treated, resulting in less complicating hydrocephalus, but, unfortunately, not all cases are recognized early and treated effectively everywhere.

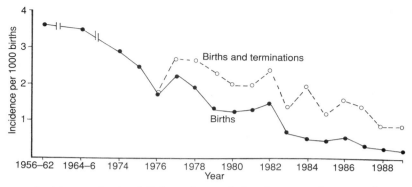

Fig. 1.1 Incidence of spina bifida and encephalocele in South East Wales. Births and terminations between 1956 and 1989.

GENETICS OF CONGENITAL HYDROCEPHALUS

Few family studies designed to throw light on both the genetics and the recurrence risk have been reported for 'uncomplicated' congenital hydrocephalus where cases with an acquired aetiology have been excluded.

'Uncomplicated' congenital hydrocephalus

Details of six studies carried out specifically on families of index cases with only congenital hydrocephalus, and five on neural tube defect (NTD) which comprised anencephaly and spina bifida (and encephalocele) and which also included index cases on 'uncomplicated' congenital hydrocephalus are shown in Table 1.1. The pooled family data on the 1739 sibs of 1110 probands had 32 cases with congenital hydrocephalus suggesting that the recurrence risk is about 1 in 55 (1.8 per cent or between 15 and 30 times the population risk). Taking the five family studies carried out on hydrocephalic patients only, there were 10 recurrences amongst 613 sibs, giving a very similar risk of 1 in 60. The risk to sibs of affected boys is twice as great (1 in 40) as that to affected girls (1 in 80). Information on the risk to cousins, who bear a third degree relationship to probands, is rather scanty but this seems to be about 1 in 300, or about four times the population risk. There is no information available on the risk to children when one of the parents had hydrocephalus but, as this is a first degree relationship, it is likely that the risk is similar to that in sibs.

The risk of recurrence suggests that the majority of cases of 'uncomplicated' congenital hydrocephalus, like most other so-called common malformations, probably have a multifactorial aetiology where the genetic component is polygenic, rendering the developing fetus liable to environmental influences. The latter, in the case of hydrocephalus, must be active rather later than those responsible for NTD but these have not yet been identified, though maternal virus infections are known to lead to some cases. The lower risk of recurrence for 'uncomplicated' hydrocephalus compared with that found for most other

Table 1.1 Family studies on 'uncomplicated' congenital hydrocephalus

Locality	Number of probands	Number of sibs			
		Total	Anencephaly	Spina Bifida	Hydrocephalus
Hungary[60]	149	121	1	0	7
Rhode Island[61]	86	54	0	0	1
Southampton[21]	15[†]	31	0	0	1
South Wales[24]	45[†]	109	1	0	2
Liverpool[25]	111[†]	206	4	0	6
Budapest[20]	91	144	0	0	0
Chicago[9]	205[*]	353	0	0	5
London[35]	24	50	0	0	1
Belfast[22]	78[†]	159	0	1	3
Sheffield[37]	250[**†]	417	4	4	4
San Francisco[40]	56[*]	95	0	0	2
Total	1110	1739	10	5	32

[*] Cases of aqueduct stenosis also included in Table 1.2
[*] Highly selected series
[†] Population with high prevalence of NTD.

common malformations is probably because some cases have a purely postnatal acquired aetiology even though no suggestive history can be obtained.

Congenital hydrocephalus due to aqueduct stenosis

Most cases of aqueduct stenosis probably have a multifactorial aetiology but it has been estimated that 2 per cent of isolated 'uncomplicated' hydrocephalus and, therefore, by extrapolation, just over 5 per cent of isolated aqueduct stenosis in males may be of the X-linked variety.[34] This is rather less than the 6–12 per cent suggested by the Australian study, when those with tumours, cysts and an obvious acquired aetiology are excluded.[23]

Two family studies carried out on hydrocephalus due to aqueduct stenosis (from London and Victoria, Australia) can be added to two other studies on hydrocephalus of various types, from Chicago and San Francisco, where the cases due to aqueduct stenosis had been identified (Table 1.2).

When the results of the London study of Howard, Till, and Carter are combined with those from San Francisco and Chicago but excluding the two families from the latter study where there seemed to be a definite X-linked mode of inheritance,[35] it is estimated that in 211 sibs, the risk for brothers of an affected male was about 1 in 22 (4.5 per cent) and for sisters only about 1 in 50 (2 per cent). The conclusions drawn from the Australian study were almost the same. In the case of an affected female, the risk to either brothers or sisters was probably no more than 1 in 100. Although, again, no data are available on the children of successfully treated adults with aqueduct stenosis, the risk to children would be expected to be similar to those for sibs.

Table 1.2 Family studies on hydrocephalus due to aqueduct stenosis

Locality	Number of Probands	Total	Number of sibs NTD	Hydrocephalus
Chicago[*9]	88	126	0	4
San Francisco[40]	20	35	0	2
London[35]	24	50	0	1
Victoria[23]	66	156	2	4
Total	198	367	2	11

[*] Two families with X-linked hydrocephalus excluded.

Relationship between 'uncomplicated' hydrocephalus and neural tube defect (NTD)

At first sight it would appear that there is also an added risk of NTD for the sibs of cases of 'uncomplicated' hydrocephalus.[36,37] However, over half the sibs with NTD have come from the Sheffield study which seems to have been based on a selected series rather than on a population study. Omitting this study the risk is reduced to 5.0/1000 instead of 8.7/1000. As the majority of probands were drawn from populations in which the incidence of NTD ranged from 4 to over 8/1000 births, this risk no longer seems extraordinary. Family studies of anencephaly and spina bifida, also largely carried out in high incidence areas, show that amongst the 9509 sibs of probands, there were 436 with NTD, about 1 in 22 (4.5 per cent), but only 26 sibs with 'uncomplicated' hydrocephalus (Table 1.3), representing a risk of 1 in 365 (0.27 per cent), or 3.3 times the population risk. However, when the second study from Sheffield[38] (based again on a selected

Table 1.3 Family studies carried out on anencephaly and spina bifida

Locality	Number of Probands	Total	Number of sibs Anencephaly	Spina Bifida	Hydrocephalus
Lund[62]	67	87	0	1	0
Rhode Island[61]	1037	1263	28	30	5
Paris[63]	254[+]	423	5	3	1
Southampton[21]	88	160	3	6	0
South Wales[24]	790	1562	36	45	1
London[48]	870	1484	36	30	2
Liverpool[25]	1327	1790	46	24	7
Budapest[20]	443	579	3	13	1
Glasgow[66]	318	904	24	27	0
Sheffield[38]	539[*]	1256	22	54	9
Total	5733	9509	203	233	26

[+] Anencephaly only
[*] Selected series of spina bifida.

series rather than on a total population and which is the only one with a relatively large number of cases of 'uncomplicated' hydrocephalus amongst the sib component) is excluded, then the risk decreases to 1 in 485 (0.20 per cent) or 2.5 times the population risk (Table 1.4).

Over a 12-year-period almost 1300 families, where the proband had a dysraphic neural tube defect, have been seen in the South Wales Genetic Clinics, and 70 where the proband had 'uncomplicated' hydrocephalus. In all these families, careful enquiries were made about the outcome of all the pregnancies of the parents concerned. The 1279 NTD probands had 2380 sibs (including pregnancies terminated after 16 weeks' gestation and stillbirths of 28 weeks' gestation or more). These included 120 who had either spina bifida or anencephaly (recurrences of 1 in 20) and four with 'uncomplicated' hydrocephalus (1 in 600). In two of the latter, this followed traumatic delivery with bleeding into the cerebrospinal fluid, leaving only two cases where the hydrocephalus was likely to have been 'congenital'. This would give a risk of only 1 in 1200, or the population risk. The 79 hydrocephalic probands had 121 sibs with no NTDs and one with hydrocephalus. The number of 'hydrocephalic' families is too small to be meaningful but the trend is in keeping with the other results.

Excluding the two Sheffield series, which seem to have atypical recurrence risks from all the others, both the relatively low risks of 'uncomplicated' hydrocephalus amongst the sibs of probands with NTD, and the low risk of NTD amongst the sibs of cases of 'uncomplicated' hydrocephalus, lend little support for the view held that NTD and 'uncomplicated' hydrocephalus have a largely common aetiology. 'Uncomplicated' congenital hydrocephalus, therefore, does not seem to be part of the anencephaly–spina bifida spectrum of NTDs.

Hydrocephalus due to distinct monogenic disorders

X-linked aqueduct stenosis

This is a rare form with an incidence of probably no more than 1 in 30 000 live and stillborn births and probably only 1 in 60 000 males, where the hydrocephalus is combined with disproportionately severe mental retardation and

Table 1.4 Comparison of recurrences in the Sheffield and the other family studies of hydrocephalus.[23,34-38]

Type of study	Number of sibs			Number of recurrences	
	Total	Sheffield excluded	Sheffield only	NTD	Hydrocephalus
NTD probands	9509	—	—	436(1:22)	26(1:365)
	—	8253	—	360(1:23)	17(1:485)
	—	—	1256	76(1:16)	9(1:140)
Hydrocephalus	613	—	—	9(1:68)	10(1:60)
	—	363	—	1(1:360)	6(1:60)
	—	—	250	8(1:31)	4(1:63)

spasticity and also adducted, flexed thumbs. In addition to aqueduct stenosis there is absence of the pyramids in the medulla and there may be other brain abnormalities such as fused thalamic bodies and agenesis of the corpus callosum.[23] X-linked hydrocephalus, which would perhaps be better termed X-linked mental retardation with aqueduct stenosis, should be borne in mind in any male with 'uncomplicated' hydrocephalus, especially one with unexpected severe mental retardation and spasticity, and seriously suspected if there is an affected brother or hydrocephalic male relative on the maternal side of the family.[33] The condition is somewhat variable in its expression and may be confined to the thumb abnormality, or mental retardation and spasticity without any obvious hydrocephalus. The majority of cases are stillborn or die in infancy. The mother of a case is likely to be a carrier and tends to be on the 'dull side'[23] (as could be other female relatives), and there will then be a 1 in 2 risk of any son being affected, and a similar risk of any daughter being a carrier.

Dandy–Walker syndrome

Although the majority of cases of Dandy–Walker syndrome seem to be sporadic and probably polygenic in aetiology, some undoubtedly have an autosomal recessive mode of inheritance,[3,39–41] with a 1 in 4 risk of recurrence in sibs.

Autosomal recessively inherited congenital hydrocephalus

A few cases of hydrocephalus must be recessively inherited as there are a number of families on record where multiple children of both sexes with hydrocephalus but without an accompanying malformation, have been born to unaffected but often consanguineous parents.[42–45] The risk of recurrence then would be 1 in 4.

Genetics of hydrocephalus associated with spina bifida (and encephalocele)

Spina bifida (myelocele, myelomeningocele, and meningocele), encephalocele and anencephaly, and its variants, but not isolated 'uncomplicated' hydrocephalus, together with 'complicated' spina bifida occulta[46] and certain vertebral abnormalities,[47] arise as a result of faulty closure of the neural groove which should start to close at about the 18th and be complete by the 26th day after conception.[33] These NTDs are all interrelated and represent different end-products of the same general process. The NTDs are part of the so-called 'common malformations'; these have a multifactorial aetiology with a genetic predisposition which is due to two or more genes and a threshold beyond which the embryos are at risk of developing the malformations if environmental triggers act during the teratogenic period.[48]

Family and epidemiological studies which are usually carried out only on the major NTDs (spina bifida, encephalocele, and anencephaly), suggest that the risk of recurrence after one previous NTD is about 1 in 22,[49] that the risk to half-sibs, nephews and nieces, and cousins is in a descending order (Table 1.5)

Table 1.5 Incidence of NTD in relatives

Person at risk	Risk
Population incidence	1 in 340[*]
Sibs after one affected	1 in 22[*]
Sibs after two affected	1 in 10[**]
Half sibs	1 in 50[*]
Children	1 in 23[***]
Aunts, uncles, nephews, nieces	1 in 70[*]
Cousins (on mothers' side)	1 in 148[*]

[*]   Based on data published by Carter and Evans on South Eastern English Population.[49]
[**]   Based on a study by Carter and Roberts[65]
[***] Based on data from South Wales, South Eastern England, and Germany.[66]

and that the recurrence risk depends, to some extent, on the population incidence of NTD. Indeed, between 1956 and 1962 when the incidence of spina bifida and encephalocele in South Wales was 3.5/1000 births, the recurrence risk was about 1 in 20.[24] Since then this risk has fallen to less than 1 in 60 now that the incidence of affected pregnancies is fewer than 1 in 1000 (Laurence, unpublished data). The family studies show that, on average, 60–70 per cent of the causation of NTD is genetic, leaving the remainder due to environmental trigger factors which seem to include a few drugs, such as sodium valproate,[50] certain steroid hormones (including oral contraceptives), (Laurence, unpublished data) maternal diabetes, and possibly hyperthermia and poor maternal nutrition. It has been shown in several studies that the latter leads to an increased risk of having a pregnancy with an NTD, and that dietary counselling and improvement in the maternal diet in time for the start of a pregnancy reduces the risk of recurrence.[51–53] Further, preconceptional supplementation with folic acid,[37,51,54] and periconceptional supplementation with a combination of vitamins and folic acid,[55] also appears to have a beneficial effect in reducing the recurrence risk. However, the general fall in the number of pregnancies affected with neural tube defects (spina bifida amongst them) in the last two decades, is unlikely to be due to any active measures which have been undertaken, such as dietary counselling and supplementation, but more likely be due to demographic changes which have taken place and to improvement in the general standard of living and particularly of maternal nutrition (Laurence, unpublished data). The dramatic fall in the number of affected infants born, on the other hand, is almost entirely due to pregnancy screening with maternal serum alpha–fetoprotein and antenatal ultrasound followed by selective abortion, rather than to prenatal diagnosis in high-risk pregnancies, as over 9 out of 10 affected pregnancies occur in families without any previous obstetric or family history of NTD.

Not all spina bifida and encephalocele has a polygenic aetiology. In a very few families the lesion seems to have a monogenic mode of inheritance[56] and some cases have a chromosome trisomy or triploidy. Encephalocele may be part of Mechel–Gruber syndrome (encephalocele, polydactyly, polycystic kidneys) and is then recessively inherited.[8]

PRENATAL DIAGNOSIS OF HYDROCEPHALUS

Early prenatal diagnostic tests should be considered for any pregnancy in which there is an increased risk of hydrocephalus. Parents may well want to have a pregnancy of an affected fetus terminated. Some, however, may wish intrauterine treatment to be carried out, though this is still controversial and the results questionable. Others might opt for premature elective caesarean section to minimize the risk of brain damage, followed by an immediate neonatal shunting operation.[57]

X-ray examination is not only undesirable in pregnancy, but is also unhelpful in the identification of hydrocephalus, except near term when it may aid a decision about the management of delivery.

With modern real-time, high resolution ultrasound equipment, an experienced skilled ultrasonographer coupled with patience and high-resolution ultrasonography, which is non-invasive and safe, can demonstrate ventricular dilatation as an area of sonolucency inside the echogenic line produced by the fetal skull as early as 15 weeks' gestation (Fig. 1.2) and usually by 20 weeks.[58] The maximum transverse diameter of the lateral ventricle should not exceed 9 mm in mid-trimester and the body of the ventricle should be largely filled by the choroid plexus. However, early hydrocephalus may not be easily demonstrable and repeat scans may have to be considered at 20, 24, and even 28 weeks, especially for those forms of hydrocephalus such as aqueduct stenosis which may not develop until later in pregnancy. The head size alone, (fetal biparietal diameter), is not a reliable guide to the presence of hydrocephalus. In hydrocephalus associated with spina bifida, marked ventricular dilatation is often present without enlargement of the skull and the biparietal diameter measurement is, on average, smaller than normal and gives readings which would suggest that the gestation is two weeks less than the actual dates.[59]

The ultrasonographic findings can be misleading. Relative ventricular widening of the normal mid-trimester brain has to be distinguished from pathological widening. Echogenic lines may give a false impression of the ventricular wall and echo-free areas may mistakenly suggest a widened ventricular space. An ultrasonic diagnosis should be followed by further examinations for confirmation before termination of pregnancy is offered if the tragedy of a mistake is to be avoided.

The presence of spina bifida, or an encephalocele, should lead to a search for hydrocephalus, and vice versa. The normal spine in the longitudinal axis is seen as a pair of continuously interrupted parallel lines which become confluent in the sacral region and diverge in the cervical areas.[58] The loss of parallelism or a

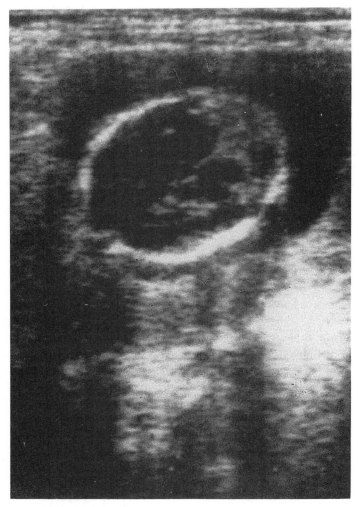

Fig. 1.2 Ultrasonogram of the skull of a 17 week hydrocephalic fetus with moderate/severely dilated ventricles.

splaying irregularity at the level of the malformation (Fig. 1.3), a kyphos, the interruption of the fetal skin surface, or an open U- or V-shaped canal (Fig. 1.4) seen instead of the normal ring structure in transverse section, should suggest the presence of a serious spina bifida.[58] This, in turn, should lead to a critical examination of the fetal head for hydrocephalus which accompanies the great majority of cases. Similarly, a misshapen head with compression of the frontal bones (Fig. 1.5) the so called 'Lemon sign', or the 'banana sign' (Fig. 1.6) of the Arnold–Chiari malformation should warn the ultrasonographer that hydrocephalus may be present.[58]

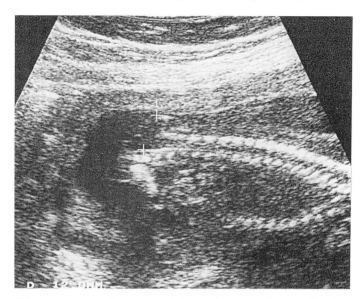

Fig. 1.3 Ultrasonogram of an 18 week fetus showing a longitudinal view of a fetal spine with a sacral spina bifida and associated sac.

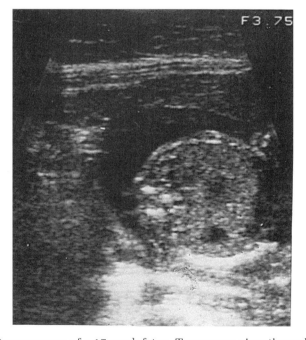

Fig. 1.4 Ultrasonogram of a 17 week fetus. Transverse view through the trunk, showing a vertebral body, open vertebral arches, and discontinuous skin which is replaced by a bulging membrane.

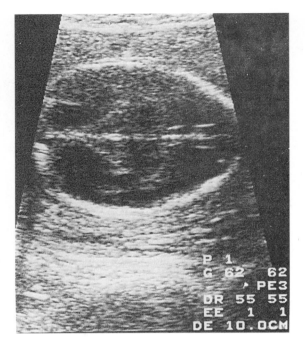

Fig. 1.5 Ultrasonogram of a 16 week fetal skull showing the 'lemon' sign —
relative narrowing of the frontal region.

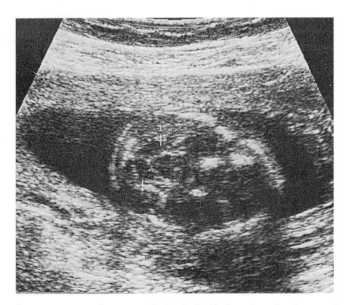

Fig. 1.6 Ultrasonogram of a 16 week fetal skull showing the 'banana' sign —
curvilinear hyperdensity suggestive of an Arnold–Chiari malformation.

First trimester chorionic villous biopsy or amniocentesis may need to be considered for fetal sexing to be carried out in a pregnancy at risk for X-linked aqueduct stenosis, if it is intended to terminate a potentially affected male pregnancy.[33] Unless the parents request it, amniocentesis followed by biochemical tests purely for the identification of open NTD is not justified, as it is an invasive procedure which carries a definite risk of sequential abortion.[33] A high precision ultrasound scan for head and spinal abnormality and a serum alpha-fetoprotein estimation at 16 weeks should suffice as any additional risk of NTD, if indeed there is one, is low.[33]

REFERENCES

1. Laurence, K.M. and Cavanagh, J.B. Progressive degeneration of the cerebral cortex in infancy. *Brain*, **91**, 261–80 (1968).
2. Laurence, K.M. The biology of choroid plexus papilloma and carcinoma of the lateral ventricle. In *Handbook of clinical neurology* (ed. Vinken, P.J. and Bruyn, G.W.) Vol. 17, Tumours of the skull and brain, pp. 555–95 North Holland Publishing Co, Aurstesdam (1974).
3. Afifi, A.K., Jacoby, C.G., Bell, W.E., and Menezes, A.H. Aqueductal stenosis and neurofibromatosis, a rare association. *Journal of Child Neurology*, **3**, 125–30 (1988).
4. Russell, D.S. *Observations on the pathology of hydrocephalus*. HMSO, London (1949).
5. Levin, H., Ritch, R., Barathier, R., Dunn, M.W., Teekhasaenee, C., and Margolis, S. Aniridia, congenital glaucoma and hydrocephalus in a male with ring chromosome 6. *American Journal of Medical Genetics*, **25**, 281–7 (1986).
6. Laurence, K.M. The pathology of hydrocephalus. *Annals of the Royal College of Surgeons*, **24**, 388–401 (1959).
7. Laurence, K.M., Dew, J.O., Dyer, C., and Downey, K.M. Amniocentesis carried out for neural tube indications in South Wales: outcome of pregnancies and findings in the abortuses. *Prenatal Diagnosis*, **3**, 187–201 (1983).
8. Smith, D.W. *Recognisable patterns of human malformations*, (3rd edn) W.B. Saunders Co, Philadelphia (1982).
9. Burton, B.K. Recurrence risk for congenital hydrocephalus. *Clinical Genetics*, **16**, 47–53 (1979).
10. Chow, C.W., McKelvie, P.A., Anderson, R.Mc.D., Phelan, E.M.D., Klug, G.L., and Rogers J.G. Austosomal recessive hydrocephalus with third ventricle obstruction. *American Journal of Medical Genetics*, **35**, 310–13 (1990).
11. Daish, P., Hardman, M.J., and Lamont, M.A. Hydrocephalus, tall stature, joint laxity, kyphosis: a new inherited disorder of connective tissue? *Journal of Medical Genetics*, **26**, 51–4 (1989).
12. Game, K., Friedman, J.M., Paradice, B., and Norman, G.M. Fetal growth retardation, hydrocephalus and hypoplastic multi-lobed lungs. *American Journal of Medical Genetics*, **33**, 276–9 (1989).
13. Pierquin, G., Deroover, J., Levi, S., Masson, T., Hayez-Delatte, F, and Van Rege Morter, N. Dandy–Walker syndrome with polydactyly: a new syndrome. *American Journal of Medical Genetics*, **33**, 483–4 (1989).
14. Winter, R.M., Campbell, S., Wigglesworth, J.S. and Nevokla, E.J. A previously undescribed syndrome of thoracic dysplasia and communicating hydrocephalus in

two sibs, one diagnosed prenatally by ultrasound. *Journal of Medical Genetics*, **24**, 204–6 (1987).

15. Laurence, K.M. Hydrocephalus and malformations of the central nervous system. In *Fetal and neonatal pathology*, (ed. Keeling, J.), pp. 463–90. Springer Verlag, Berlin (1987).

16. Bickers, D.S. and Adams, R.D. Hereditary stenosis of the aqueduct of Sylvius as a cause of congenital hydrocephalus. *Brain*, **72**, 246–62 (1949).

17. Laurence, K.M. Genetic aspects of 'uncomplicated' hydrocephalus and its relationship to neural tube defect. *Zeitschrift für Kinderchirurgie*, **39**, (Suppl. II), 96–9 (1984).

18. Fernell, E., Hagberg, B., Hagberg, G., and Van Wendt, L. Epidemiology of infantile hydrocephalus in Sweden: 1. Birth prevalence and general data. *Acta Paediatrica Scandinavica*, **75**, 975–81 (1986).

19. MacMahon, B., Pugh, T.F., and Ingels, T.H. Anencephalus, spina bifida and hydrocephalus. *British Journal of Preventive and Social Medicine*, **7**, 211–19 (1953).

20. Czeizel, A. and Reversz, C. Major malformation of the central nervous system in Hungary *British Journal of Preventive and Social Medicine*, **24**, 205–22 (1970).

21. Williamson, E.M. Incidence and family aggregation of major congenital malformations of the central nervous system. *Journal of Medical Genetics*, **2**, 161–72 (1965).

22. Adams, C., Johnston, W.P. and Nevin, N.C. Family study of congenital hydrocephalus. *Developmental Medicine and Child Neurology*, **24**, 493–8 (1982).

23. Halliday, J., Chow, C.W., Wallace, D., and Danks, D.M. X-linked hydrocephalus: a survey of a 20 year period in Victoria, Australia. *Journal of Medical Genetics*, **23**, 23–31 (1986).

24. Carter, C.O., David, P.A., and Laurence, K.M. A family study of central nervous system malformations in South Wales. *Journal of Medical Genetics*, **5**, 81–106 (1968).

25. Smithells, R.W., D'Arcy, E.E., and McAllister, E.F. Outcome of pregnancies before and after birth of infants with nervous system malformations. *Developmental Medicine and Child Neurology*, Suppl. 15, 6–10 (1968).

26. Böök, J.A. The incidence of congenital disease and defects in a south Swedish population. *Acta Genetica (Basel)*, **2**, 289–311 (1951).

27. McKeown, T. and Record, R.G. Malformations in a population observed for five years after birth. In *Ciba Symposium: Congenital malformations*, (ed. Wolstonholme, G.E.W. and O'Connor, C.M.), pp. 2–27. Churchill, London (1960).

28. Record, R.G. and McKeown, T. Congenital malformations of the central nervous system. I. Survey of 930 cases. *British Journal of Preventive and Social Medicine*, **3**, 183–219 (1949).

29. Stephenson, A.C., Johnston, H.A., Stewart, M.I.P., and Golding, D.R. Congenital malformations. *Bulletin of the World Health Organization*, **34**, Suppl. 1–125 (1966).

30. Wiswell, T.E., Tuttle, D.J., Northam, R.S., and Simonds, G.R. Major congenital neurologic malformations: a 17 year study. *American Journal of Diseases of Childho.d*, **144**, 61–7 (1990).

31. Elwood, J.M. and Elwood, J.H. *The epidemiology of anencephalus and spina bifida*. Oxford University Press, Oxford (1980).

32. Laurence, K.M. Declining incidence of neural tube defects in the U.K. *Zeitschrift für Kinderchirurgie*, **44** (Suppl. 1), 51, (1989).

33. Laurence, K.M. Genetics and prevention of neural tube defects and 'uncomplicated' hydrocephalus In *Principles and practice of medical genetics*, (ed. Emery, A.E.H. and Rimoin, D.L.). 323–46 Edinburgh, Churchill Livingstone, (1990).

34. Sex-linked hydrocephalus with severe mental defects. *British Medical Journal*, **1**, 168 (1962).

35. Howard, F.M., Till, K., and Carter, C.O. A family study of hydrocephalus resulting from aqueduct stenosis. *Journal of Medical Genetics*, **18**, 252–5 (1981).

36. Lorber, J. Family history of spina bifida cystica. *Paediatrics*, **35**, 589–95 (1965).

37. Lorber, J. and De, N.C. Family history of congenital hydrocephalus. *Developmental Medicine and Child Neurology*, **12** (Suppl 2), 94–100 (1970).

38. Lorber, J. Family history of congenital hydrocephalus. In *Der Hydrocephalus internus im frühen Kindesalter*, (ed. Voth, D.), pp 61–7. Enke, Stuttgart (1983).

39. Benda, C.E. Dandy–Walker syndrome or the so-called atresia of the foramen of Magendie. *Journal of Neuropathology and Experimental Neurology*, **13**, 14–29 (1954).

40. Bay, C., Kerzin, L., and Hall, B.D. Recurrence risk in hydrocephalus birth defects. *Org, Art, Series*, **15** (5c), 95–105 (1975).

41. D'Argostini, A.N., Kenohan, J.W., and Brown, J.R. Dandy–Walker syndrome. *Journal of Neuropathology and Experimental Neurology*, **22**, 450–70 (1963).

42. Buttiens M., Fryns J.P., and Van den Berghe, H. An apparently new autosomal recessive syndrome with facial dysmorphology. *Clinical Genetics*, **36**, 451–5 (1989).

43. Dignan P.St J. and Warkany, J. Congenital malformations: hydrocephaly. *Mental Retardation* **6**, 44 (1973).

44. Fowler, M.R., Dow, R., White, T.A., and Greer, C.H. Congenital hydrocephalus — hydrocephaly in 5 siblings with autopsy studies. A new disease. *Developmental Medicine and Child Neurology*, **14**, 173–88 (1971).

45. Mehne, R.G. Three hydrocephalic newborns each of a successive pregnancy of a white female. *Archives of Paediatrics*, **78**, 67–71 (1961).

46. Laurence, K.M., Bligh, A.S., Evans, K.T., and Shurtleff, D.B. Vertebral abnormalities in parents and sibs of cases of spina bifida cystica and anencephaly. *Proceedings of the 13th International Congress of Paediatrics*, Vol. V, pp. 415–21 Wiener Medizinischen Akademie Verlag, Wien(1971).

47. Wynne-Davies, R. Congenital vertebral anomalies: aetiology and relationship to spina bifida cystica. *Journal of Medical Genetics*, **12**, 280–8 (1976).

48. Carter, C.O. Clues to the aetiology of neural tube malformations. *Developmental Medicine and Child Neurology*, **16,** (Suppl. 32), 3–15 (1974).

49. Carter, C.O. and Evans. K. Spina bifida and anencephaly in Greater London. *Journal of Medical Genetics*, **10**, 209–34 (1973).

50. Ardinger, H.H. Verification of the fetal Valproate syndrome phenotype. *American Journal of Medical Genetics*, **29**, 171–86 (1988).

51. Laurence, K.M., Campbell, H., and James, N. The role of improvement in the maternal diet and preconceptional folic acid supplementation in the prevention of neural tube defects. In *Prevention of spina bifida and other neural tube defects*, (ed. Dobbing, J.) pp. 85–125. Dobbing Academic Press, London (1983).

52. Laurence, K.M., James, N., Miller, M., and Campbell, H. The increased risk of recurrence of neural tube defects to mothers on poor diets and the possible benefit of dietary counselling. *British Medical Journal*, **281**, 1542–4 (1980).

53. Laurence, K.M., James, N., Miller, M.H. Tennant, G.B. and Campbell, H. Double blind randomised controlled trial of preconceptional folate therapy to prevent neural tube defects. *British Medical Journal*, **282**, 1509–11 (1981).

54. Vogal, R.G., Saches, L.R., Heredero, B.L., Rodrigues, P.L., and Martinez, A.J. Primary prevention of NTD with folic acid supplementation: Cuban experience. *Prenatal Diagnosis*, **10**, 149–52 (1990).

55. Smithells, R.W., Sheppard, S., Schorah, C.J., Seller, M.J., Nevin, N.C., Harris, R., Read, A.P., and Fielding, D.W. Possible prevention of neural tube defects by periconceptional vitamin supplementation. *Lancet*, **i**, 339–40 (1980).

56. Fuhrmann, W., Seeger, W., and Bohm, R. Apparently monogenic inheritance of anencephaly and spina bifida in a kindred. *Human genetik*, **13**, 241–3 (1971).

57. Shurtleff, D.B. Prenatal diagnosis: prevention and management for improved pregnancy outcome. In *Myelodysplasias and extrophies*. (ed. Shurtleff, D.B.) pp. 65–87. Grune & Stratton, Orlando (1986).

58. Romero, R., Pilu, G., Jeanty, P., Chidini, A., and Hobbins, J.C. *Prenatal diagnosis of congenital anomalies*. Appleton, Lange, Connecticut (1988).

59. Wald, N.J., Cuckle, H.S., Boreham, J., and Stirrat, G. Small biparietal diameter of fetuses with spina bifida: implication for antenatal diagnosis. *British Journal of Obstetrics and Gynaecology*, **87**, 219–21 (1980).

60. Varadi, V., Toth, Z., Torok, O. and Papp, Z. Heterogeneity and recurrence risk for congenital hydrocephalus (ventriculomegaly), a prospective study. *American Journal of Medical Genetics*, **29**, 305–10 (1988).

61. Yen, S. and McMahon, B. Genetics of anencephaly and spina bifida. *Lancet*, **ii**, 623–6 (1968).

62   Böök, J.A. and Rayner, S. A clinical and genetical study of anencephaly. *American Journal of Human Genetics*, **2**, 61–84 (1950).

63. Frezal, J., Kelly, K., Guillemot, M.L., and Laing, M. Anencephaly in France. *American Journal of Medical Genetics*, **16**, 336–50 (1964).

64. Richards, I.D.G., McIntosh, H.T., and Sweenie, S. Genetic study of anencephaly and spina bifida in Glasgow. *Developmental Medicine and Child Neurology*, **14**, 626–39 (1972).

65. Carter, C.O. and Roberts, J.J.A.F. Risk of recurrence after two children with central nervous system malformations. *Lancet*, **i**, 306–8 (1967).

66. Laurence, K.M. and Beresford, A. Continence, friends, marriage and children in 51 adults with spina bifida. *Developmental Medicine and Child Neurology*, **17** (Suppl. 35), 123–8 (1975).

2 Anatomy and physiology of cerebrospinal fluid

M.W.B. Bradbury

INTRODUCTION

The normal cerebrospinal fluid (CSF) is a clear, colourless fluid with the appearance of clear water. Its clarity is due to the minimal content of protein. It is contained within the ventricular system of the brain and within the subarachnoid space surrounding both brain and spinal cord. It is one of the extracellular fluids of the brain. The other is the cerebral interstitial fluid which fills the spaces between the nerve cells and glial cells of the central nervous system itself (CNS) and hence is not directly accessible to examination or measurement.

Since there are no permeability barriers between CSF in either the ventricles or in the subarachnoid space and adjacent CNS tissue, substances in solution can diffuse in either direction. Similarly, if there is a hydrostatic pressure gradient between CSF and the interstitial space, fluid will move in the direction which will reduce that gradient. In a steady state, CSF from any site is likely to be of similar composition and at similar pressure to interstitial fluid in CNS tissue adjacent to that CSF.

Cerebral interstitial fluid and CSF together form a special 'milieu interieur' or internal environment for the brain. The composition of both fluids is protected from chemical disturbances in blood plasma and in extracellular fluids outside the brain by a system of permeability barriers which make brain, spinal cord, and their CSF into something of a closed system. These barriers are at the level of the endothelium of brain capillaries and of other intracerebral vessels (blood–brain barrier), at the level of the epithelium of the choroid plexuses, and at the outer layers of the arachnoid mater (the last two comprising the blood–CSF barrier), see below. Not only do these barriers protect CNS tissue from potentially damaging influences outside the brain, but they retain wanted compounds in the brain, for example neurotransmitters, and allow homeostasis of certain substances in the cerebral extracellular fluids to provide a constant and appropriate environment for normal function of the nerve cells. Hydrogen ions, potassium, calcium, and magnesium, are among the solutes in the cerebral interstitial fluid and CSF which are maintained at a remarkably constant concentration in the face of severe and prolonged disturbances in blood plasma.

THE DISTRIBUTION, VOLUME, AND CONTAINMENT OF CSF

The ventricular system of the brain is derived from the hollow central region of the embryonic neural tube. It is continuous inferiorly with the central canal of the spinal cord. The two lateral ventricles, one in each hemisphere, communicate through the interventricular foramina of Monro with the third ventricle shaped like a vertical slit between the thalamus on each side and the hypothalamus inferiorly (Fig. 2.1). The cerebral aqueduct originates from it caudally and runs through the mid-brain to communicate with the fourth ventricle. The floor of the IVth ventricle is diamond-shaped and consists of parts of both pons and medulla oblongata. In its roof behind is the cerebellum. Three openings allow discharge of CSF into the subarachnoid space, a midline foramen of Magendie and two lateral apertures of Lushka.

The subarachnoid space containing CSF surrounds the whole brain and spinal cord (Fig. 2.2). The depth of the layer of CSF between CNS tissue and bone depends somewhat on posture, and the volume of fluid is greater where it fills sulci or fissures in the brain. Wherever the brain and cranium are not closely applied, there are large volumes of fluid, named subarachnoid cisterns, which are continuous with each other through the general subarachnoid space. A large cistern, the cerebellomedullary or cisterna magna, lies in the angle between the cerebellum and the medulla oblongata. There are important cisterns which lie in the midline under the base of the brain. These basal cisterns include the pontine

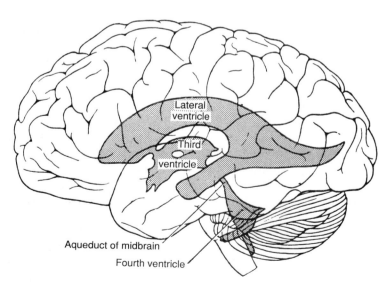

Fig. 2.1 Projection of the ventricles on the left surface of the brain. (From *Gray's anatomy.*)

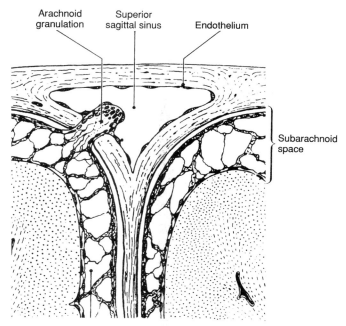

Fig. 2.2 Diagram of the meninges and subarachnoid space with arachnoid villi protruding through the collagenous dura mater as a villus. (From Millen and Woollam, 1962.[26])

cistern, containing the basilar artery, and the interpeduncular cistern, containing the arterial circle of Willis. Caudally, the subarachnoid space around the spinal cord extends into the lumbar sac at the base of the vertebral column where a volume of CSF surrounds lumbar and sacral nerve roots and the filum terminale, the vestigial end of the spinal cord.

The volume of CSF within the lateral ventricles, which is the greater part, has been measured in fixed brains by making casts with resin. In neurologically normal adults of both sexes, aged between 29 to 73 years, this volume was rather variable but averaged 23 ml.[1] Ventricular volume measurements by use of a radioisotope and gammacamera or by computerized tomography are subject to large errors. Magnetic resonance imaging (MRI) gives more accurate *in vivo* ventricular volume measurements in man. Condon *et al.*[2] found an average of 25 ml for five men and five women. The mean total intracranial CSF volume was 123 ml, indicating 98 ml of subarachnoid fluid in the skull. In a more extensive series, Grant *et al.*[3] looked at the effect of age. In men, average ventricular volume increased from 14 to 20 ml between 20–60 years, whilst total volume increased from 110 to 196 ml. The total volume was 14 per cent less in females than in males at 20 years, and also increased markedly with age. All studies have emphasized the variability between individuals.

The volume of CSF in the lumbar sac is about 30 ml so that the total volume is likely to be usually more than the 140 ml given by Weston.[4]

Meninges

From without inwards these are the thick dura mater, the arachnoid mater, and the pia mater (Fig. 2.3). The inner two membranes are more cellular and more delicate than the dura mater. In contrast to the dura, they are probably derived from neurectoderm and are sometimes referred to as the leptomeninges. The subarachnoid CSF lies between the two leptomeninges. The pia mater is closely applied to the external surface of the brain and of the spinal cord.

Dura mater

The cerebral dura mater lines the cranial cavity. It is sometimes described as having two layers, an outer or periosteal layer and an inner or meningeal layer.

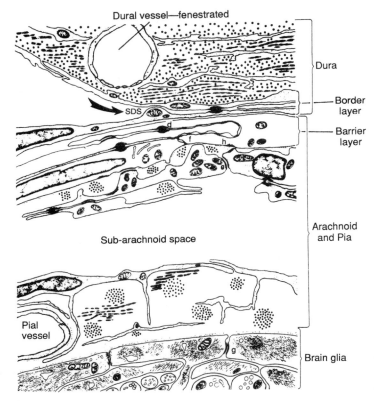

Fig. 2.3 Summary diagram of layers of cells, types of cells and cell junctions in the meninges. 'SDS' is widening of the subdural (actually intradural) space produced during preparation of the tissue. Junctions are labelled d, desmosomes; h, hemidesmosomes; t, tight junctions; and g, gap junctions.[5]

This is only effectively so when the layers separate to enclose a venous sinus. The dura is a tough membrane and is largely composed of white collagen fibres densely aggregated in laminae running at oblique angles to each other. There are fibroblasts and some elastic fibres. Meningeal arteries lie on the periosteal surface of the dura immediately under the skull. These give rise to anastomotic arteries in the same plane. Penetrating arteries arise from the latter and run inwards to supply a rich capillary plexus located within the dura near the underlying arachnoid. Many of the capillaries are 'fenestrated', i.e. highly permeable. The dura also contains lymphatics.

Where the dura meets the arachnoid mater, there are one or more layers of flattened cells which have been called a 'dural mesothelium'. According to Nabeshima *et al.*,[5] these cells are flattened fibroblasts and have no tight junctions between them. They prefer the name 'dural border cells'. (Fig. 2.3). They consider that the plane of separation is always through these loose border cells. In monkeys this layer contains enlarged intercellular spaces filled with fuzzy material. A similar situation exists in man where the dural border cells form several loose layers with much extracellular space. The innermost dural border layer is more firmly attached to the outer arachnoid barrier layer than it is to the other dural cells.[6] Hence, it would seem that the so-called 'sub-dural space' is actually intradural.

The spinal dura mater is a loose sheath which represents the meningeal layer of the cerebral dura only, there being a separate periosteum within the vertebral canal. The space between dura and periosteum is called epidural. It contains loose connective tissue, fat, and a venous plexus.

Arachnoid mater

The outer barrier consists of 3–6 layers of flattened elongated cells with numerous mitochondria. There are many tight junctions and desmosomes between the cells in these layers, making them into a cellular barrier of low permeability. On its inner part, the cells of the arachnoid become looser as they abut the CSF in the subarachnoid space. There are collagen fibres between the cells of the inner layers. Sheet-like trabeculae cross from the arachnoid to the pia. They contain collagen fibres and sometimes small vessels which are surrounded by leptomeningeal cells continuous at the outer end of each trabecula with the arachnoid cells and at the inner end with the pial cells.[7]

Pia mater

There is an outer layer of flattened thin cells which probably makes a continuous sheet. Dissociated pial cells and bundles of collagen fibres lie between this outer layer and the basement lamina which separates the pia from the outer glial limiting layer of the cerebral cortex. Hutchings and Weller[8] consider that the plane of separation between pia and basement lamina represents a sub-pial space.

Relation of blood vessels and nerves to the meninges

As arteries pierce the dura and enter the subarachnoid space, they acquire a leptomeningeal coat from the arachnoid mater. This coat surrounds the vessels as they lie in the space and then becomes continuous with pia mater. Inside the leptomeningeal sleeve and outside the smooth muscle of the vessel, as it lies in the subarachnoid CSF, is a real or potential perivascular compartment (Fig. 2.4) There is also a perivascular space around arteries and veins where they are within the cerebral cortex (Virchow–Robin). These contain CSF, interstitial fluid, and perhaps cellular elements. The cellular elements are not prolongations of the leptomeninges, as once thought, as they do not stain for vimentin as is characteristic for pial and arachnoid cells.[7] The intracerebral perivascular spaces are continuous with the perivascular spaces outside the brain and perhaps with the potential sub-pial space.[7,8] The perivascular spaces terminate externally where the vessel pierces through the dura. This modern view of the morphology of various fluid spaces relates interestingly to current concepts of the bulk flow of cerebral interstitial fluid and CSF, see below.

The points at which cranial and spinal nerves or nerve roots pass outwards through the arachnoid and dural membranes are potential sites at which CSF may move out of the subarachnoid space. In general, the dura mater becomes continuous with the epineurium of the nerve and the arachnoid with the perineurium. The subarachnoid space is prolonged around spinal nerve roots and, where the space ends, there is loose tissue which may allow the escape of

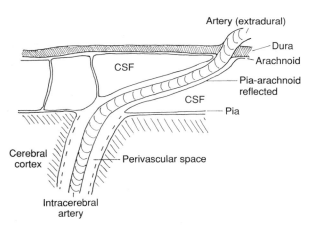

Fig. 2.4 Diagram of the relation of the leptomeninges, arachnoid and pia mater. Note that the perivascular (Virchow–Robin) space around the intracerebral artery is in continuity with the perivascular region and the artery in the subarachnoid space but not with the subarachnoid CSF; the intervening leptomeningeal sheath is considered to be highly permeable. (Based on the electromicrographs of Weller and colleagues.[7,8])

CSF either into the endoneurium or into the extracellular spaces where dura meets epineurium. There are also arachnoid villi in this region, see below.

Prolongations of the subarachnoid space are also associated with certain cranial nerves, and, in some cases, rather special anatomical arrangements allow drainage of CSF, see below.

The choroid plexuses and the ependyma

The choroid plexuses are highly vascular invaginations of pial tissue into the lateral, IIIrd and IVth ventricles. The vascular plexuses are covered with a single–layered secretory epithelium, one surface of which is in contact with ventricular CSF. The ependyma lines the ventricular cavities and separates ventricular CSF from brain tissue, it is continuous with the choroid epithelium and both take origin from the initially single-layered wall of the neural tube. However, the choroid epithelium and the ventricular ependyma are rather different in their relations, fine structure, and physiology, including permeability properties.

Choroid plexuses

The external curved line on the medial surface of each hemisphere through which the pial tissue invaginates is called the choroid fissure. Within the lateral ventricles the plexus in each ventricle extends posteriorly from the interventricular foramen to curve into the inferior horns of the ventricles, reaching the anterior end of the hippocampus. At the interventricular foramina, the choroid plexuses of the lateral ventricles are continuous with the choroid plexus in the roof of the IIIrd ventricle. The latter forms two parallel longitudinal folds.

The choroid plexus of the IVth ventricle is roughly T shaped and projects into the ventricle from its roof in the lower part below cerebellum. The double vertical limb of the T projects into the ventricle medially. The horizontal limbs pass into the lateral recesses of the ventricle and protrude through the lateral apertures into the subarachnoid space.

Within the lateral ventricles in life, the plexuses appear as red, glistening frond-like structures with a complex vasculature (Fig. 2.5). Microscopically, the visible fronds are covered with villous folds or processes (Fig. 2.6) each containing a capillary plexus and fine afferent and efferent vessels. The epithelium consists of a single layer of tightly packed cuboidal cells with slightly curved surfaces and cilia on the ventricular side. The cells contain numerous rod-shaped mitochondria, lipid inclusions, and other vesicular formations (Fig. 2.7). The epithelium has several features which are characteristic of fluid transporting epithelia in general. The ventricular surface has a brush-border, consisting of microvilli. These are extensions of the apical cell membrane and cytoplasm but lack the regularity seen in the brush-border of the intestine. Again as with other transporting epithelia, there are elaborate foldings and interdigitations between cells at their basal regions. Tight junctions (zonulae occludentes) occur between cells at their apical ends. These junctions

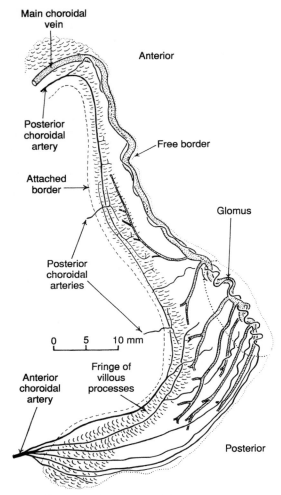

Fig. 2.5 Diagram to illustrate the principal features of the human choroid plexus. Lateral ventricle — right side. (From Millen and Woollam, 1962.[26])

though tight to horseradish peroxidase of 40 000 molecular weight are permeable to the much smaller ionic lanthanum. They are thus tight junctions of the so called 'leaky' type, again characteristic of fluid secretion. The epithelium, however, differs from that of the gut and the renal tubules in that fluid is secreted at the apical end with the microvilli and the junctions, rather than being absorbed at the apical and secreted at the basal end. Hence, the choroid epithelium has been called 'backward facing'.

There tends to be a capillary in the apex of each villous fold close to the epithelium, whilst arterioles, venules, and connective tissue elements are more

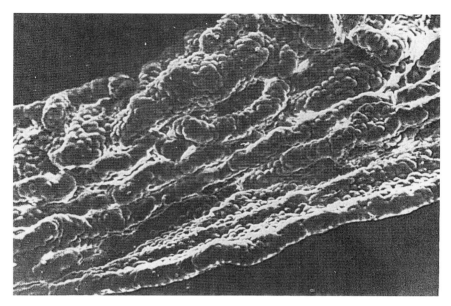

Fig. 2.6 Scanning electron micrograph of the ventricular surface of choroid plexus from a rat. The plexus consists of more or less longitudinal folds of variable length. Each rounded protrusion is a choroid plexus cell. (×350) (From Peters *et al.*, 1976.[27])

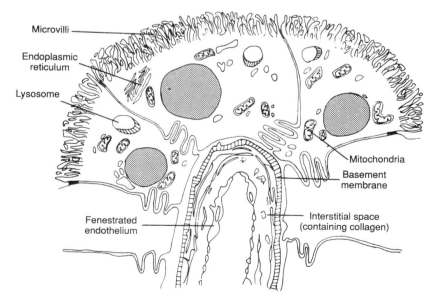

Fig. 2.7 Drawing of the choroid epithelium. Note numerous microvilli at the ventricular surface, tight junctions, basal infoldings of the lateral membranes, and mitochondria. The endothelium of the capillary is fenestrated.

numerous at the base. Immediately under the epithelium is a basement membrane which is separated from the capillary endothelium by a thin stroma containing collagen fibres and scattered pial cells. The endothelial cells of the capillary are 'fenestrated', i.e. contain very thin attenuated areas. Such structures, associated with high permeability at least to small and medium-sized molecules, are characteristic of capillaries across which high water flow can occur.

Ventricular ependyma

In the adult, the ventricles are lined by a single layer of cubical or columnar cells, the layer being continuous with the epithelium (ependyma) of the choroid plexus. These cells tend to be larger and less densely packed than those of the plexuses. Their ventricular surfaces have microvilli and cilia, but there are fewer mitochondria and cytoplasmic inclusions. Although there may be some tight junctions between adjacent cells they do not form a complete seal and molecules up to the size of large proteins can freely pass through intercellular channels from CSF into interstitial fluid or in the reverse direction.

The ependyma generally lies on a layer of glial processes beyond which are the astrocytes themselves. The structure of the ependyma is not uniform throughout the ventricular system. In general, the cells tend to be more flattened over white matter and more cuboidal or columnar over grey nuclei.

Arachnoid villi and other exit sites

Arachnoid villi and granulations

Villi and granulations are essentially the same structure, the term granulation being applied to villi which are more developed, more complex, and visible to the naked eye. The villus is an intrusion of web-like arachnoid tissue into and often through the dura mater. It has a 'stalk' within the dura but blossoms into a rounded or cauliflower-like protuberance within the dural sinus (Fig. 2.8). The interior contains a network of arachnoid cells separating a labyrinth of channels about 4–12 µm in width. These channels are in continuity with the subarachnoid space and contain CSF. The external surface of the villus is covered with an endothelium which is continuous with the endothelium of the venous sinus. The endothelium separates CSF within the villus from venous blood. How CSF crosses the endothelium to drain into venous blood is a matter for some controversy and will be discussed below.

In adult man, arachnoid villi are present in dural sinuses generally but are most numerous in the superior sagittal sinus. At birth they are not obvious, but by the age of 18 months, they appear where the parieto-occipital and central veins open into the superior sagittal sinus. By the age of 3, they occur over a considerable area and spread along the lateral sinuses.

Arachnoid villi also occur within the spinal dura. Here they are related to the prolongations of the subarachnoid space around nerve roots, the subarachnoid

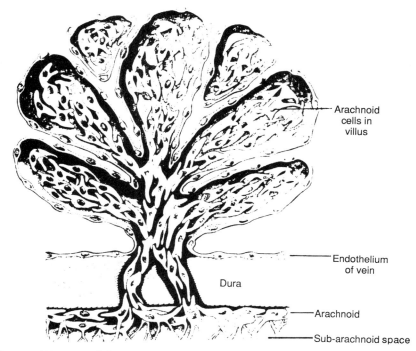

Arachnoid
cells in
villus

Endothelium
of vein

Dura

Arachnoid

Sub-arachnoid space

Fig. 2.8 Diagram of the structure of an arachnoid villus, based on studies in the sheep and the dog. Arachnoid cells project into the villus through two holes in the dura. (From Potts *et al.*, 1972.[28])

angle. In this region they have been described as being of three types: entirely internal to the dura, within the dura or passing beyond it into a venous sinus of the dorsal root venous plexus.

Other exit points of CSF

Where the subarachnoid space is prolonged around cranial and spinal nerves before they pass beyond the enclosing arachnoid and dura maters, there are potential sites at which CSF may escape into interstitial spaces outside the arachnoid mater, (reviewed by Bradbury[9]). Most functional and structural studies on such escape of CSF have been made in animals other than man, but there is evidence that routes of this kind are present in primates and in man. Even if they normally contribute little to the total volume of CSF drainage, such routes may play a bigger role in abnormal conditions. Additionally, they provide a route for entry of large molecules, for example protein, from brain into the lymphatic system and hence may have immunological implications.

Quantitatively the most important of such exit routes in non-primate mammals, is that related to the olfactory nerves and the nose. Extensions of the subarachnoid space around the olfactory nerves allow passage of CSF into the submucous spaces of the nose. The olfactory nerve fila within the cribriform plate are surrounded by a space which is continuous on the brain side with the subarachnoid space and on the nose side with the perineural space, the arachnoid merging into the perineurium at the level of the bone. In the nose, the perineurium becomes thin and loose, permitting CSF to enter the submucosal interstitial space. The nasal submucosa contains profuse plexuses of both blood and lymph capillaries.

The optic nerves are completely surrounded by marked prolongations of the subarachnoid space. These allow CSF to connect with the interstitial fluid of the perineural sclera and the posterior sclera of the globe. There may also be connections between the perineural sclera and the highly vascular choroid via the border tissue of Elschnig. This may allow some CSF to pass into the highly permeable capillaries of the choroid.

Cerebrospinal fluid may also be in continuity with the epineural spaces of the VII and VIIIth nerves. In the ear there is additionally, a connection between the subarachnoid space and the perilymph via the perilymphatic duct (cochlear aqueduct).

As already described CSF may be discharged into the interstitial spaces within or outside the dura around spinal nerve roots via local arachnoid villi. There may also be non-specific seepage in this region.

FORMATION OF CEREBROSPINAL FLUID

It is generally agreed that the majority of CSF production is due to secretion by the choroid plexuses.[10,11] It has seemed probable that some fluid is contributed from the brain across the ventricular ependyma or directly into the subarachnoid space or by both routes. There is some experimental evidence supporting extra-choroidal CSF production, but it has proved very difficult to definitely separate other sites of formation from the choroid plexuses and to precisely measure their contribution. In the author's opinion, the best estimates indicate that 10–30 per cent of CSF production comes elsewhere than from the choroid plexuses.

Rate of production of CSF

CSF production in laboratory animals and in man may be estimated by a variety of methods. Simplest of all is to insert a needle in the lumbar sac or cisterna magna and to collect and weigh all extruded fluid over a long period of steady flow. This method is subject to the criticism that the technique is likely to reduce CSF pressure unless the point of outflow is kept raised. In that case not all the fluid produced will be collected. Theoretically, the best method is to perfuse artificial CSF between two sites in the system, for example a lateral ventricle to the cisterna magna, and to control the pressure at the outflow site, (cisterna magna), at the normal level. Addition of fluid to the perfusate may be estimated by measuring the dilution of a non-diffusible marker molecule in the outflow compared with the amount in the inflowing perfusate. An appropriate marker is dextran of 2×10^6 molecular weight, labelled with Evans blue. There is no potential influence of an abnormal hydrostatic pressure and fluid not recovered from the outflow will not affect the estimate of production.

$$F_{CSF} = F_{PF}.(C_{IN} - C_{OUT})/C_{OUT}$$

where F_{CSF} and F_{PF} are the flows of added CSF and inflowing perfusate, respectively, and C_{IN} and C_{OUT} are the concentrations of the non-diffusible marker in inflowing and outflowing perfusate respectively. The method is too invasive for routine use in patients. A compromise in man is to withdraw a set volume of CSF and to measure the pressure reduction. The time, until normal pressure is restored, is then recorded. Cerebrospinal fluid production is then the volume withdrawn divided by the time for restitution of the previous normal pressure. The technique is simple, but the approach to the normal pressure is asymptotic and may not be easy to time precisely.

Mean results for rate of CSF production in man, estimated by the first two methods, vary between 0.35 and 0.4 ml min^{-1}. This represents a replacement of about 0.2–0.25 per cent of the total CSF volume per minute, or a half time for the system of 5–6 hours.

Secretion by the choroid epithelium

It was realized by a number of workers, but most cogently pointed out by Davson in the 1950s, that the composition of CSF is such that it cannot be accounted for by ultrafiltration from blood plasma. The arguments have been reiterated by Davson *et al.*[10] The concentrations of sodium, magnesium chloride, and hydrogen ion in CSF are higher than is to be anticipated in an ultrafiltrate. Those of potassium, calcium, and bicarbonate are lower. Much greater discrepancies occur when plasma concentrations of these ions are disturbed and their respective concentrations are held constant. The protein concentration in CSF is about 400–500 times less than in blood plasma. As we have seen, the capillaries of the choroid plexuses are of a highly permeable type whilst the epithelium is tighter and has many characteristics of fluid-secreting epithelia.

Mechanism of CSF secretion

It has been known for some time that two specific drugs cause a potent inhibition of CSF formation. The carbonic anhydrase inhibitor, acetazolamide, administered either systemically or into the ventricular CSF of experimental animals reduces CSF production by 50–60 per cent. This indicates that hydration of CO_2 to produce carbonic acid and hence H and HCO_3 ions is important in the secretory mechanism. Introduction of an inhibitor of the Na–K-pump, such as the digitalis alkaloid ouabain, into the ventricular system causes up to 100 per cent inhibition of CSF formation. This indicates that the Na–K-pump is the main motive force for CSF secretion. Indeed a high concentration of the enzyme Na–K–ATPase has been localized in the ventricular microvillus surface of the choroid epithelium by both autoradiography after ^{13}H ouabain binding and by direct histochemistry of the enzyme.

It has not yet proved technically possible to experimentally analyse the details of the mechanism of secretion in the human organ or indeed in a mammalian choroid plexus. However, Wright and his colleagues have been able to mount the choroid epithelium of the IVth ventricle of the bull-frog as a membrane between two chambers containing physiological saline. This enabled them to measure ion fluxes with radiotracers in both directions across the epithelium under different conditions. These studies were supplemented with measurements of the effects of ions, intracellular mediators, etc on short circuit current and of various agents on membrane potential and membrane resistance in relation to both the ventricular and basal side of the epithelial cell. A working model of secretion was built up from such experiments,[14,15] (Fig. 2.9).

When the epithelium is considered as a whole, there is a net transport of sodium, chloride, bicarbonate, and water towards the ventricular CSF, and a

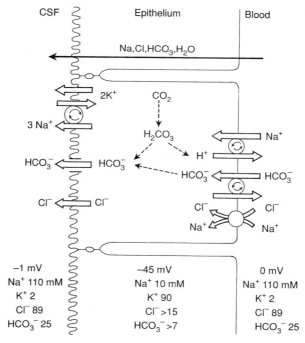

Fig. 2.9 A working model of ion transport mechanisms across the choroid membrane. There is net transport of, Na^+, Cl^-, and HCO_3^- towards CSF. The inside negativity, due to outward potassium diffusion and the electrogenicity of the pump, together with intracellular accumulation of chloride and bicarbonate, causes these anions to move across the brush border into CSF. (From Saito and Wright, 1983.[14])

small net transport of potassium in the opposite direction from CSF to blood. The primary pump dependent on ATP moves three sodium ions across the ventricular plasma membrane into the CSF; two potassium ions are moved in the opposite direction and largely diffuse back into CSF via potassium channels. Bicarbonate and chloride ions follow the excess of positively charged ions into CSF, again presumably via their respective ion channels. The net movement of solute into the ventricle induces local build up of osmolality, probably in the spaces between the microvilli, causing water to follow down its osmotic gradient and hence to the formation of 'new' CSF. Intracellular sodium, bicarbonate, and chloride need to be replenished. Sodium moves from the blood down its electrochemical gradient via Na–H transporters in the basal plasma membrane. Intracellular H ions for this exchange are generated in the cell from hydration of CO_2 to carbonic acid — probably acetazolamide deprives the mechanism of intracellular hydrogen ion and hence starves the Na–K-pump of the sodium ions normally provided by the exchanger. Chloride and more sodium ions enter the cell via Na–H and Na–Cl cotransporters again in the basal membrane. Intracellular chloride is, in fact, accumulated beyond its equilibrium potential from energy derived from the sodium ions going the same way on the same transporter but down their electrochemical gradient. There is also an HCO_3 exchanger in the basal membrane, the proposed function of which is to allow more bicarbonate into the cell on top of that generated from hydration of CO_2.

It has been further proposed that the rate of secretion of CSF is limited by the permeability of the ventricular plasma membrane to bicarbonate. Conditions which increase intracellular cyclic AMP, for example the drug theophylline, an inhibitor of the enzyme which destroys cAMP, increase the bicarbonate conductance of this membrane and hence CSF production by providing more anion. Cholera toxin, which powerfully stimulates CSF production, additionally increases cAMP in the choroid plexus so may also act in this way.

Caution is required in applying results found in an amphibian epithelium to the mammalian and human situation. Undoubtedly, the importance and site of the Na–K pump are the same in the frog and mammal. Also the hydration of CO_2 and a high intracellular chloride level seem to play a role in both cases.

Control of CSF production

The limited evidence available supports a view of persistent steady production of CSF in the face of varying conditions rather than of large adaptive changes frequently occurring in response to particular physiological needs. Similar statements were made about cerebral flow until it became possible to measure regional cerebral blood flow during normal cerebral function. Repetitive measurements of secretion from each plexus separately during particular brain tasks are not yet possible, but may yield surprises when achieved.

Production of CSF is fairly independent of CSF pressure between 280 mm H_2O and –100 mm H_2O. Similarly, secretion appears to be independent of mean arterial blood pressure, until this is reduced to below about 60 mm Hg. If ventricular pressure and arterial pressure are both varied, it seems that it is the difference between the two, the perfusion pressure, which determines the threshold below which CSF production is reduced, i.e. this reduction occurs at a higher threshold of arterial BP when CSF pressure is raised.[16] Reduced perfusion pressure might act either by diminishing choroid plexus blood flow, and hence the supply of metabolites necessary for secretion, or by lessening capillary filtration, and hence the supply of solutes and water for secretion itself. A reduction in fluid production may also be caused by severe hypoglycaemia.

In view of the role of carbon dioxide and hydrogen ions in both determining cerebral blood flow and in the mechanism of CSF secretion, it is of interest to know how hypercapnia and hypocapnia influence fluid production. The effects of high CO_2 are rather unpredictable, whereas respiratory alkalosis has generally been found to reduce CSF formation, an effect potentiated by the administration of the carbonic anhydrase inhibitor, acetazolamide.

High doses of the glucocorticoid dexamethasone diminish CSF formation, probably by inhibiting the Na–K–ATPase. This effect may contribute to the beneficial influence of this steroid on cerebral oedema.

All the choroid plexuses receive a well-developed innervation by autonomic nerves, both adrenergic and cholinergic.[13] These fibres make contact with both plexus blood vessels and with the epithelial secretory cells. It seems clear that sympathectomy increases fluid production, whereas sympathetic stimulation reduces it, indicating a normal inhibitory tone.

Vasoconstriction is linked to α-adrenergic receptors on the blood vessels. There is controversy as to whether stimulation of β-adrenergic receptors and of cholinergic receptors on the epithelial cells are associated with inhibition or enhancement of CSF secretion. It is not known whether these controversial effects have a role in the physiology or pathophysiology of the CSF. However, the presence of autonomic influences, taken together with the possible role of cyclic nucleotides in the control of the secretory process, suggests that CSF secretion might well be amenable to pharmacological manipulation.

Extrachoroidal production of CSF

Since fluid can move easily from the interstitial spaces of brain into CSF and in the reverse direction, it seems likely that any net filtration or secretion of fluid at the brain capillaries will find its way into the CSF spaces. The question has been approached by studying CSF production in animals with some or all of the choroid plexuses removed or by isolating, for perfusion, a part of the ventricular system which does not contain choroid plexus tissue. Such experiments have suggested that 30–60 per cent of the fluid may come from elsewhere other than the plexuses, but are technically difficult and susceptible to problematic interpretation. The work of Cserr and her colleagues, who have examined bulk flow of fluid within the brain, have provided more physiological information. The movement of large molecular weight tracers, for example Evans' blue–albumin, dextrans, and peroxidase, was studied after microinjection deep within the rat brain, usually into the caudate nucleus.[17] Each marker slowly diffused outwards making a small blob, but then moved preferentially in streams within the brain. These streams moved centrifugally in perivascular spaces and also occurred between fibre tracts and under the ependyma. Later it was shown that a series of radioactive molecules, between 900 and 69 000 molecular weight, all moved out of brain as a whole at precisely the same rate, a behaviour quite incompatible with diffusion.

Such findings, taken together with observations of a high concentration of the Na–K–ATPase in the abluminal plasma membrane of brain endothelial cells, led to the concept of cerebral interstitial fluid being slowly secreted by the capillaries and hence moving slowly through the brain to discharge mainly via the perivascular spaces into the subarachnoid space. The rate of disappearance of large molecules from the brain allows an estimate to be made of this rate of interstitial fluid drainage.[18] In the rat, 11 per cent of CSF was computed as deriving from brain interstitial fluid; in the rabbit, the estimated value was 6 per cent — both much lower than the estimates given from other methods and recorded above.

Both Cserr's experiments and the modern view of the perivascular anatomy indicate that interstitial fluid-CSF in the intracerebral perivascular spaces initially passes into the extracerebral perivascular space. The leptomeningeal sheathing enclosing this space is highly permeable and allows water and solutes of any molecular weight into the subarachnoid space. Cells may, however, be temporarily retained in the perivascular region. On top of the long–term centrifugal movement of interstitial fluid in the perivascular space, there may well be transient to-and-fro (sloshing) movements. During systole, arteries and arterioles in the brain expand which may be anticipated to displace perivascular fluid. During diastole, the vessels' diameter will reduce and fluid will run back into the spaces.

CIRCULATION AND DRAINAGE OF CSF

Circulation within the cranium

Cerebrospinal fluid secreted by the choroid plexuses passes relatively rapidly through the ventricular system, because of its comparatively small volume, to flow out through the median and lateral apertures into the cisterna magna. Mixing within the ventricles is encouraged by the numerous cilia on the ependymal lining. the cilia may generate quite complex currents within the fluid and break up non-stirred layers adjacent to the ependyma, thus assisting diffusion of solutes between CSF and brain.

From the cisterna magna the fluid passes around the brain and forward in the system of basal cisterns. From the base of the brain, the CSF flows laterally and upwards around the cerebral hemispheres to reach the large dural sinuses, particularly the superior sagittal (Fig. 2.10). Preferential routes are in the lateral

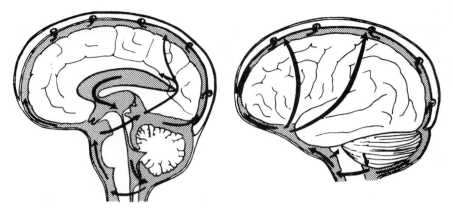

Fig. 2.10 Normal pathways of CSF circulation, with absorption through the arachnoid villi, shown in sagittal section and from a lateral view. (From Milhorat, 1972.[29])

(Sylvian) fissures, anteriorly over and between the frontal lobes and posteriorly in relation to the occipital lobes and tentorium. Radioisotope scanning after cisternal injection, indicates that it takes 1–2 hours for fluid to reach the basal cisterns, 3–5 hours to reach the lateral fissure, and 10–12 hours to spread over the cerebral subarachnoid space. By 24 hours, radioiodinated albumin becomes concentrated along the superior sagittal sinus and is clearing from the basal cisterns.

CSF in the spinal subarachnoid space

Experiments in man and in animals in which dyes or radiotracers have been introduced at different levels in the spinal subarachnoid space and where the subject or animal have been kept immobile in the horizontal position suggest that there is very little consistent movement of CSF in either a caudal or head-ward direction. This is not to say that transient sizable movements in a backward or forward direction do not occur in relation to factors which disturb venous pressure, see below. However, there are arachnoid villi in the spinal dura which presumably allow exit of some CSF. Marmarou *et al.*[19] measured resistance to drainage in the anaesthetized cat in the presence and absence of spinal block induced by a balloon at the level of the 6th cervical vertebra (C6). These experiments suggested that about 16 per cent of CSF total absorption occurs through the spinal meninges. If the situation is comparable in man, one may suppose that there is a scarcely perceptible movement of CSF in a caudal direction around the spine with subsequent small loss from the system.

Passage through the arachnoid villi

Although it is generally agreed that the villi provide the main route for exit of CSF from the subarachnoid space into blood, the mechanism has until recently remained obscure and is still not fully elucidated. Physiological experiments indicate that the villi allow bulk flow of fluid, solutes, and contained particles up to the size of red blood cells from the subarachnoid space to blood in response to a hydrostatic pressure gradient.[20] There is rectification, flow in the opposite direction not being possible, perhaps because a greater pressure on the venous side causes the villus to collapse against the sinus wall (Fig. 2.11). There is no involvement of colloid osmotic pressure as originally envisaged by Weed. An opening pressure of about 50 mm H_2O is required to start the flow, and under normal conditions this is about the difference between CSF pressure and pressure in the superior sagittal sinus.

Although the channels within the contained arachnoid labyrinth are of the right size, i.e. about 5 μm across, to account for the physiologically observed movement of fluid and contained particles from CSF to blood, there is controversy as to how the venous endothelium which appears tight allows this passage. There are two possibilities. Either a few intercellular channels carry the flow, or vacuoles and channels open up within and across the endothelial cells in

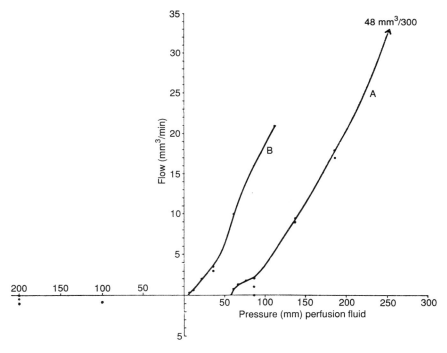

Fig. 2.11 Flow–pressure curves through a dural disc bearing arachnoid villi, mounted between two chambers *in vitro*. Curve A represents the flow–pressure relationship for an artificial CSF. Curve B was obtained after the addition of a surfactant to the fluid. The critical opening pressure was virtually eliminated. (From Welch and Friedman, 1960.[20])

response to pressure. It may be noted that very few intercellular channels would be required to accommodate the slow net production of CSF, and that these might be easily missed in electron microscopy. There is evidence for giant vacuoles being involved in the exit of aqueous humour across the endothelium of the analogous canal of Schlemm in the eye. Whatever the ultrastructural route, it must be emphasized that all functional studies, *in vitro* and *in vivo*, point to hydrostatic pressure-mediated flow through a resistance, see below.

Role of other drainage routes

It has already been discussed that CSF may escape across the meninges in relation to prolongations of the subarachnoid space around certain cranial and spinal nerves.[9] In a number of nonprimate mammals, the most important of such routes is that involving the olfactory nerves and the nose. CSF passes through the cribriform plate into the submucosal interstitial fluid. Here water, ions, and solutes up to 40 000 molecular weight enter blood capillaries and are carried away into the general circulation. Larger molecules, including labelled albumin, are taken into nasal lymphatics and are drained through the deep cervical lymph nodes and trunks to enter the great veins at the base of the neck. This route is present in primates, including man, but in keeping with the relatively small size and importance of the olfactory apparatus in these species, appears to play a minor role in CSF drainage.

It is probable that other potential sites of escape of CSF, i.e. those in relation to the optic nerves, the ear, and the spinal nerve roots, are functional in man. It is to be noted that these are not directly connected to lymphatics but allow CSF to exit into extracellular spaces outside the tight arachnoid barrier. Once outside, water, ions, and small molecules are likely to enter blood capillaries, whereas larger molecules may be picked up by lymphatics (Fig. 2.12). The fact that the regional lymph nodes have potential access to protein draining from the central nervous system may have immunological importance which is out of proportion to the amount of material involved. It is also open to question as to whether CSF or any of its components pass across the arachnoid in general. Certainly, materials so transferred would then have ready access to both blood and lymph capillaries in the dura mater.

Resistance to drainage of CSF and its measurement

Resistance, R, to outflow of CSF, F, may be expressed by the relation

$$R = (P_{CSF} - P_{SS})/F$$

where F_{CSF} and P_{SS} are the hydrostatic pressures in the CSF and in the superior sagittal sinus, respectively. If outflow is progressively raised by infusion of artificial CSF and provided P_{SS} remains constant and flow laminar, a linear relation between plateau CSF pressure and flow is to be anticipated. The slope of the line will be the resistance to drainage.

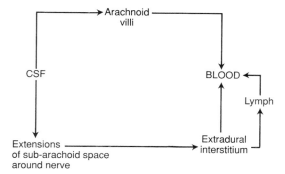

Fig. 2.12 Diagram illustrating the fact that CSF, which does not pass through the arachnoid villi directly into the blood, but escapes into the extracellular spaces within or beyond the dura, is taken into the blood capillaries in the case of water and small molecular weight solutes and lymph capillaries in the case of the larger molecules.

A number of studies of this type have been made in laboratory animals and in man. Ideally, sterile artificial CSF is infused at a constant rate through one needle, for example in the lumbar sac, and the pressure is recorded from a second needle in an adjacent position. Infusion at a given rate is maintained until the CSF pressure reaches a constant plateau (or the pressure may be predetermined and fluid infused rapidly until this pressure is reached). The infusion rate is then increased again to maintain a higher steady pressure (Fig. 2.13).

Resistance to outflow may be estimated by another method. The compliance of the CSF compartment, i.e. the increment in volume in response to a small increment in pressure, may be measured by bolus injection of artificial CSF or saline. The return of the raised pressure to normal depends on exit of CSF from the system and hence may be used to estimated resistance to outflow. The pressure–time curve is converted to a volume–time curve. These enable outflow to be related to pressure. In normal mammals and subjects the volume–time curve is exponential, indicating a single process.

Outflow resistances measured, by the same two methods in the same animal or subject, do not generally agree well. It is considered that the constant infusion method gives better values. In 58 patients, aged between 15 and 83 years ,and not considered to have neurological disease and in the supine horizontal position, the mean resistance to outflow was 94.5 ± 21.3 mm H_2O/ml min^{-1} (SD).[21] In the adult hydrocephalus syndrome, resistance to outflow is consistently raised. In the child, the resistance to drainage is probably of similar size to that in the adult, both resting CSF pressure and CSF production being somewhat less. Where investigated, communicating hydrocephalus in the child is generally associated with some demonstrable change in the relationship between CSF pressure and outflow rate.

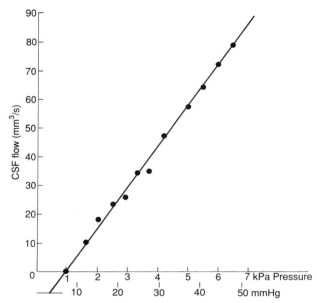

Fig. 2.13 Relationship between steady-state pressure and flow in a human subject, determined by measuring pressure in the lumbar sac during a series of step increases in the infusion rate of sterile artificial CSF. The reciprocal of the slope is the resistance to drainage. (From Ekstedt, 1978.[21])

CSF PRESSURE AND PRESSURE–VOLUME RELATIONS

Normal CSF pressure

The pressure obtained from a needle in the lumbar sac with the patient in the lateral recumbent position is frequently measured as part of a neurological investigation. Ekstedt has argued that, when CSF hydrodynamics are being investigated, it is better to have the patient in the supine position since the patient is more comfortable and instabilities due to adventitious movements are reduced. In 58 reference patients, from 15 to 83 years of age, a mean value of 141 ± 19 mm H_2O was obtained, with pressures, in 90 per cent of the subjects, lying between 117 and 179 mm H_2O.[21] There was no influence of age within the age limits of the group. Pressures above 200 mm H_2O have generally been considered as abnormal.

Cerebrospinal fluid pressure is highly dependent on the venous pressure within the cranium and the vertebral canal. It is normally some 40–50 mm H_2O greater than the superior sagittal venous pressure. The dependence is due to the flexibility of the venous walls. The differential is due to the resistance to outflow of CSF being produced at its normal steady rate. The relation between the pressures does not apply in the opposite direction, and generally venous pressure in the skull is not affected by CSF pressure.

In children and babies CSF pressure is definitely lower. Values of near zero (atmospheric) have been reported in the newborn; 40–50 mm H_2O in infants; and 40–100 mm H_2O in children. In immature rats during the first postnatal week, resistance to CSF outflow appears to be 7-fold higher than in older rats. This apparent increase in resistance can be accounted for by the fact that, in contrast to the situation in the adult, venous pressure increases with CSF pressure.[22]

Posture and CSF pressure

A very simple model of the CSF spaces might demonstrated by a closed rigid tube, about 700 mm in length, and containing water at a pressure of 140 mm H_2O in the horizontal position. It is self-evident that, if the tube is rotated through 90° to the vertical position, the pressure at the centre of the tube will remain at 140 mm H_2O. At the bottom it will be $140 + 700/2 = 490$ mm H_2O, and at the top it will be $140 – 700/2 = –210$ mm H_2O. Thus at 210 mm below the top of the tube (top of the skull) the pressure will be zero. This model undoubtedly provides the main physical basis for the changes in hydrostatic pressure observed in CSF after movement from the recumbent to the upright sitting position and vice versa. The pressure changes in CSF during postural alterations are, however, complicated by the fact that the physiological tube is not completely sealed and is not rigid. Fluid may be lost through the arachnoid villi and may be gained by CSF production, if there is no corresponding loss by drainage. A greater factor is the flexibility of the walls of venous sinuses in the cranium and of the epidural veins within the vertebral canal, which allows transmission of the venous pressure to the CSF (Fig. 2.14). At any height in the system, CSF pressure is likely to be some 40–50 mm H_2O greater than the venous pressure at the same height. If CSF pressure transiently becomes greater than venous pressure by more than the normal differential, this pressure will be transmitted to the intracranial veins, etc., and blood will be displaced out of them into the veins outside the skull and vertebral column; and, if transiently lower, venous blood will move into the craniovertebral system.

In the vertical sitting position, measured CSF pressure is zero at the level of about C1–C4, in keeping with the model. A 'hydrostatic indifference point' has been described, at which CSF pressure is the same in the horizontal and vertical sitting positions, at the level of T1–T4. Welch (cited in reference 2) has pointed out that the level of the hydrostatic indifference point is, in the sitting position, approximately at the level at which venous pressure is atmospheric. The observations fit with the hypothesis that the systemic venous pressure sets a floor or tonic CSF pressure upon which are added pressures resulting from forces characteristic of or intrinsic to the craniospinal system.

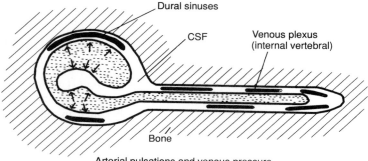

Fig. 2.14 Diagram illustrating how the cranium and vertebral canal form a largely closed container. Changes in the arterial or venous pressure will be transmitted to the CSF.

Fluctuations in CSF pressure

Ventilation

Rhythmic changes in lumbar CSF pressure of about 40 mm H_2O occur at the same frequency as ventilation. CSF pressure falls with inspiration and rises during expiration, (Fig. 2.15). These fluctuations closely mirror similar fluctuations in central venous pressure. Interestingly, the phase of the CSF waves is reversed in the presence of spinal block. This has been attributed to the fact that the isolated lumbar sac receives transmitted oscillations from veins below the diaphragm where pressure rises with inspiration and falls with expiration.

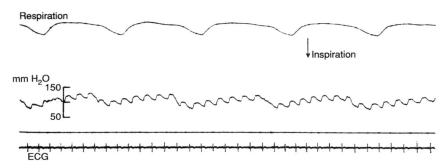

Fig. 2.15 Normal respiratory fluctuations in the pressure of the lumbar CSF. Expiration causes an increase in pressure, and inspiration a decrease. The higher frequency rhythm is due to arterial pulsation. (From Lakke and Schut, 1969.[30])

Arterial Pulsation

In addition to the slow pressure waves due to ventilation, there is a higher frequency, lower amplitude (about 20 mm H_2O) pressure pulse in phase with the ECG. There is controversy as to whether expansion of arterial vessels due to ventricular systole is directly transmitted to CSF or whether there is forward thrust of blood through capillaries leading to pulsatile distension of venous vessels. Suffice to say there is an effective increase in brain volume due to raised blood content very soon after ventricular systole. The size of the volume disturbance is, of course, proportional to the total blood flow through the particular region. Hence the brain is a much greater amplitude generator than the spinal cord (Fig. 2.14). Studies with X-ray contrast media in the CSF indicate that there is a normal 'stroke volume' movement of CSF from the cranial to the spinal compartment of about 1 ml during systole.

Compliance of the CSF compartment and its measurement

Rapid injection of a bolus of saline into the lumbar sac causes a rise in CSF pressure which subsides as already described. By repeating the injections with increased volumes of the bolus, a pressure–volume curve can be constructed. The curve can be extended into the lower pressure region by removal of standard volumes of CSF.

Attempts have been made to fit the positive part of the pressure–volume relation with an exponential model.[23] A pressure volume index (*PVI*) has been defined by the relation:

$$PVI = V(\log_{10} P_2/P_1);$$

where V is the volume injected, P_1 the resting pressure, and P_2 the pressure immediately after injection. The *PVI* is the theoretical volume required to produce a ten-fold rise in pressure.

Over the range of negative and positive volume increments, the curve has the shape of the pH curve for titration of a buffer with a strong acid or alkali, i.e. shallow slope in the central region with a sharply increasing slope at the extremes of volume disturbance,[24] (Fig. 2.16). The shallow 'good buffering' region probably largely represents gradual displacement of venous blood from the craniovertebral compartment with increasing pressure. The slope steepens sharply at either extreme, because no more venous blood can be accommodated at the lowest CSF volumes and no more venous blood can be displaced at the highest CSF volumes.

Interestingly, as volume and pressure rise, the pulse amplitude greatly increases,[25] (Fig. 2.17). This is of course a result of the reduction in compliance of the system at high pressures. Such big increases in pulse pressure occur in experimental and human hydrocephalus and may be a significant fact in its genesis.

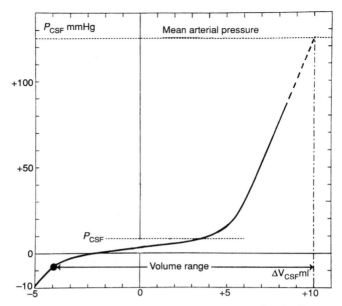

Fig. 2.16 The average CSF volume–pressure curve in the dog between the limits of −10 mm Hg and the mean arterial blood pressure. The last part of the curve (---) has been obtained by extrapolation. (From Lofgren *et al.*, 1973.[24])

Transient bulk movements of CSF

Transient bulk flows of CSF within the craniovertebral system must depend on generation of transient pressure gradients within the system. Such gradients are likely to depend on similar distributions of pressure in the systemic venous blood. Coughing and sneezing initially increase venous pressure and hence CSF pressure in the upper parts of the body. Thus, there will be sloshing of CSF between the cranial and vertebral compartments, the initial flow being caudally. Similarly, ventilation causes differential effects on venous pressure in the upper and lower parts of the body, hence there will be tidal flows of CSF. These will become much greater during hyperventilation. Rapid changes in posture also cause mixing between CSF in the cranial and spinal compartments. The inference is that in the relatively immobile, recumbent subject, lumbar CSF is a fairly stagnant pool, whereas the conditions described above cause ready mixing with CSF from the cranial compartment. Withdrawal of CSF will of itself cause compensatory flows.

The arterial pulse also plays some role in mixing of the CSF. If abnormal in size or in its direction of propagation, it may contribute to disturbances in the size and shape of the ventricles or of the central canal of the spinal cord, for example hydrocephalus or syringomyelia, respectively.

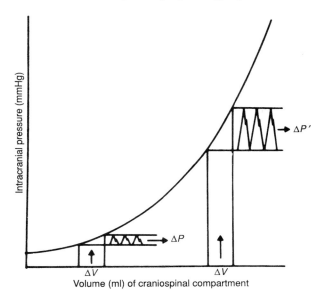

Fig. 2.17 Relation of intracranial pressure (*ICP*) to volume change, *V*, in the combined intracranial and intraspinal compartment. The pulse amplitude is depicted as the response to the same transient increase in brain–blood volume at two different levels of compliance in the system. (From Avezaat *et al.*, 1979.[25])

PHYSIOLOGICAL ROLE OF CSF

Chemical functions

The tightness of the blood–brain barrier prevents polar compounds of medium or large molecular weight passing from interstitial fluid to blood across the cerebral capillary wall as well as in the opposite direction. If such compounds arise in brain due to normal metabolism, or due to a pathological process, they can be removed by diffusion into the CSF, followed by its drainage. This 'sink action' can act as a clearance mechanism and is probably aided by bulk flow of fluid through the brain, as already discussed.

The flow of CSF of a regular ionic composition over the brain as a whole, and especially over the cerebral cortex, assists in the maintenance of a constant ionic concentration within the interstitial fluid surrounding the cortical cells and other brain cells.

Hydraulic functions

The most important of these is the function of the CSF as a space reservoir. Brain, blood, and CSF are contained within the almost rigid box of the cranium and the vertebral canal (Fig. 2.14). Large changes in pressure may potentially occur in response to any change in intracranial blood volume or in the brain volume itself. The CSF introduces some 'give' into the system. Thus an increase in blood volume due to vasodilatation, or even some degree of brain swelling, can be compensated for by displacement of CSF out of the system through the arachnoid villi into blood. Similarly, any diminution in blood or in brain volume can be buffered by build up of CSF due to secretion without equivalent drainage.

Additionally, since the density of brain is only very slightly greater than that of CSF, the weight of the brain does not bear on the bony floor of the cranium. Cerebrospinal fluid may also act to some extent as a hydraulic buffer against rapid impact of the brain against the skull. Thus, if the moving head is suddenly brought to a stop, as in a motor accident, the moving brain cannot hit the skull until some CSF is first displaced. The viscous resistance of the subarachnoid spaces to this displacement will at least tend to slow the brain movement.

REFERENCES

1. Last, R.J. and Tompsett, D.H. Casts of the cerebral ventricles. *British Journal of Surgery*, **40**, 525–43 (1953).
2. Condon, B., Patterson, J., Wyper, D., Hadley, D., Grant, R., Teasdale, G., and Rowan, J. Use of magnetic resonance imaging to measure intracranial cerebrospinal fluid volume. *Lancet*, **i**, 1355–7 (1986).
3. Grant, R., Condon, B., Lawrence, A., Hadley, D.M., Patterson, J., Bone, I., and Teasdale, G.M. Human cranial CSF volumes measured by MRI; sex and age influences. *Magnetic Resonance Imaging*, **5**, 465–8 (1987).
4. Weston, P.G. Sugar content of the blood and spinal fluid of insane subjects. *Journal of Medical Research*, **35**, 199–207 (1916).
5. Nabeshima, S., Reese, T.S., Landis, D.M.D., and Brightman, M.W. Junctions in the meninges and marginal glia. *Journal of Comparative Neurology*, **164**, 127–70 (1975).
6. Schachemayr, W. and Friede, R.L. The origin of subdural membranes. 1. Fine structure of the dura–arachnoid interface in man. *America Journal of Pathology*, **92**, 53–68 (1978).
7. Alcolado, R., Weller, R.O., Parrish, E.P., and Garrod, D. The cranial arachnoid and pia mater in man. Anatomical and ultrastructural observations. *Neuropathology and Applied Neurobiology*, **14**, 1–17 (1988).
8. Hutchings, M. and Weller, R.O. Anatomical relationships of the pia mater to cerebral blood vessels in man. *Journal of Neurosurgery*, **65**, 316–25 (1986).
9. Bradbury, M.W.B. Overview of passage routes of interstitial fluid to the lymphatics: history and current concepts. In *Pathophysiology of the blood–brain barrier* (ed. Johansson, B.B., Owman, C., and Widner, H.). pp. 403–12. Elsevier, Amsterdam (1990).
10. Davson, H., Welch, K. and Segal, M.B. *Physiology and pathophysiology of the cerebrospinal fluid*. Churchill Livingstone, Edinburgh (1987).
11. McComb, J.G. Recent research into the nature of cerebrospinal fluid formation and absorption. *Journal of Neurosurgery*, **59**, 369–83 (1983).
12. Wright, E.M. Transport processes in the formation of the cerebrospinal fluid. *Reviews in Physiology, Biochemistry and Pharmacology*, **83**, 1–34 (1978).

13. Lindvall, M. and Owman, L. Autonomic nerves in the mammalian choroid plexus and their influence on the formation of cerebrospinal fluid. *Journal of Cerebral Blood Flow and Metabolism*, **1**, 245–66 (1981).

14. Saito, Y. and Wright, E.M. Bicarbonate transport across the frog choroid plexus and its control by cyclic nucleotides. *Journal of Physiology (London)*, **336**, 635–48 (1983).

15. Saito, Y. and Wright, E.M. Regulation of bicarbonate transport across the brush border membrane of the bull-frog choroid plexus. *Journal of Physiology (London)*, **350**, 327–42 (1984).

16. Weiss, M.H. and Wertman, N. Modulation of CSF production by alterations in cerebral perfusion pressure. *Archives of Neurology*, **35**, 527–9 (1978).

17. Cserr, H.F., Cooper, D.N., and Milhorat, T.H. Flow of cerebral interstitial fluid as indicated by the removal of extracellular markers from the rat caudate nucleus. *Experimental Eye Research (Suppl.)*, **25**, 461–73 (1977).

18. Szentistvanji, I., Patlak, C.S., Ellis, R.A., and Cserr, H.F. Drainage of interstitial fluid from different regions of rat brain. *American Journal of Physiology*, **246**, F835–F844 (1984).

19. Marmarou, A., Shulman, K., and LaMorgese, J. Compartmental analysis of compliance and outflow resistance of the cerebrospinal fluid system. *Journal of Neurosurgery*, **43**, 523–34 (1975).

20. Welch, K. and Friedman, V. The cerebrospinal fluid valves. *Brain*, **83**, 554–69 (1960).

21. Ekstedt, J. CSF hydrodynamic studies in man. 2. Normal hydrodynamic variables related to CSF pressure and flow. *Journal of Neurology, Neurosurgery and Psychiatry*, **41**, 345–53 (1978).

22. Jones, H. and Gratton, J.A. The effect of cerebrospinal fluid pressure on dural venous pressure in young rats. *Journal of Neurosurgery*, **71**, 119–23 (1989).

23. Marmarou, A., Shulman, K., and Rosende, R.M. A non-linear analysis of the cerebrospinal fluid system and intracranial pressure dynamics. *Journal of Neurosurgery*, **48**, 332–44 (1978).

24. Lofgren, J., von Essen, C., and Zwetnow, N.N. The pressure–volume curve of the cerebrospinal fluid space in dogs. *Acta Neurologica Scandinavica*, **49**, 557–74 (1973).

25. Avezaat, C.J., van Eijndhoven, J.H.M., and Wyper, D.D.J. Cerebrospinal fluid pulse pressure and intracranial volume–pressure relationships. *Journal of Neurology, Neurosurgery, and Psychiatry*, **42**, 687–700 (1979).

26. Millen, J.W., and Woollam, D.H.M. *The anatomy of the cerebrospinal fluid*. Oxford University Press (1962).

27. Peters A., Palay S.L., and Webster H.de F. *The fine structure of the nervous system: the neurones and supporting cells*. Saunders, Philadelphia and London (1976).

28. Potts, D.G., Reilly, K.F., and Deonaire V. Morphology of the arachnoid villi and granulations. *Radiology*, **105**, 333–41 (1972).

29. Milhorat, T.H. *Hydrocephalus and the cerebrospinal fluid*. Williams and Wilkins, Baltimore (1972).

30. Lakke, J.P.W.F., and Schut, D. Electromagnetic examination of CSF pressure response to jugular compression. I. Determination of normal values. *Excerpta Medica Foundation, Amsterdam*, **22**, section 8, abstract 96, p. 19 (1969).

3 Aetiology and pathology of hydrocephalus

R.O. Weller, S. Kida, and B.N. Harding

INTRODUCTION

Accounts of hydrocephalus have been recorded since earliest times, and even Hippocrates recommended decompression by trepanation for the treatment of hydrocephalus.[1] Further graphic descriptions of hydrocephalus were given in the 16th century by Vesalius who recognized the difference between internal and external hydrocephalus.[2]

Serious attempts to treat hydrocephalus did not begin until the present century when it was recognized that hydrocephalus was due to impedance or complete obstruction of the cerebrospinal fluid circulation.[2,3] With the introduction of effective valve systems[4] combined with ventriculoatrial and ventriculoperitoneal shunts, the prognosis for survival and intellectual development of hydrocephalic children improved. For example, in 1962, Laurence and Coates[5] examined 81 survivors from their series of 182 unoperated cases of hydrocephalus and found that only 38 per cent were of normal intelligence (IQ of 85+). MacNab,[6] on the other hand, cites the results of the early insertion of valves in children who developed hydrocephalus following closure of myelomeningoceles: 79 per cent were of normal intelligence.

Despite improvements in shunting techniques and increasing sophistication in the investigation of hydrocephalus by computerized tomography (CT) and magnetic resonance imaging (MRI), the treatment of hydrocephalus remains a problem and there is still a high complication rate.[1] It is essential, therefore, that the wide variety of pathological lesions that result in hydrocephalus is appreciated and that the effects of hydrocephalus upon the brain at its various stages of development are fully characterized.

The presence of periventricular oedema and tissue damage in the acute stages of hydrocephalus was initially identified in experimental pathological studies[7-9] and in biopsies of human cases of hydrocephalus.[10] Such changes in the periventricular tissues became widely appreciated with the introduction of CT scanning.[11] Pathological studies also emphasized that brain damage occurred during the acute stages of hydrocephalus and subsequently led to gliosis, particularly in the periventricular white matter.[7,9,10,12]

Definition of hydrocephalus

Classically, external and internal hydrocephalus have both been recognised.[2] External hydrocephalus is a condition in which infants with rapidly enlarging heads have a CT scan that shows widening of the subarachnoid space with mild or no ventricular dilatation.[13] In the majority of cases, external hydrocephalus is an age-related, self-limited condition occurring in infants with open cranial sutures and associated macrocephaly; it usually resolves without intervention by 2–3 years of age.[13] Internal hydrocephalus, which will be discussed in this chapter, can be defined as dilatation of the intracranial ventricles. When older tracer methods were used for investigation, a blockage located cephalad to the fourth ventricle was said to cause 'non-communicating' hydrocephalus, whereas a block at the fourth ventricle foramina or in the subarachnoid space produced 'communicating hydrocephalus'.[14] With the introduction of CT and MRI, these terms appear to have been largely abandoned. It is now recognized that hydrocephalus in the fetus, infancy, and in adults falls into several major categories.

A. Imbalance between production and drainage of cerebrospinal fluid

This may occur due to the blockage of cerebrospinal fluid pathways within the ventricles, subarachnoid space, or arachnoid granulations, or, on rare occasions, be due to the overproduction of cerebrospinal fluid.

B. Developmental abnormalities

In this group the ventricular dilatation is not due to an imbalance of CSF production and drainage but to anatomical abnormalities in the brain.

C. Destruction of brain tissue with associated cerebral atrophy and ventricular dilatation (ex vacuo hydrocephalus)

This is seen particularly in children following pre- or perinatal brain damage, and in adults with Alzheimer disease or multi-infarct dementia.

D. Mixed hydrocephalus with a combination of A and C

This type of hydrocephalus occurs particularly following perinatal brain damage,[15,16] and in adults in whom there is a combination of normal pressure hydrocephalus and brain destruction due to multi-infarct dementia[17] or Alzheimer's disease.

HYDROCEPHALUS IN THE FETUS, INFANCY, AND CHILDHOOD

A summary of the major causes of hydrocephalus in children is set out in Table 3.1 and the subsequent description of these disorders follows the pattern established in this table.

As the aetiology and pathology of hydrocephalus in fetal life, infancy, and childhood differ from that seen in adults, they will be discussed in separate sections of this chapter.

I.   Imbalance between production and drainage of CSF — (A) Impedance of CSF drainage

Ventricular system — occlusion

Tumours

Hydrocephalus resulting from intrinsic and extrinsic tumours are largely dealt with in the section on adult hydrocephalus (pp. 72–80). Astrocytomas of the pons (Fig. 3.1), and primitive neuroectodermal tumours (PNET) of the cerebellum (medulloblastoma) (Fig. 3.2), are more common in children than in adults. Such tumours frequently occlude the fourth ventricle and subarachnoid space causing hydrocephalus (Fig. 3.2). The giant cell astrocytoma (Fig. 3.3) in patients with tuberous sclerosis should also be mentioned, it evolves from subependymal nodules or 'candle-gutterings' and may expand to obstruct the foramen of Monro.[18] Pineal tumours are also a cause of ventricular distention in children. Most are germinomas or teratomas which compress the quadrigeminal plate and compromise the aqueduct.

Malformations

A great variety of malformations can be associated with hydrocephalus in childhood. Accurate recognition of these anomalies has been considered of great importance to physicians in affording them evidence of inherited disorders with important implications for genetic counselling. A few words of caution are relevant here. One must be careful not to confuse the co-natal with the con-genital. Recent advances in embryology and teratology have led to an increasing realization of the complex interaction between intrinsic and extrinsic, inherited and acquired factors in the causation of structural anomalies. Furthermore, the pathologist can no longer rely solely on the presence or absence of specific indicators, such as inflammation or gliosis, to support a given aetiological hypothesis. The extended ontogeny of the CNS, the long period over which damage can occur, and the profound maturational changes to the various cell systems which take place, as well as the varying delay before clinicopathological

Table 3.1   Aetiology of hydrocephalus in children

I	**Imbalance between production and drainage of CSF**

(A)   Impedance of CSF drainage (p. 49)

    (1)   *Ventricular system — occlusion* (pp. 50–65)

        (a)   Tumours — intrinsic to the ventricle:
choroid plexus papilloma, ependymoma, colloid cyst, giant-cell astrocytoma, primitive neuroectodermal tumours (PNET).

            Tumours — extrinsic — compressing or distorting the ventricles:
gliomas (cerebellar, brainstem, hypothalamic), craniopharyngioma, pineal tumours (germinoma, teratoma).

        (b)   Malformations:

            (i)   membranous obstruction of the foramen of Monro,

            (ii)   obliteration of the third ventricle,

            (iii)   obstruction to the aqueduct of Sylvius:
atresia, stenosis, septum, vascular anomaly,

            (iv)   obstruction of the foramina of Luschka and Magendie:
atresia, Dandy–Walker malformation, arachnoid cyst.

        (c)   Inflammation and haemorrhage and their consequences:
coaption of the lateral ventricle, obliteration of the foramen of Monro, gliosis of the aqueduct and septum, obstruction of the foramina of Luschka and Magendie, sequestration of the fourth ventricle.

    (2)   *Subarachnoid space*: (pp. 65–6)

        (a)   Foramen magnum: Chiari type I and type II malformations

        (b)   Diffuse obliteration: cerebrovascular dysplasias

        (c)   Subarachnoid fibrosis: post-haemorrhagic, meningitic, mucopolysaccharidosis.

    (3)   *Arachnoid granulations*: (pp. 66–8)

        (a)   Congenital absence

        (b)   Functional: change in venous pressure, cranial dysplasias.

(B)   Over production of CSF — choroid plexus papilloma. (pp. 68–70)

(C)   Reduced production of CSF — ciliary dysplasia. (p. 70)

II.   **Developmental abnormalities**: (pp. 71–2)
Malformations in which ventricular dilatation is an essential feature but with uncertain pathogenesis

III.   **Hydrocephalus due to destruction of brain tissue**. (p. 72)
Prenatal hypoxic — ischaemic
Perinatal hypoxic — ischaemic
Postnatal infection, degeneration

IV.   **Mixed due to I and III**

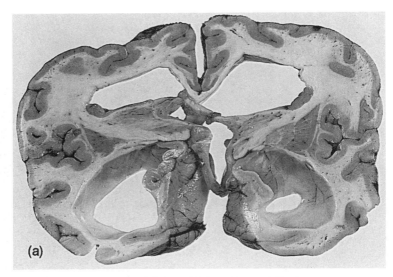

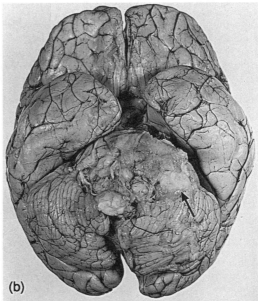

Fig. 3.1 Marked hydrocephalus resulting from infiltration of the brainstem and fourth ventricle by a malignant glioma (arrow). (a) Coronal section; (b) inferior surface.

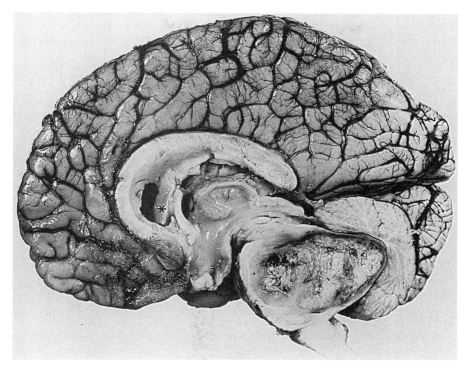

Fig. 3.2 A medulloblastoma involving pons and cerebellum causes hydrocephalus and fenestration of the septum (*). Medial surface of hemisected brain.

analysis is obtainable are all obstacles placed in the path of the morphologist trying to extrapolate back to the original noxa. In practical terms, however, a small proportion of cases of childhood hydrocephalus are clearly inherited and these are indicated throughout the text.

1. Membranous occlusion of one foramen of Monro: This is a rare cause of unilateral dilatation of one lateral ventricle.[19] Most reports are surgical or radiological.[20] Diagnosis has been achieved as early as the 29th week of gestation.[21] Pfeiffer and Friede[22] describe occlusion by a glio–ependymal bridge without evidence of inflammation and in association with other subtle developmental anomalies.

2. Obliteration of the third ventricle: This is an exceptional condition. Neonatal onset hydrocephalus with a narrow third ventricle has been demonstrated by ultrasound in two siblings;[23] post-mortem examination in one of them

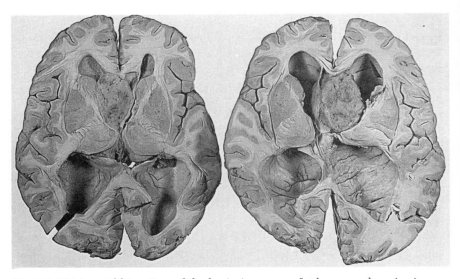

Fig. 3.3 Horizontal bisection of the brain in a case of tuberous sclerosis. A giant-cell astrocytoma blocks both foramina of Monro.

revealed extensive fusion of the thalami. A unique example of congenital fusion of the thalamus, atresia of the aqueduct and upper fourth ventricle, and rhomboencephalosynapsis (absent vermis and fused dentate nuclei) is reported in a 6-month-old boy with progressive hydrocephalus from birth.[24]

3. Obstruction to the Aqueduct of Sylvius: As the narrowest part of the ventricular system, the aqueduct is a prime location for an obstruction to CSF flow. The aqueduct is a curved tube of irregular calibre with two constrictions separated by a central dilatation or ampulla. According to Woollam and Millen[25] the area of its narrowest part in adult subjects ranges from 0.4 to 1.5 mm^2, while in normal children[26] the mean was found to be 0.5 mm^2, the smallest observation being 0.1 mm^2.

The nomenclature for aqueductal anomalies has remained controversial from both a descriptive and a pathogenetic viewpoint. Different authors vary in their use of terms, and even within one aqueduct there may be considerable variations.[27] But at the heart of the argument has been the desire to separate the apparently malformative, and thus possibly inherited, from the evidently acquired, and thus sporadic and preventable. The terms employed in this text have been found to be the most useful and unambiguous. They are based on morphology, for it has become increasingly clear that the distinction between congenital and acquired aqueduct stenosis is probably artificial. Neurulation, the infolding of the neural plate, leads to the formation of the neural tube, an initially hollow structure which gradually narrows to become the aqueduct.[28] It follows that all aqueduct obliterations are, in the strict sense, acquired. One must look for other clues towards an external interference. The presence of gliosis as an indication of previous infection or inflammation[2] has recently been discounted. Experimental inoculation of mumps virus in hamsters[29] can produce aqueduct atresia with no evidence of inflammation at late stages. In man an astroglial response to tissue destruction is only effectively mounted during the second half of gestation. Gliosis is thus an indicator of the timing rather than the type of the noxious event. A more radical view is that aqueduct stenosis itself is secondary to an initial communicating hydrocephalus.[30] A number of lines of evidence favour this concept. Williams[31] from a study of resin casts of aqueducts from children with spina bifida demonstrated flattening of the tectal plate resulting from compression by the expanding hydrocephalic hemispheres, findings further supported by Emery[32] who also showed shortening, dorsal displacement, and angulation of the aqueduct in a large series of children with hydrocephalus and myelomeningocele. Clinicopathological studies in X-linked hydrocephalus would also be compatible with this concept. In animals, communicating hydrocephalus followed by aqueduct stenosis has been described in the hydrocephalic mutant mouse 'oh'[33] and in the rheovirus inoculation model in mice.[34]

(i) Atresia (forking, dysgenesis): In this rare condition, part of the aqueduct is not visible by naked eye examination, but microscopy reveals tiny rosettes or canals lined by ependymal cells grouped together in the midline or scattered across the midbrain tegmentum (Fig. 3.4). The normal contour of the aqueduct is

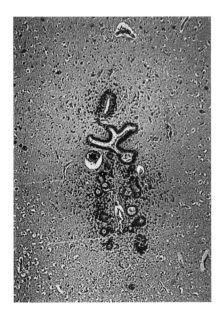

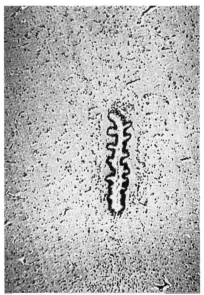

Fig. 3.4 Aqueduct atresia. Microscopic section of aqueduct. Numerous scattered aqueductules. Haematoxylin– eosin. (×25)

Fig. 3.5 Aqueduct stenosis. The tiny canal has intact ependyma. Haematoxylin–eosin. (×25)

absent, but there is no excessive gliosis surrounding the aqueductules. Aqueduct atresia may be an isolated phenomenon or may be associated with spina bifida, Arnold–Chiari malformation, or craniosynostosis.[2,35] Clinical reports of aqueduct obstruction in children following mumps meningoencephalitis,[36,37] and experimental induction of aqueduct atresia using myxovirus in hamsters,[29] suggest mumps infection as one possible aetiological factor.

There are still unresolved problems of nomenclature. Dorothy Russell[2] argued intensely against the use of atresia as being illogical in the presence of small patent channels, she considered 'forking' more appropriate. Friede[38] has pointed out the inconsistency of this term with the known ontogeny of the aqueduct, as well as the confusion caused by the presence of a ventral fork in normal subjects.[39] A recent suggestion is 'dysgenesis'[35] which although an improvement on the earlier nomenclature also carries pathogenetic implications which may not prove to be justified. In view of our knowledge of virus-induced aqueduct block in animals, aqueduct obliteration seems, to the authors, a more appropriate term at present.

(ii) Stenosis: Simple stenosis implies a greatly reduced lumen but with an intact ependymal lining and without gliosis (Fig. 3.5). Bickers and Adams[40] first described a rare X-linked form of hydrocephalus and aqueduct stenosis, now estimated to account for 2 per cent of all cases of congenital hydrocephalus.[41] At least 30 families are on record.[42,43,44] Only boys are affected, most stillborn or exhibiting macrocephaly at birth, but there is considerable intersibling variation and some mildly affected brothers survive to adulthood.[45,46] A quarter of patients have adduction–flexion deformity of the thumbs.[47] The aqueduct is markedly narrow in some cases[42,43] but normal size in others (Fig. 3.6b),[44,46,48] favouring the argument that stenosis results from hydrocephalus. Bilateral absence of the pyramids is frequently observed.[49] Autosomal recessive aqueduct stenosis has also been reported.[50]

(iii) Septum: Despite the classical view that septum of the aqueduct is a maldevelopmental cause of hydrocephalus,[2] more recent evidence suggests a closer relationship to aqueduct gliosis (see below).

(iv) Vascular malformation: Aneurysms of the Great vein of Galen situated over the quadrigeminal plate compress the midbrain tectum and may effectively occlude the aqueduct.[51] Rare vascular malformations in the aqueduct may also be a source of non-communicating hydrocephalus.[52,53]

4. Foramina of Luschka and Magendie: Each of the three fourth ventricular outlets is more than sufficient for CSF drainage,[54] so that all three must be compromised to produce hydrocephalus. A few reports of isolated atresia[55] demonstrate membranous pouches (Fig. 3.7) covering the foramina which histologically consist of a thin glioependymal membrane.[56,57] Atresia of the fourth ventricular foramina was originally considered the cause of hydrocephalus in Dandy–Walker malformation,[58] but this is clearly incorrect since in many cases one or more foramina are patent.[59,60] Three features are necessary for diagnosis: partial or

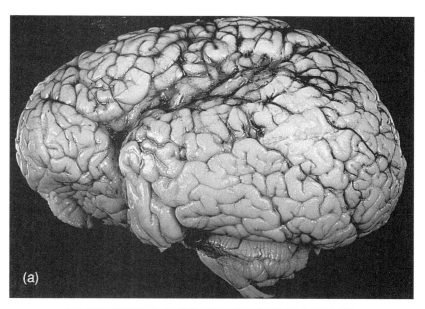

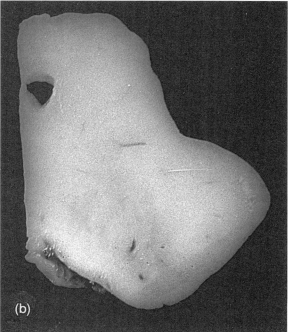

Fig. 3.6 X-linked hydrocephalus. (a) The brain has an excessively convoluted surface, known as polygyria. (b) Horizontal section of part of the midbrain to show the patency of the aqueduct.

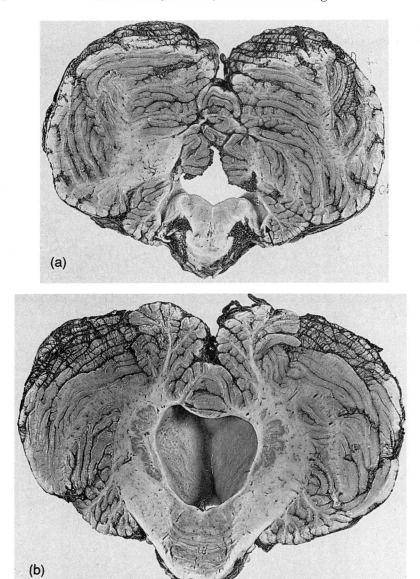

Fig. 3.7 Atresia of the foramina of Luschka. The lateral outlets are dilated and closed over by a glioependymal membrane (arrow). (a) Horizontal section at the level of the pontomedullary junction. (b) At the level of the pons the fourth ventricle is markedly dilated and its wall shows granular ependymitis.

complete agenesis of the cerebellar vermis, enlargement of the posterior fossa, and cystic dilatation of the fourth ventricle (Fig. 3.8). Neonatal hydrocephalus is the usual clinical presentation, but dilatation of the lateral ventricles is very variable and may be quite mild. The vast majority of cases are sporadic but

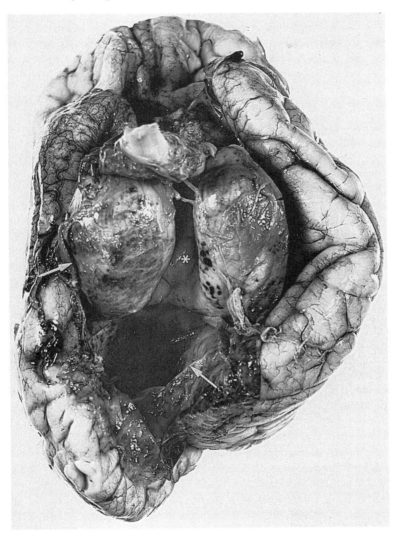

Fig. 3.8 Dandy–Walker malformation. Inferior view showing absence of the vermis (*) and cystic dilatation of the fourth ventricle. The thin membraneous cyst wall (arrowheads) has torn during the prosection.

sibling cases are known.[61] A wide range of somatic and neural malformations are associated with the disorder[15] which appear to be the result of a developmental arrest of the hindbrain, probably originating in the first trimester.

Infratentorial arachnoid cysts are frequently associated with hydrocephalus (Figs 3.9(a), (b)). In the series of Galassi et al.[62] the childhood cases presented at birth, or soon after, with macrocephaly. Adult patients had evidence of a posterior fossa lesion. Hydrocephalus appeared to result from a combination of obstruction of the fourth ventricular outlet foramina by the cyst wall and compression of the aqueduct and fourth ventricle by the expanding cyst.

Inflammation and haemorrhage and their consequences

Intrauterine and neonatal infection with a variety of organisms, protozoa, bacteria, and fungi, is a notable source of ventriculitis and resulting hydrocephalus. Congenital toxoplasmosis (Fig. 3.10) follows transplacental infection after the second gestational month. The clinical features, present soon after birth include microcephaly, intracerebral calcifications, and chorioretinitis. Progressive hydrocephalus is the result of both parenchymal destruction and block of the aqueduct by necrotic debris as well as acute ependymitis and chronic gliosis. In neonatal leptomeningitis, caused principally by Gram-negative enterobacteria, streptococci, and staphylococci, or sometimes pseudomonas, acute fibrino-purulent exudate may plug the aqueduct or fourth ventricular outlets. Ventriculitis (Fig. 3.11), abscess, infarction, and cavity formation, together with later scarring and organization produce ventricular diverticuli or loculations which may be subject to hydrocephalic distention.[2,63,64] Neonatal fungal infection with Candida albicans is another cause of purulent leptomeningitis, ventriculitis, and hydrocephalus.[65,66]

Intraventricular haemorrhage, the most common CNS disorder in neonates,[67] is a frequent cause of hydrocephalus in childhood[68] through a variety of mechanisms involving both the ventricular walls and the leptomeninges (see below). Subependymal germinal matrix is the usual origin of intraventricular haemorrhage in low birthweight premature infants, while choroid plexus haemorrhage or haemorrhage complicating periventricular leucomalacia (white matter infarction) are found in mature newborns. Acute hydrocephalus may result from occlusion of the foramen of Monro (Fig. 3.12), the aqueduct, or the fourth ventricular outlets by blood clot at the time of the ictus. Post-haemorrhagic hydrocephalus in infancy has been studied sequentially with ultrasound and CT scans: it may be non-progressive[69] or increasing intracranial pressure (ICP) may require shunting.[70] Subarachnoid fibrosis blocking the basal cisterns (see below) is the most usual cause, but organization of the haematoma and gliosis may block ventricular foramina or aqueduct, while fibrotic thickening of the leptomeninges may occlude the foramina of Luschka and Magendie (Fig. 3.13).[71,72] Partial obliteration of one lateral ventricle with contralateral dilatation is also possible. Such transventricular adhesions have been called coarctation or

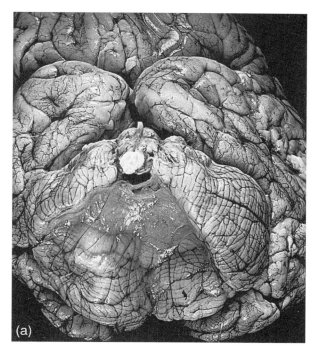

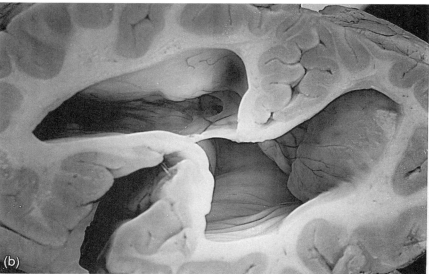

Fig. 3.9 Basal midline arachnoid cyst causing fourth ventricle hydrocephalus. (a) Inferior view of the cerebellum and cyst. (b) Coronal section of the hemispheres.

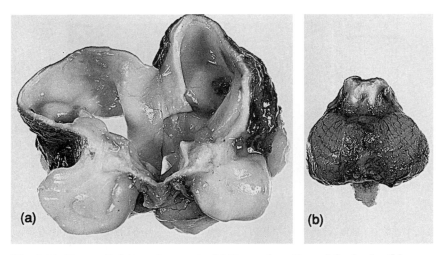

Fig. 3.10 Congenital toxoplasmosis. (a) Coronal section of the brain. (b) Cerebellum and hind brain. The midbrain was necrotic and the aqueduct occluded.

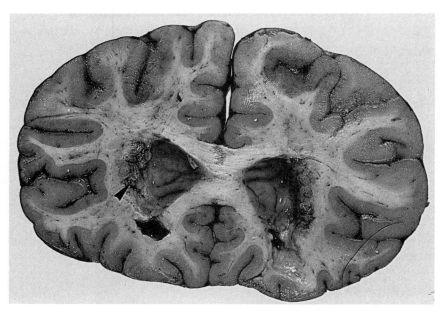

Fig. 3.11 Dilated frontal horns with ragged inflamed walls indicating ventriculitis (arrowhead). Hydrocephalus resulting from acute haemophilus meningitis with basal cistern block.

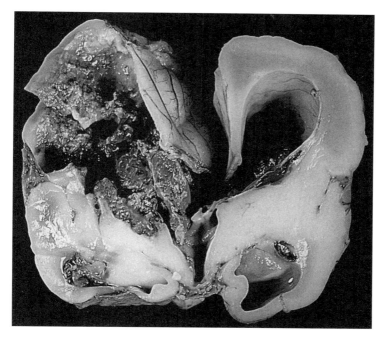

Fig. 3.12 Neonatal hydrocephalus. The right lateral ventricle is dilated as a consequence of block of the foramina of Monro resulting from haemorrhage into the left ventricle (from germinal plate haemorrhage and haemorrhagic white matter necrosis).

coaption[73] and usually occur between the corpus callosum and caudate nucleus. Along the line of obliteration one finds gliosis and ependymal rosettes and sometimes haemosiderin-laden macrophages.[15,74] Transventricular adhesions and unilateral hydrocephalus may also result from shunting procedures.[75] Sequestration or isolation of the fourth ventricle has been reported after insertion of a ventricular shunt in children with obstruction of the fourth ventricle foramen secondary to intraventricular haemorrhage.[76,77] The superadded aqueduct obstruction appears to be related to ependymitis consequent upon the presence of foreign material within the ventricular system.

In aqueduct gliosis the expected outline of the aqueduct remains discernible as an interrupted ring of ependymal cells, tubules, and rosettes (Fig. 3.14). Dense fibrillary gliosis envelops the aqueductules and partially or completely fills the aqueductal lumen. Widespread ventriculitis and ependymitis supports the view that aqueduct gliosis is either post-inflammatory or a consequence of intraventricular haemorrhage with organization of pus or blood clot and proliferation of the subependymal glia.[2,15,71] Probably closely related pathogenetically, is the rare septum of the aqueduct. A thin membrane obstructs the lower

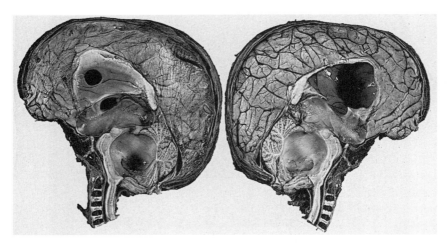

Fig. 3.13 Hemisection of brain and calvarium showing massive hydrocephalus with fourth ventricular outlet block resulting from post-meningitic leptomeningeal fibrosis.

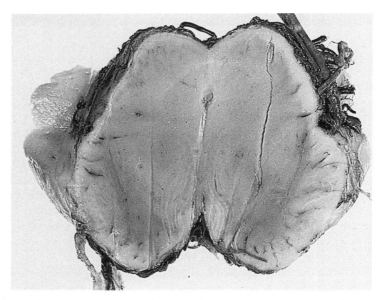

Fig. 3.14 Gliotic obstruction of the aqueduct. Horizontal section of the midbrain.

part of the aqueduct (Fig. 3.15). It consists, histologically, of glial tissue surrounded by an interrupted ring of ependymal cells and rosettes.[15] Turnbull and Drake,[78] from four personal cases and the small literature, suggest that the

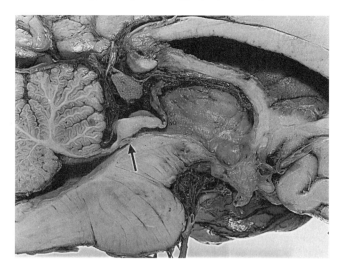

Fig. 3.15 Septum of the aqueduct. A septum is situated at the lower end of the aqueduct (arrow): midline sagittal section. Note the marked dilatation of the third ventricle but normal size of the fourth ventricle.

membrane originates from a glial plug stretched by prolonged pressure from above.

Subarachnoid space

Foramen magnum

Deformation and displacement of the hindbrain which plugs the foramen magnum and blocks movement of CSF between spinal and intracranial compartments may be partly responsible for the hydrocephalus which occurs in the Chiari malformations. In Chiari type I there is herniation of the cerebellar tonsils into the vertebral canal in the absence of a space occupying lesion. A cause of late onset hydrocephalus, presentation is usually in adult life with neck pain, cerebellar ataxia, pyramidal syndrome, or dissociated sensory loss. Chiari type I is occasionally associated with sudden death in infancy[79] and sleep apnoea.[80] Many patients have syringomyelia[81] and craniocervical bony malformations, particularly occipital dysplasia.[82] Familial occurrence,[83] including dominant inheritance, has been reported.[84]

Chiari type II, better known as the Arnold-Chiari malformation (Fig. 3.16), is a frequent cause of hydrocephalus in infancy in association with a myelomeningocele. The malformation consists essentially of elongation of the inferior vermis and brainstem and their displacement into the spinal canal.[15] While the subarachnoid space around the hindbrain at the foramen magnum is obliterated, the exit foramina of the fourth ventricle are open and herniated into the spinal canal. Ascending spinal meningitis (complicating the spina bifida defect) may produce a ventriculitis while the cerebral leptomeninges are spared. A variety of deformations and malformations of the hindbrain is also present and obstruction of the aqueduct may also contribute to the hydrocephalus. Atresia, forking, and gliosis have all been recorded,[85,86] while in a large series of children Emery[87] described shortening and angulation of the aqueduct suggesting a valve-like mechanism.

As with other examples of infantile hydrocephalus, the distended cerebral hemispheres have an abnormal excessively convoluted gyral pattern (Fig. 3.6(a)), variously termed polygyria,[15] stenogyria,[88] or redundant gyration.[38] Histologically, cortical laminar anatomy is normal but quantitative analysis shows a marked increase in sulcal length per unit area of cortex compared with controls.[89]

Diffuse obliteration of the cerebral subarachnoid spaces

This may be responsible for the hydrocephalus which occurs in the cerebro-ocular dysplasias, a group of familial disorders characterized by a distinctive form of cerebral cortical dysplasia,[90] recently termed lissencephaly type II,[91] diffuse cerebellar cortical dysplasia, retinal malformation and muscular dystrophy.[92] Mesodermal proliferation and massive glioneuronal heterotopia thicken the leptomeninges and fuse it to the underlying malformed cortex obliterating the subarachnoid spaces. The whole ventricular system shows marked or even massive dilatation (Fig. 3.17). The high frequency of familial cases suggests autosomal recessive inheritance,[92,93] but other workers postulate a chronic fetal meningoencephalitis with maternal horizontal transmission.[94] Hydrocephalus and encephalocele can be detected as early as 18 weeks' gestation allowing therapeutic abortion and pathological confirmation.[15] In a unique case, Norman et al.[95] have reported a 19 week fetus with hydrocephalus due to abnormal leptomeningeal vessels obstructing CSF flow in the posterior fossa.

Subarachnoid fibrosis

Several studies have shown that this is the commonest cause of infantile hydrocephalus.[68] Organization of purulent exudate or haemorrhage produces densely fibrotic, sometimes rust-coloured meninges, including scattered inflammatory infiltrates or haemosiderin-laden macrophages. The basal cisterns and exit foramina are often most severely affected (Fig. 3.18). Leptomeningeal fibrosis is also responsible for the hydrocephalus which occurs in mucopolysaccharidosis.[96]

Arachnoid granulations

Congenital aplasia of arachnoid granulations and cilia have been recorded in three hydrocephalic children by Gilles and Davidson[97] and Gutierrez et al.[98]

Functional changes in CSF absorption by the arachnoid granulations appear to be the underlying mechanism for hydrocephalus found in certain types of cranial dysplasias (Fig. 3.19), craniosynostosis,[99] achondroplasia,[100] Apert, Crouzon, and Pfeiffer syndromes.[101–103] Studies in hydrocephalic subjects with craniosynostosis or achondroplasia, utilizing simultaneous recording of pressures in the

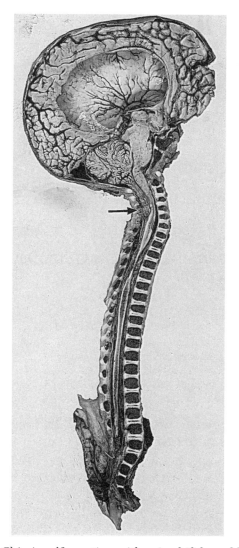

Fig. 3.16 Arnold–Chiari malformation with spina bifida and hydrocephalus. In this preparation where both calvarium and brain are fixed before being bisected, note the elongation and herniation of cerebellar vermis (arrow) and brainstem into the upper cervical canal and their close apposition to the foramen magnum.

lateral ventricle, superior sagittal sinus, and jugular vein during experimentally-induced manipulations of the intracerebral pressure, suggest that the superior sagittal sinus venous pressure resulting from anatomical obstruction is increased

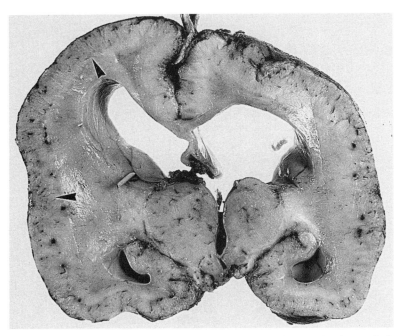

Fig. 3.17 Cerebro-ocular dysplasia. Coronal section. There is hydrocephalus, argyria, and greatly thickened cortex (arrowheads).

independent of changes in intracranial pressure and is the cause of hydrocephalus.[104,105] In a minority of cases aqueduct obstruction may also be present.[106]

I.   Imbalance between production and drainage of CSF — (B) Overproduction of CSF

The notion that progressive hydrocephalus may result from hypersecretion by a choroid plexus papilloma[107,108] was initially challenged by Dorothy Russell[2] who considered the accompanying adhesive basal meningitis of far greater pathogenetic importance. Nevertheless, diffuse enlargement throughout the ventricular system and basal cisterns may be associated with choroid plexus papillomas situated in the lateral (Fig. 3.20) or occasionally fourth ventricle.[109,110] Rare bilateral examples[111,112] are also referred to as villous hypertrophy.[108] Hydrocephalus is especially prevalent in infantile examples of choroid plexus papilloma and may be diagnosed *in utero.*[112]

Evidence for hypersecretion of CSF comes from measurements of CSF flow (upwards of 1 ml/min[113]) and from the results of surgical intervention, namely massive abdominal distention after intra-abdominal shunting[112,114] and rapid reduction of the hydrocephalus following surgical excision of the papilloma.[115,116]

Persistence of hydrocephalus after plexotomy[117] has been ascribed to basal arachnoiditis and obstruction of the basal cisterns, probably resulting from

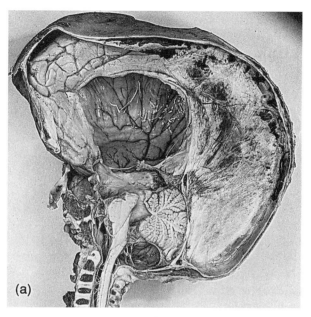

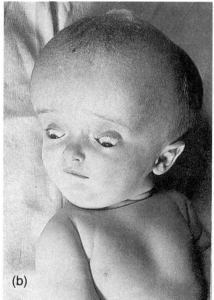

Fig. 3.18 (a) Hemisection of calvarium and brain. The whole ventricular system including the aqueduct and the basal cisterns are greatly distended as a result of post-meningitic adhesive arachnoiditis. (b) The patient showed striking macrocephaly and setting-sun sign.

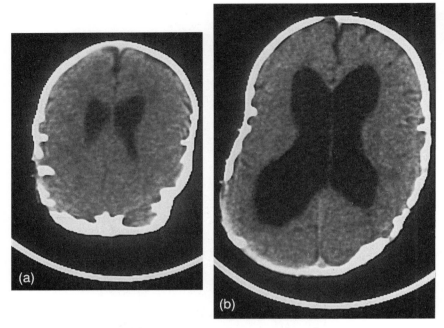

Fig. 3.19 Hydrocephalus complicating Crouzon syndrome. (a) CT scan at one and a half months. (b) Note the progression of the hydrocephalus, age eighteen months. The synostosis and skull distortion are well displayed.

spontaneous haemorrhage from the papilloma.[2,113,118] Casey and Vries[119] document a unique example of hydrocephalus and CSF overproduction in the absence of an observable abnormality in the choroid plexus.

I.   Imbalance between production and drainage of CSF — (C) Reduced propulsion of CSF

Both continuous secretion from the choroid plexus and transmission of the cervical pressure wave are responsible for the bulk flow of CSF in man. A contributory role for the beating of ependymal cilia is less certain, although their presence throughout the ventricular system and their beating action in man is well established.[120] A mutant mouse (hpy/hpy) exhibits a generalized disorder of cilia, male sterility, and hydrocephalus,[121] and rare reports of hydrocephalus in childhood have been associated with ciliary disorders. These include a 12–year–old boy with primary ciliary dyskinesia, a generalized disorder of ciliary beating related ultrastructurally to absence of the outer dynein arms of each cilium,[122] and a case of neonatal onset hydrocephalus, bronchiectasis, and ciliary aplasia.[123]

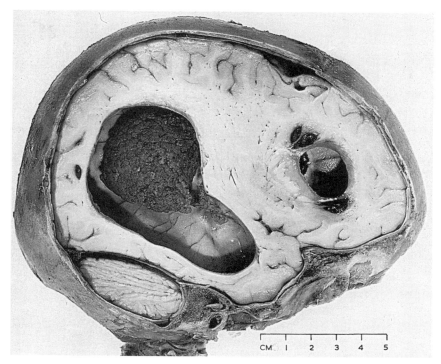

Fig. 3.20 Hydrocephalus associated with a large choroid plexus papilloma.

II. Developmental abnormalities

Significant degrees of ventricular dilatation are found in a number of rare developmental disorders though the causes of hydrocephalus remain obscure. Hydrocephalus is a cardinal feature along with hydramnios and lethality in the hydrolethalus syndrome;[124] it is present in the severe forms of Smith–Lemli–Opitz syndrome[125] and occasionally in Meckel syndrome. All these are autosomal recessive disorders. Hydrocephalus is also notable in the X-linked dominant oro–facial–digital syndrome.[126] Two Australian families have been reported with a hydranencephalic–hydrocephalic syndrome and a unique proliferative vasculopathy.[127,128] Also described from Australia is a small group of infants with cerebral lactic acidosis due to a deficiency of pyruvate dehydrogenase, they show a characteristic pattern of malformations including microcephaly, hypoplastic pyramids, heterotopia of the olives, and hydrocephalus.[129] Similar cases (Fig. 3.21) have been examined personally.[15] It should also be mentioned that ventricular dilatation is present in the abnormal hemisphere in hemimegalencephaly, in the occipital lobes in callosal agenesis, and of the holosphere in some cases of holoprosencephaly.

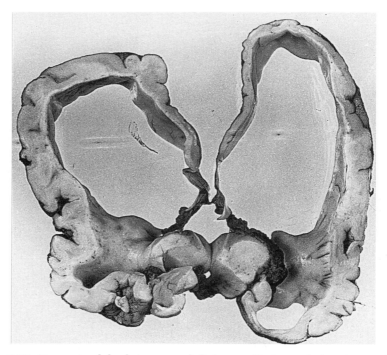

Fig. 3.21 Pyruvate dehydrogenase deficiency. Hydrocephalus in a microcephalic brain.

III.   Hydrocephalus due to destruction of brain tissue

Ventricular enlargement is a consequence of many destructive and degenerative disorders in uterine and post-natal life, but detailed discussion is beyond the scope of this chapter. In essence, the pathogenetic basis for many is hypoxia–ischaemia, such as the hydranencephaly–porencephaly defects of intrauterine origin (Fig. 3.22) and necrosis of the white matter which is a feature of the perinatal period (Fig. 3.23). Many rare degenerative disorders can also produce hydrocephalus '*ex vacuo*' whether they principally affect the cortex, as in Alpers — progressive neuronal degeneration of childhood disease[130] — or neuronal storage diseases,[96] the white matter in certain leucodystrophies,[38] or the deep grey nuclei in Leigh's disease or striatal degenerations (Fig. 3.24).[131,132]

AETIOLOGY OF HYDROCEPHALUS IN THE ADULT (TABLE 3.2)

Hydrocephalus in adults may present with a progressive rise in intraventricular and intracranial pressure with the onset of headache, drowsiness, and eventual loss of consciousness, or as the syndrome of normal pressure hydrocephalus

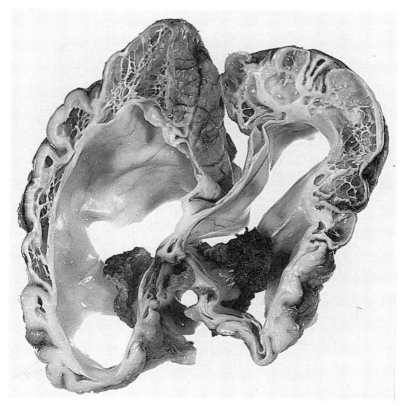

Fig. 3.22 Multicystic encephalopathy with extreme hydrocephalus '*ex vacuo*'.

(intermittently raised pressure hydrocephalus). It is mainly the lesions which obstruct or distort the ventricular system, thus causing impedance of CSF flow, that result in progressive high pressure hydrocephalus, whereas pathology in the subarachnoid space may result in normal pressure hydrocephalus.

I.   Imbalance between production and drainage of CSF

(A) Impedance of CSF drainage

Ventricular system — occlusion

Tumours and malformations

Cerebrospinal fluid flow may be impeded or blocked by intrinsic tumours or malformations within the ventricular system or by extrinsic lesions compressing or distorting the ventricular system (Table 3.2). The resulting dilatation may affect one ventricle only[133,134] or just one part of one lateral ventricle.[135] Occlusion of the foramina of Monro can occur due to the presence of a variety of

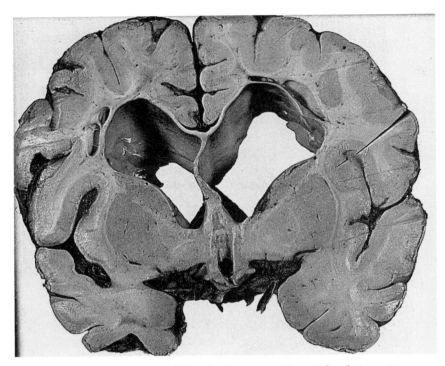

Fig. 3.23 Marked ventricular dilatation in association with white matter atrophy and periventricular cyst formation, the result of severe perinatal hypoglycaemia.

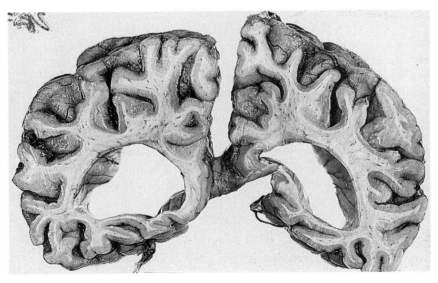

Fig. 3.24 Hydrocephalus in mucopolysaccharidosis — Sanfillipo type A.

Table 3.2   Aetiology of hydrocephalus in adults

I.	**Imbalance between production and drainage of CSF**

(A)   Impedance of CSF drainage(pp. 73–8)

    (1)   *Ventricular system — occlusion*

        (a)   Tumours — intrinsic to the ventricle:
choroid plexus papilloma, ependymoma, colloid cyst of the third ventricle. Neurocytoma of foramen of Monro, primitive neuroectodermal tumours e.g. neuroblastoma, medulloblastoma.

                Tumours — extrinsic — compressing or distorting the ventricles:
gliomas, e.g. thalamic, brainstem, cerebellar. Pituitary adenomas, craniopharyngioma. Acoustic Schwannomas. Lipomas.
Spinal tumours - unknown mechanism.

        (b)   Malformations
arteriovenous, venous.

        (c)   Inflammation
bacterial or fungal ventriculitis or abcess. Otitic hydrocephalus, multiple sclerosis.

    (2)   *Subarachnoid space — fibrosis.*

        Meningitis - pyogenic, tuberculous, fungal. Sarcoidosis. Subarachnoid haemorrhage. Cholesteatoma & suprasellar cyst contents.

    (3)   *Arachnoid granulations:*

        Post-subarachnoid haemorrhage; congenital absence.

(B)   Over production of CSF

    Rarely, if ever, causes hydrocephalus in adults.

II.   **Hydrocephalus due to destruction of brain tissue** (Hydrocephalus *ex vacuo*) (pp. 78–9)
Trauma, aging, Alzheimer disease, multi-infarct dementia. Alcoholism, Huntington disease. Creutzfeld – Jakob disease. Pick disease.

III.   **Mixed aetiology (pp. 79–80)**
Intermittently raised pressure (normal pressure) hydrocephalus and destructive lesions as in II above.

tumours within the ventricles,[136] which include relatively benign and treatable tumours or malformations such as giant cell subependymal astrocytomas (Fig. 3.3), choroid plexus papilloma (Fig. 3.20), neurocytoma,[137] and colloid cysts which are probably derived from the primitive stomatodaeum.[138] Colloid cysts may present with intermittent headaches and can be readily identified by their bright enhancement on CT scan. Usually they are thin-walled colloid-filled cysts, but if haemorrhage occurs the cyst enlarges and becomes thick-walled and fibrous with dense adhesions to the ventricular wall.[16] Ependymomas and primitive neuroectodermal tumours arising in the cerebrum (cerebral neuroblastomas) or in the cerebellum (medulloblastomas) (Fig. 3.2) are more common in children, but they do occur in adults and may spread widely through the ventricular system and the subarachnoid space around the spinal cord causing hydrocephalus.[16,136]

Extrinsic tumours may distort the ventricular system. Astrocytomas or glioblastomas of the thalamus may compress the third ventricle resulting in unilateral or bilateral dilatation of the lateral ventricles, and brainstem astrocytomas may occlude the aqueduct or fourth ventricle (Fig. 3.1). Pituitary adenomas, craniopharyngiomas (Fig. 3.25) and suprasellar cysts[139] may extend upward from the base of the skull to occlude the third ventricle and thus cause hydrocephalus. Similarly, acoustic Schwannomas growing in the cerebello–pontine angle may distort the brainstem and cause hydrocephalus by occlusion

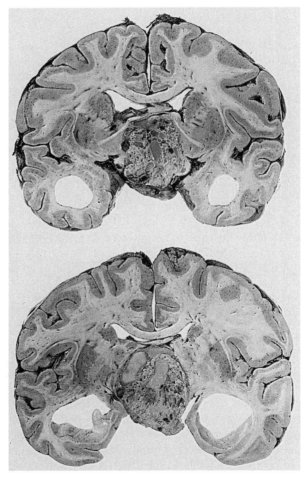

Fig. 3.25 A solid and cystic craniopharyngioma obliterates the third ventricle. Coronal section of the brain.

of the fourth ventricle. Metastatic tumours may grow within the ventricles or distort the ventricular system and thus cause hydrocephalus.[16] Although it is a rare event, spinal tumours may result in hydrocephalus both in children[140] and in adults.

Inflammation

Inflammatory lesions may result in hydrocephalus either by bacterial ventriculitis or by compression of the ventricular system due to bacterial or fungal abscesses.[16] Otitic hydrocephalus is a sequel of otitis media, and may result from thrombotic obstruction of the sigmoid sinus due to the spread of inflammation from the middle ear or mastoid air spaces.[141] Other rare inflammatory causes of hydrocephalus include mass effects due to plaques of demyelination in the brainstem in multiple sclerosis.[142]

Impedance of CSF flow through the subarachnoid space and arachnoid granulations

Apart from the cisterna magna, pontine, and interpeduncular cisterns, most of the subarachnoid space over the surface of the brain and spinal cord is divided into small compartments by numerous trabeculae of collagen and leptomeningeal cells extending from the arachnoid mater to the pia mater.[143–145] Experimental studies suggest that these compartments lead to a highly directionalized flow of cerebrospinal fluid.[146] In man, much of the cerebrospinal fluid drains into the superior sagittal sinus and other venous sinuses through arachnoid granulations and villi which are, in effect, an extension of the subarachnoid space.[147,148] In a number of animal species, however, there is an alternative, if not major route of drainage of cerebrospinal fluid into nasal lymphatics (p. 38).[149] Hydrocephalus may follow inflammation of the meninges, either as a late complication of purulent meningitis, or as a result of tuberculous meningitis or sarcoidosis. During the acute stages of purulent meningitis, the subarachnoid space may be filled with inflammatory cells, bacteria, and proteinaceous exudate,[16,143] and in tuberculous meningitis and sarcoidosis[150] there is granulomatous inflammation of the leptomeninges and the walls of meningeal vessels. Hydrocephalus is a well-recognized late complication of such meningeal inflammation and appears to be due to organization and fibrosis of the meninges with occlusion of the subarachnoid space. Fungal meningitis may also result in hydrocephalus.[151] Inflammation and subsequent thrombotic occlusion of cerebral arteries in the subarachnoid space may cause focal or widespread infarction as a complication of meningitis. Ventricular dilatation following meningitis, therefore, may be a combination of occlusion of the subarachnoid space and of tissue loss due to focal infarction both in children and in adults.

Another cause of hydrocephalus is subarachnoid haemorrhage. Ventricular dilatation occurs in the acute stages, probably due to obstruction of the cerebrospinal fluid pathways by fresh blood, and hydrocephalus may also follow as a late sequela due to organization and fibrosis within the subarachnoid space.[16] The distribution of fresh blood in recent subarachnoid haemorrhages is usually obvious, however, some months or years after the event the only evidence of past subarachnoid haemorrhage may be an orange-brown discoloration of the meninges and the presence of haemosiderin within macrophages and leptomeningeal cells over the surface of the brain.

Severe sterile granulomatous inflammation and fibrosis within the subarachnoid space may be seen following the release of keratin and cholesterol crystals from suprasellar epidermoid cysts, craniopharyngiomas, epidermoid cysts in the cerebello–pontine angle (cholesteatomas), and epidermoid cysts elsewhere in the cerebrospinal axis. If widespread, the fibrotic occlusion of the subarachnoid space may result in hydrocephalus.

It is not only fibrosis that interferes with the flow of cerebrospinal fluid through the subarachnoid space, for hydrocephalus may result from the metastatic spread of carcinoma or glioma cells. The presence of such cells can be detected in CSF samples[16] or by histology as they may float free within the cerebrospinal fluid spaces or be attached to the surfaces of the arachnoid and pia.[16]

Despite the clear association of leptomeningitis and subarachnoid haemorrhage with hydrocephalus and fibrosis of the meninges, occlusion of the arachnoid granulations as a cause of hydrocephalus is less certain.[152]

II. Hydrocephalus due to destruction of brain tissue (hydrocephalus ex vacuo)

Destruction of brain tissue may result in a significant reduction in the volume of the brain. In many instances the destruction is focal, as with areas of infarction, but in a significant number of diseases there is a diffuse loss of brain tissue with cerebral atrophy affecting large areas of the brain (Fig. 3.22). It is in these patients that the ventricular dilatation that accompanies cerebral atrophy may be confused with hydrocephalus resulting from obstruction of cerebrospinal fluid flow.

Progressive loss of brain tissue occurs with ageing. Loss of neurones from the cortex results in shrinkage of the gyri and widening of the sulci. The ventricular system is often dilated and the lateral angles of the lateral ventricles become rounded. The hippocampi fail to fill the temporal horns and the aqueduct may be distended.[153,154] A greater degree of ventricular dilatation may be seen in a number of diseases associated with diffuse brain damage and dementia (Table 3.2). In Alzheimer's disease, cortical atrophy and ventricular dilatation are associated with the presence of argyrophilic senile plaques and neurofibrillary tangles in the cerebral cortex (Fig. 3.26),[154,155] whereas in multi-infarct dementia, the tissue destruction is due to a myriad of small infarcts often the result of multiple embolic episodes or associated with hypertension.[154] Ventricular dilatation has been recorded in chronic alcoholics, although the nature of the tissue damage is difficult to determine. Diffuse axonal injury in severe head injuries, and the hypoxia which may complicate brain trauma,

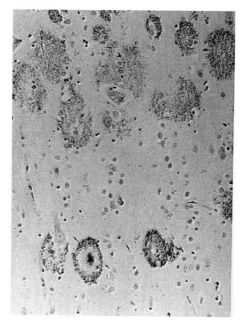

Fig. 3.26 Alzheimer's disease. Senile plaques show amyloid deposited as a central core and more diffusely in the plaque. Immunocytochemistry for A4 protein (C958) ×365.

frequently results in some degree of cerebral atrophy and ventricular dilatation which is visible for some months after the injury.[156] Other dementias are associated with ventricular dilatation, such as Huntington's disease in which there is bilateral atrophy and gliosis of the caudate nucleus, putamen and globus pallidus,[154,157] and Pick's disease, in which the cerebral atrophy is associated with neuronal loss and the presence of globular argyrophilic inclusions of neuro-fibrillary material within neurones in the frontal and temporal regions.[154] The transmissible dementia, Creutzfeldt–Jakob disease, in which there is spongiform change in the cerebral and cerebellar cortices and in the deep grey matter of the cerebral hemisphere, is associated with neuronal loss, gliosis, cerebral atrophy and ventricular dilatation in the later stages of the disease.[154,158]

Mixed aetiology

Frequently associated with clinical features of dementia, gait disturbance, and urinary incontinence, intermittently raised pressure hydrocephalus is potentially a treatable disorder.[159] The aetiology and pathogenesis of the condition is unknown in approximately 50 per cent of cases,[160] but underlying causes, such as past subarachnoid haemorrhage, head injury, or meningitis which result in fibrous adhesions in the basal cisterns and subarachnoid space, are found in other cases. The cerebrospinal fluid pressure may not be significantly raised on a single recording but 24-hour records usually reveal periods in which the pressure is elevated.

A proportion of patients who have been diagnosed as suffering from intermittently raised pressure hydrocephalus respond well to ventricular shunting. Measurements of resistance to cerebrospinal fluid outflow may be valuable predictors of the outcome of shunting procedures.[160] It appears, however, that gait disturbance rather than dementia may be the most important symptom of normal pressure hydrocephalus.[161]

Failure of patients with apparent intermittently raised pressure hydrocephalus to respond to shunting procedures may be due to the presence of underlying brain damage associated with the cause of the hydrocephalus or of independent associated Alzheimer's disease or multi-infarct dementia.[162] In some cases, patients may respond initially to shunting but subsequently signs of dementia return despite a fully functioning shunt. In these cases, there may be a true mixture of normal pressure hydrocephalus and progressive dementia due to Alzheimer's disease or multi-infarct dementia.[163] In addition to CSF pressure monitoring, small biopsies can be taken for histological examination at the time of shunt insertion. The detection of Alzheimer senile plaques or the presence of small infarcts in the biopsies may help with the assessment of underlying destructive brain damage present in patients with intermittently raised pressure hydrocephalus.

EXPERIMENTAL HYDROCEPHALUS

There is a wide variety of techniques for producing hydrocephalus in experimental animals. Initially, the hydrocephalus produced by these techniques confirmed that cerebrospinal fluid was produced by the choroid plexus and that impedance of the cerebrospinal fluid flow was the cause of hydrocephalus.[3] As it became apparent that brain damage was associated with the ventricular dilatation, hydrocephalus in experimental animals was used to define the type, extent, and mechanisms of such damage. With the widespread institution of therapy by shunting the dilated ventricles, attention has focused on the effects on the brain of inserting shunts into hydrocephalic ventricles. Much of the basic data are produced from experimental studies. Choice of the experimental model depends upon the object of the study.

Techniques for the production of experimental hydrocephalus

The many and varied techniques used to produce hydrocephalus in experimental animals are set out in Table 3.3. Initially, techniques concentrated on causing obstruction of cerebrospinal fluid flow by the injection of irritative agents such as Indian ink,[164] Pantopaque,[165] or kaolin[166] into the cisterna magna. Sterile meningitis resulted in subsequent fibrosis, scarring and occlusion of the subarachnoid space. Unfortunately, such irritative agents also entered the ventricular system causing damage to the ependyma and underlying white matter,[165]

Table 3.3   Techniques for the induction of experimental hydrocephalus

Obstruction of CSF flow

(i)   Injection of sclerogenic material into the subarachnoid space and ventricular system, e.g. Indian ink, Pantopaque, Kaolin, Silastic.

(ii)   Infusion of non-sclerogenic material into the posterior fossa, e.g. silicone oil.

Destructive technique

(i)   Irradiation of pregnant females.

Toxic methods

(i)   Foetus (pregnant females):
        using trypan blue, methyl mercuric chloride.

(ii)   Suckling and young animals:
        using 6-aminonicotinamide, tellurium.

(iii)   Adults:

Vitamin A deficiency

(iv)   Hypersensitivity to foreign proteins.

Virus infections

(i)   Mumps in suckling animals.

(ii)   Rheovirus in suckling animals.

Genetic defects - hereditary hydrocephalus

(i)   Mouse mutants.

(ii)   Rat mutants.

so that such models were unsuitable for the study of the brain damage caused by the hydrocephalus. The injection of inert viscous silicone oil into the posterior fossa, however, caused no inflammation or brain damage and was more suitable for the study of the brain damage resulting from hydrocephalus.[7,9] Other methods of obstruction of CSF flow have been used particularly in larger animals; these include occlusion of the aqueduct by gauze[3] or by an inflated Foley catheter.[8] Despite reservations, kaolin injections are both simple and popular for the production of experimental hydrocephalus.

Reflecting the mixed aetiology of obestruction of cerebrospinal fluid flow and brain destruction in human hydrocephalus, there are a number of experimental studies which have used irradiation (100 gray) of pregnant rats at day 9.5 of gestation, this results in stenosis of the aqueduct and hydrocephalus in a proportion of the offspring.[167] Toxic agents such as trypan blue,[168] and methyl mercuric chloride,[169] or tellurium[170] administered to pregnant rats result in hydrocephalus in the offspring. Injection of 6-aminonicotinamide into suckling mice on the fifth post-natal day causes hydrocephalus, which in the early stages (7–9 days after injection) is characterized by aqueductal stenosis due to oedematous ependymal and subependymal cells.[171] At a later stage, the oedema subsides, the ependymal cells degenerate, and the aqueduct is stenosed. Vitamin

A deficiency in adult rabbits results in hydrocephalus with raised CSF pressure,[172] the animals respond to Vitamin A administration with lowering of ventricular pressure, but, again, the mechanism is unclear. There is also some suggestion that hydrocephalus may result from a hypersensitivity reaction to the presence of foreign proteins in the ventricles.[173]

Perhaps one of the most significant discoveries in relation to the cause of hydrocephalus in the fetus and newborn is the finding that mumps virus injected into suckling hamsters causes ependymitis with destruction of the ependyma. This is followed by aqueductal stenosis and hydrocephalus in 95 per cent of the animals by the age of three months.[174] Similar results are seen with rheovirus in several species.[175]

In recent years, a number of hereditary hydrocephalus models have been described. These include spontaneous mutations such as the mouse strain SUMS bred in Southampton.[176,177] The hydrocephalus is inherited as an autosomal recessive trait with variable penetrance. Ventricular enlargement is detectable at 3 days after birth and many of the animals die with gross hydrocephalus by 3 weeks.[177] Although the exact cause of the hydrocephalus is unknown, it can be used as a model to study tissue damage and the effects of ventriculitis.[177] Other models such as hydrocephalus with hop-gait have defined genetic abnormalities; in this case a mutation on the proximal end of chromosome 7.[178] Hereditary hydrocephalus is described in the rat.[179-181] Some are similar to the mouse models and others have evidence of prenatal stenosis of the aqueduct.[180]

Brain damage resulting from hydrocephalus

Quite apart from the brain damage which may result from the causes of hydro-cephalus (Tables 3.1 and 3.2), raised CSF pressure and ventricular dilatation do themselves cause damage to neurological tissue. Clinical evidence suggests that delay in the treatment of progressive hydrocephalus results in low intellectual scores or poor school attainment.[5,6,182] However, the cause and extent of the brain damage was difficult to determine before the development of appropriate experimental models and clinical evaluation by CT and MRI.

Classical accounts[2] report the ventricular enlargement, which can be very extensive in children, and the gross thinning of the cerebral mantle, whereby the total thickness of the cortex and white matter may be less than 1 mm, parti-cularly in the occipital lobes. Hydrocephalic brains often appear globular due to the almost spherical ventricles, and the gyral pattern may be distorted and flattened (Figs 3.1(b) and 3.6(a)). Coronal sectioning of the brain shows that it is mainly attenuation of the cerebral mantle that accommodates the enlargement of the ventricles, whereas the central grey matter areas are often intact even if depressed and separated by a large third ventricle. The corpus callosum in many hydrocephalic brains is very thin and the ependymal surface may be granular due to defects in the ependyma and small glial excrescences protruding from the subependymal regions (granular ependymitis) (Fig. 3.7(b)). Synechiae may be seen in the form of thin sheets or bands crossing the ventricular lumen. If bacterial infections have complicated the hydrocephalus, pus may be seen in the ventricles or there may be adhesions due to scarring following infection. The aqueduct may be occluded (non-communicating hydrocephalus) or widely dilated, depending upon the site of the cerebrospinal fluid block. In cases of past meningitis or subarachnoid haemorrhage, there may be patchy or extensive thickening of the arachnoid on the outer aspects of the cerebral hemispheres and brain stem.[16]

There are many variables which determine the degree of brain damage resulting from the hydrocephalus, such as the age of the patient, the degree of myelination in the periventricular white matter, the stage of maturity of the skull, and the cause of the hydrocephalus.[10] Clinical features and CT findings, however, show that it is not possible to relate the ventricular size to subsequent intellectual development.[183] The results of experimental studies have determined the sequence of events in acute and chronic brain damage in hydrocephalus, and correlative biopsy studies in human children[10,12] have allowed a relationship between pathological tissue damage and subsequent intellectual development to be established.

Acute hydrocephalus

The acute stages of hydrocephalus are characterized by oedema of the periventricular white matter. In histological preparations and by electron microscopy[7,9,10] the interstitial oedema fluid appears to be low in protein and excites little inflammatory reaction. CT scan studies have shown that the now familiar periventricular low density regions in the white matter in acute hydrocephalus are the result of insudation of cerebrospinal fluid from the ventricles.[184] It occurs within 12 hours after restriction of the normal flow of CSF and is concentrated initially near the angles of the lateral ventricles.[8,185] Histological studies in the white matter of dogs after the induction of hydrocephalus, by the injection of silastic into the prepontine cisterns or fourth ventricle, have shown that the area of extracellular oedema is comparable to the region of increased signal intensity on T2-weighted images on MRI.[186]

The tissue damage detectable by histology and by electron microscopy in the periventricular white matter depends partly upon the rate of ventricular enlargement,[187] partly upon the severity of the hydrocephalus, and partly upon the length of time that the hydrocephalus has been present.[7,9] In man and in experimental animals, the acute stages of hydrocephalus are characterized by splitting and disruption of the ependyma,[7] and by cerebrospinal fluid oedema of the periventricular white matter. Myelinated nerve fibres or non-myelinated nerve fibres in very young infant brains are widely separated by clear fluid (Figs 3.27 and 3.28). Very little inflammatory reaction is seen, and in the early stages only isolated degenerating axons can be recognized.[7,10] If ventricular dilatation and high CSF pressure persists, axonal damage continues and there is tissue breakdown, macrophage invasion, and reactive astrocytosis (Fig. 3.28).[9] If the hydrocephalus enters a more chronic stage the CSF oedema subsides, but the tissue

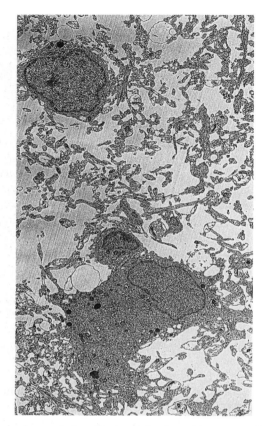

Fig. 3.27 Acute hydrocephalus. Periventricular white matter from the occipital lobe of a 29-day-old child showing extensive oedema with clear fluid between axonal and astrocyte processes. A reactive astrocyte is seen at the bottom of the picture. Electron micrograph ×3000 [Reproduced by permission of the Editor from: Weller, R.0. and Shulman, K.J. *Neurosurgery*, **36**, 255 (1972). (Fig. 1)].

damage that has occurred during the acute phases, and may continue in the chronic phase, is reflected in the severe gliosis and loss of axons and myelin in the periventricular white matter (Fig. 3.28).[10,12] If damage is very severe, as it can be in infantile and adult experimental animals, periventricular tissue may be so badly damaged that it remains oedematous with extensive loss of myelinated fibres[7,9,] or may virtually disappear (Fig. 3.28).

The cause of the damage to the periventricular white matter is not clear. It may be due to ischaemia, as there is considerable disturbance of metabolism in association with decreased blood flow, by some 50 per cent, in both acute and chronic stages of experimental hydrocephalus.[188] In these studies, autoregulation was preserved and the water content of the brain tissue increased temporarily,

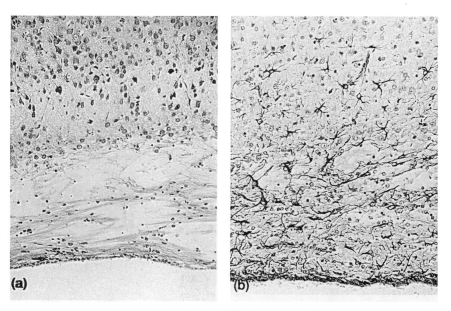

Fig. 3.28 Acute hydrocephalus in the SUMS mouse. All illustrations are at the same magnification (×140) and taken from the same area of the brain, i.e. the cerebral mantle superiorly; there is severe ventricular dilatation. In (a) the ventricle is at the bottom of the picture and the cerebral cortex at the top. An intact ependyma is seen but the white matter between the ependyma and the cortex is spongy and vacuolated with nerve fibres in the white matter widely separated by clear fluid-filled spaces. The cortex is unaffected by the oedema. Stained with Klüver Barrera. (b) Same area as (a) showing stellate reactive astrocytes in the damaged white matter stained darkly for glial fibrillary acidic protein. Although a few reactive astrocytes are seen in the deep cortex, the superficial cortex (top) is almost unaffected. Stained with immunoperoxidase for fibrillary acidic protein (GFAP).

but only within the periventricular white matter. Other studies have also suggested a disturbed microcirculation in hydrocephalic brains.[189] In some cases, the amount of tissue damage may be almost undetectable. It is also possible that the presence of cerebrospinal fluid oedema in the periventricular white matter is a cause of the tissue damage due to expansion of the extracellular compartment. Although this may cause problems in diffusion of nutrients and metabolites, such interstitial oedema does not appear to have a direct effect on cells, since transplanted fetal brain cells survive well in oedematous white matter in hydrocephalic rat brains.[190]

In mildly hydrocephalic rats, there may be no white matter oedema and no detectable axon degeneration, but proliferation of subependymal cells in these animals is an indication that the tissue is still reacting.[191]

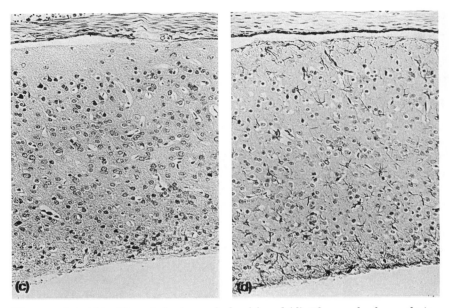

Fig. 3.28 (*contd.*)   *Chronic hydrocephalus* (c) and (d). The cerebral mantle is now much thinner than in (a) and (b). In (c) the ventricle is at the bottom of the picture; the ependyma has disappeared and there is virtually no white matter remaining. The meningeal surface of the brain is seen at the top of the picture. Stained with Klüver Barrera. (d) Same area as (c) showing some gliosis of the remaining white matter (bottom) but few darkly stained astrocytes in the cerebral cortex. Stained with immunoperoxidase for glial fibrillary acidic protein (GFAP).

The ependyma may be stretched and flattened[191] in hydrocephalus or, in the more severely affected brain, tears may spontaneously occur in the linings of the ventricles.[7,192] Eventually, gaps appear between individual cells and they may form small isolated nests of ependymal cells.[7,10] In experimental studies, such ependymal defects are covered within the first 48 hours by small cells resembling subependymal cells.[193] As repair continues, the cells develop processes, and such a mechanism may lead to the astrocytic nodules seen around many hydrocephalic ventricles.

In post-natal hydrocephalus, the central grey matter and the cerebral cortex do not appear to be directly damaged to the same extent as the periventricular white matter. Despite the significant rise in the free water content of the white matter in experimental hydrocephalus, there was no change in either the total water content or free or bound water content in the cortical grey matter.[193] Such findings are confirmed by histological studies of hydrocephalic mice in which there may be almost total destruction of the white matter due to extensive oedema, yet the central grey matter of the cortex shows only mild reactive astrocytosis (Fig. 3.28).

Hydrocephalus in the fetus may disturb neuronal proliferation and migration[194] and may thus have a greater effect upon grey matter areas than is seen in post-natal and adult brains.

Effects of shunting on the brain

In addition to the problems that arise from the revision of shunts in children and infections that complicate shunting, reaction to shunt tubing may occur when it is implanted into periventricular tissue for long periods. Ependyma may be lost and subependymal gliosis may ensue.[195] Evagination of periventricular glial scar tissue into the perforations of the shunt tubing may be a cause of shunt obstruction.[195]

Significant changes may also occur in the white matter of hydrocephalic brains following shunt insertion. Although the ventricles may return to a normal size following shunting, the expanded white matter may remain spongy and oedematous and the ventricles may be surrounded by a thick rigid layer of subependymal gliosis.[10] A progressive state of 'slit-ventricle' may be induced in experimental animals by creating a low-pressure state through external ventricular drainage. The white matter becomes disorganized and the ependymal lining partly stripped, with gliosis of the subependymal areas and adjacent white matter.[196] Such changes may result in decreased compliance of the periventricular tissue.[196]

Alternative pathways of CSF drainage in hydrocephalus

The major pathways of cerebrospinal fluid in man appear to be through arachnoid granulations (see pp. 36–8).[32,33] It has been shown in a number of species, however, that cerebrospinal fluid also drains into nasal lymphatics[197] and along cranial perineural lymphatic channels.[197] In addition, some 5 per cent of CSF in normal rabbits appears to pass into the spinal canal.[197] It is not clear to what extent any of these pathways play a role in the drainage of CSF in human or animal hydrocephalus. Under normal circumstances, pressure gradients are seen to favour diffusion of extracellular fluid diffusely through white matter[31,198] with drainage into the ventricular CSF.[199] These gradients appear to be reversed in hydrocephalus, with resulting periventricular CSF oedema and a greatly increased flow of fluid into blood vessels of the periventricular white matter.[200] It does appear, however, that this pathway, and the increased flow of fluid down the spinal cord, often with dilatation of the central canal are insufficient to arrest hydrocephalus.[197,198]

ACKNOWLEDGEMENTS

We would like to thank Margaret Harris for typing the manuscript.

REFERENCES

1. Ring-Mrozik, E. and Angerpointner, T.A. Historical aspects of hydrocephalus. *Progress in Pediatric Surgery*, **20**, 158–87 (1986).
2. Russell, D.S. Observations on the pathology of hydrocephalus. *MRC Special Report Series No. 265*, HMSO, London (1949).
3. Dandy, W.E. and Blackfan, K.D. Internal hydrocephalus. An experimental, clinical and pathological study. *American Journal of Diseases of Children*, **8**, 406–82 (1914).
4. Pudenz, R.H. The surgical treatment of infantile hydrocephalus. In *Disorders of the developing nervous system*, (ed. Fields, W.S. and Desmond, M.M.), pp. 468–89. C.C. Thomas, Springfield, Illinois, (1961).
5. Laurence, K.M. and Coates, S. The natural history of hydrocephalus; detailed analysis of 182 unoperated cases. *Archives of Disease in Childhood*, **37**, 345–62 (1962).
6. MacNab, G.H. The development of the knowledge and treatment of hydrocephalus. *Developmental Medicine and Child Neurology*, **11**, (Suppl.) 1–9 (1966).
7. Weller, R.O. and, Wisniewski, H. Histological and ultrastructural changes in experimental hydrocephalus: I: Adult Rabbit. *Brain*, **92**, 819–28 (1969).
8. Clark, R.G. and Milhorat, T.H. Experimental hydrocephalus. Part 3: Light microscopic findings in acute and subacute obstructive hydrocephalus in the monkey. *Journal of Neurosurgery*, **32**, 400–13 (1970).
9. Weller, R.O., Wisniewski, H., Shulman, K., and Terry, R.D. Experimental hydrocephalus in young dogs: Histological and ultrastructural study of the brain tissue damage. *Journal of Neuropathology and Experimental Neurology*, **30**, 613–27 (1971).
10. Weller, R.O. and Shulman, K. Infantile hydrocephalus: Clinical, histological and ultrastructural study of brain damage. *Journal of Neurosurgery*, **36**, 255–6 (1972).
11. Naidich, T.P., Epstein, F., Lin, J.P. *et al.* Evaluation of pediatric hydrocephalus by computer tomography. *Radiology*, **119**, 337–45 (1976).
12. Weller, R.O. and Williams, B.N. Cerebral biopsy in the assessment of brain damage in hydrocephalus. *Archives of Disease in Childhood*, **10**, 763–8 (1975).
13. Maytal, J., Alvarez, L.A., Elkin, C.M., and Shinner, S. External hydrocephalus: radiologic spectrum and differentiation from cerebral atrophy. *American Journal of Roentgenology*, **148**, 1223–330 (1987).
14. Paine, R.S., Luessenhop, A.J., Avery, G.B., and Kachmann, R. Hydrocephalus. *Clinical Proceedings of the Children's Hospital (Washington)*, **22**, 93–117 (1966).
15. Harding, B.N. Malformations. Chap. 10 In *Greenfield's Neuropathology, (5th edn)*, (ed. Adams, J.H. and Duchen, L.W.), pp. 521–638, Edward Arnold, London (1992).
16. Weller, R.O. *Systemic pathology*, (3rd edn), *Nervous system, muscle and eyes*, Churchill Livingstone, Edinburgh (1990).
17. Newton, H., Pickard, J.D., and Weller, R.O. Normal pressure hydrocephalus and cerebrovascular disease: findings of post-mortem. *Journal of Neurology, Neurosurgery and Psychiatry,* **52**, 804 (1989).
18. Gomez, M.R. *Tuberous sclerosis.* Raven Press, New York (1979).
19. Wilberger, J.E. Jr., Vertosick, F.T. Jr., and Vries, J.K. Unilateral hydrocephalus secondary to congenital atresia of the foramen of Monro. Case Report. *Journal of Neurosurgery*, **59**, 899–901 (1983).

20. Husag, L., Wieser, H.G., and Probst, C. Unilateraler Hydrozephalus bei membranösem Verschuss des Foramen Monroi. *Acta Neurochirugica*, **33**, 183–212 (1976).

21. Nakamura, S., Makiyama, H., Miyagi, A., Tsubokawa, T.U., and Shinohara, H. Congenital unilateral hydrocephalus. *Child's Nervous System*, **5**, 367–70 (1989).

22. Pfeiffer, G. and Friede, R.L. Unilateral hydrocephalus from early developmental occlusion of one foramen of Monro. *Acta Neuropathologica*, **64**, 75–7 (1984).

23. Chow, C.W., McKelvie, P.A., Anderson, R.McD., Phelan, E.M.D., Klug, G.L., and Rogers, J.G. Autosomal recessive hydrocephalus with third ventricle obstruction. *American Journal of Medical Genetics*, **35**, 310–13 (1990).

24. Kepes, J.J., Clough, C., and Villanueva, A. Congenital fusion of the thalami (atresia of the third ventricle) and associated anomalies in a 6 month old infant. *Acta Neuropathologica*, **13**, 97–104 (1969).

25. Woollam, D.H.M. and Millen, J.W. Anatomical considerations in the pathology of stenosis of the cerebral aqueduct. *Brain*, **76**, 104–12 (1953).

26. Emery, J.L. and Staschak, M.C. The size and form of the cerebral aqueduct in children. *Brain*, **95**, 591–8 (1972).

27. Drachman, D.A. and Richardson, E.P. Jr. Aqueductal narrowing, congenital and acquired. *Archives of Neurology*, **5**, 552–9 (1961).

28. Turkewitsch, N. La constitution anatomique de l'Aquaeductus cerebri de l'Homme. *Archives d' Anatomie, d' Histologie et d' Embryologie*, **21**, 323–57 (1936).

29. Johnson, R.T. and Johnson, K.T. Hydrocephalus following virus infection: the pathology of aqueductal stenosis developing after experimental mumps virus infection. *Journal of Neuropathology and Experimental Neurology*, **27**, 591–606 (1968).

30. Borit A. Communicating hydrocephalus causing aqueductal stenosis. *Neuropediatrics*, **7**, 416–22 (1976).

31. Williams, B. Is aqueduct stenosis a result of hydrocephalus? *Brain*, **96**, 399–412 (1973).

32. Emery, J.L. Deformity of the aqueduct of Sylvius in children with hydrocephalus and myelomeningocoele. *Developmental Medicine and Child Neurology*, **16** (Suppl. 32), 40–8 (1974).

33. Borit, A. and Sidman, R.L. New mutant mouse with communicating hydrocephalus and secondary aqueductal stenosis. *Acta Neuropathologica*, **21**, 316–31 (1972).

34. Masters, C., Alpers, M., and Kakulas, B. Pathogenesis of Rheovirus Type 1 hydrocephalus in mice. Significance of aqueductal changes. *Archives of Neurology*, **34**, 18–28 (1977).

35. Baker, D.W. and Vinters, H.V. Hydrocephalus with cerebral aqueductal dysgenesis and craniofacial anomalies. *Acta Neuropathologica*, **63**, 170–3 (1984).

36. Bistrian, B., Phillips, C.A., and Kaye, I.S. Fatal mumps meningoencephalitis. Isolation of virus premortem and postmortem. *Journal of the American Medical Association*, **222**, 478–9 (1972).

37. Spataro, R.F., Lin, S-R., Horner, F.A., Hall, C.B., and McDonald, J.V. Aqueductal stenosis and hydrocephalus; rare sequelae of mumps virus infection. *Neuroradiology*, **12**, 11–13 (1976).

38. Friede, R.L. *Developmental neuropathology*, (2nd Edn). Springer-Verlag, Berlin (1989).

39. Beckett, R.S., Netsky, M.G., and Zimmerman, H.M. Developmental stenosis of the Aqueduct of Sylvius. *American Journal of Pathology*, **26**, 755–71 (1950).

40. Bickers, D.S. and Adams, R.D. Hereditary stenosis of the aqueduct of Sylvius as a cause of congenital hydrocephalus. *Brain*, **72**, 246–62 (1949).

41. Baraitser, M. *The genetics of neurological disorders*, (2nd edn). Oxford University Press, Oxford (1990).

42. Edwards, J.H., Norman, R.M., and Roberts, J.M. Sex-linked hydrocephalus. Report of a family with 15 affected members. *Archives of Disease in Childhood*, **36**, 481–5 (1961).

43. Holmes, L., Nash, A., Zu Rhein, G., Levin, M., and Opitz, J.M. X-linked aqueductal stenosis: clinical and morphological findings in two families. *Pediatrics*, **51**, 697–704 (1973).

44. Landrieu, P., Ninane, J., Ferrière, G., and Lyon, G. Aqueductal stenosis in X-linked hydrocephalus: a secondary phenomenon? *Developmental Medicine and Child Neurology*, **21**, 637–52 (1979).

45. Edwards, J.H. The syndrome of sex-linked hydrocephalus. *Archives of Disease in Childhood*, **36**, 486–93 (1961).

46. Willems, P.J., Brouwer, O.F., Dijkstra, I., and Wilminik, J. X-linked hydrocephalus. *American Journal of Medical Genetics*, **27**, 921–8 (1987).

47. Faivre, J., Lemarec, B., Bretagne, J., and Pecker, J. X-linked hydrocephalus, aqueductal stenosis, mental retardation, and adduction–flexion deformity of the thumbs. Report of a family. *Child's Brain*, **2**, 226–33 (1976).

48. Hanau, J., Franc, B., Faivre, J., and Foncin, J.F. Hydrocéphalie genetique liée au sexe. Étude anatomique. *Revue Neurologique*, **134**, 437–42 (1978).

49. Chow, C.H., Halliday, J.L., Anderson, R.McD., Danks, D.M., and Fortune, D.W. Congenital absence of pyramids and its significance in genetic diseases. *Acta Neuropathologica*, **65**, 313–17 (1985).

50. Howard, F.H., Till, K., and Carter, C.O. A family study of hydrocephalus resulting from aqueduct stenosis. *Journal of Medical Genetics*, **18**, 252–5 (1981).

51. Russell, D.S. and Nevin, S. Aneurysm of the great vein of Galen causing internal hydrocephalus: report of two cases. *Journal of Pathology and Bacteriology*, **51**, 375–83 (1940).

52. Rowbotham, G.F. Small aneurysm completely obstructing lower end of aqueduct of Sylvius. *Archives of Neurology and Psychiatry*, **40**, 1241–3 (1938).

53. Courville, C.B. Obstructive internal hydrocephalus incidental to small vascular anomaly of the midbrain. *Bulletin of Los Angeles Neurological Society*, **26**, 41–5 (1961).

54. Barr, M.L. Observations on the foramen of Magendie in a series of human brains. *Brain*, **71**, 281–9 (1948).

55. Vuia, 0. Malformation of the paraflocculus and atresia of the foramina Magendie and Luschka in a child. *Psychiatrie, Neurologie, Neurochirurgie (Amsterdam)*, **76**, 261–6 (1973).

56. Holland, H.C. and Graham, W.L. Congenital atresia of the foramina of Luschka and Magendie with hydrocephalus. Report of a case in an adult. *Journal of Neurosurgery*, **15**, 688–94 (1958).

57. Gardner, W.J., McCormack, C.J., and Dohn, D.F. Embryonal atresia of the fourth ventricle; the cause of 'arachnoid cyst' of the cerebellopontine angle. *Journal of Neurosurgery*, **17**, 226–37 (1960).

58. Dandy, W.E. and Blackfan, F.D. Internal hydrocephalus, an experimental clinical and pathological study. *American Journal of Diseases of Children*, **8**, 406–82 (1914).

59. Benda, C.E. The Dandy–Walker syndrome or the so-called atresias of the foramen of Magendie. *Journal of Neuropathology and Experimental Neurology*, **13**, 14–29 (1954).

60. Hart, M.N., Malamud, N., and Ellis, W.G. The Dandy–Walker syndrome. A clinicopathological study based on 28 cases. *Neurology*, **22**, 771–80 (1972).

61. Jenkyn, L.R., Roberts, D.W., Merlis, A.L., Rozycky, A.A., and Nordgren, R.E. Dandy–Walker malformation in identical twins. *Neurology*, **31**, 337–41 (1981).

62. Galassi, E., Tognetti, F., Frank, F., Fagioli, L., Nasi, M.T., and Gaist, G. Infratentorial arachnoid cysts. *Journal of Neurosurgery*, **63**, 210–17 (1985).

63. Friede, R.L. Cerebral infarcts complicating neonatal leptomeningitis. Acute and residual lesions. *Acta Neuropathologica*, **23**, 245–53 (1973).

64. Rhoton, A.L. Jr and Gomez, M.R. Conversion of multilocular hydrocephalus to unilocular. Case report. *Journal of Neurosurgery*, **36**, 348–50 (1972).

65. De Vita, V.T., Utz, J.P., Williams, T., and Carbone, P.P. Candida meningitis. *Archives of Internal Medicine*, **117**, 527–35 (1966).

66. Miller, M.J. Fungal infections. In *Infectious diseases of the fetus and newborn infant*, (ed, Remington, J.S. and Klein, J.O.), pp. 464–506. Saunders, Philadelphia, (1983).

67. Harding, B.N. The Brain. In *Diseases of the fetus and newborn,* (ed. Reed, G.B., Claireaux, A.E., and Bain, A.D.), pp. 169–216. Chapman Hall, London (1989).

68. Gilles, F.H and Shillito, J.Jr. Infantile hydrocephalus: retrocerebellar subdural haematoma. *Journal of Pediatrics*, **76**, 529–37 (1970).

69. Hill, A. and Volpe, J.J. Normal pressure hydrocephalus in the newborn. *Pediatrics*, **68,** 623–9 (1981).

70. Levene, M.I. and Starte, D.R. A longitudinal study of post-haemorrhagic ventricular dilatation in the newborn. *Archives of Disease in Childhood*, **56**, 905–10 (1981).

71. Larroche, J.C. Post haemorrhagic hydrocephalus of infancy. Anatomical study. *Biology of the Neonate*, **20**, 287–99 (1972).

72. Deonna, T., Payot, M., Probst, A., and Prod'hom, L.S. Neonatal intracranial haemorrhage in premature infants. *Pediatrics*, **56**, 1056–64 (1979).

73. Bates, J.I. and Netsky, M.G. Developmental anomalies of the horns of the lateral ventricles. *Journal of Neuropathology and Experimental Neurology*, **14**, 316–25 (1955).

74. Norman, R.M. and McMenemey, W.H. Transventricular adhesion in association with birth injury of the caudate nucleus. *Journal of Neuropathology and Experimental Neurology*, **14,** 85–91 (1955).

75. Oi, S. and Matsumoto, S. Slit ventricles as a cause of isolated ventricles after shunting. *Child's Nervous System*, **1**, 189–93 (1985).

76. Foltz, E.L. and Shurtleff, D.B. Conversion of communicating hydrocephalus to stenosis or occlusion of the aqueduct during ventricular shunt. *Journal of Neurosurgery,* **24**, 520–9 (1966).

77. Hawkins, J.C. III, Hoffman, H.J., and Humphreys, R.P. Isolated fourth ventricle as a complication of ventricular shunting. Report of 3 cases. *Journal of Neurosurgery*, **49,** 910–13 (1978).

78. Turnbull, I.M. and Drake, C.G. Membranous occlusion of the aqueduct of Sylvius. *Journal of Neurology*, **24**, 24–33 (1966).

79. Friede, R.L. and Roessmann, U. Chronic tonsillar herniation. An attempt at clarifying chronic herniations at the foramen magnum. *Acta Neuropathologica*, **34**, 219–35 (1986).

80. Ruff, M.E., Oakes, W.J., Fisher, S.R., and Spock, A. Sleep apnea and vocal cord paralysis secondary to type I Chiari malformation. *Pediatrics*, **80**, 231–4 (1987).

81. Banerji, N.K. and Millar, J.H.D. Chiari malformation presenting in adult life. Its relationship to syringomyelia. *Brain*, **97**, 157–68 (1974).

82. Shady, W., Metcalfe, R.A., and Butler, P. The incidence of craniocervical bony anomalies in the adult Chiari malformation. *Journal of the Neurological Sciences*, **82**, 193–203 (1987).

83. Gimenez-Roldani, S., Benito, C., and Mateo, D. Familial communicating syringo-myelia. *Journal of the Neurological Sciences*, **36**, 135–46 (1978).

84. Coria, F., Quintana, F., Rebollo, M., Combarros, O. and Berciano, J. Occipital dysplasia and Chiari type I deformity in a family. *Journal of the Neurological Sciences*, **62**, 147–58 (1983).

85. MacFarlane, A. and Maloney, A.F.J. The appearance of the aqueduct and its relationship to hydrocephalus in the Arnold–Chiari malformation. *Brain,* **80**, 479–91 (1957).

86. Cameron, A.H. The Arnold–Chiari and the neuroanatomical malformations associated with spina bifida. *Journal of Pathology and Bacteriology*, **73**, 195–211 (1957).

87. Emery, J.L. Deformity of the aqueduct of Sylvius in children with hydrocephalus and myelomeningocoele. *Developmental Medicine and Child Neurology,* **16** (S32), 40–8 (1974).

88. Muller, J. Congenital malformations of the brain. In T*he clinical neurosciences, Vol. 3, Neuropathology,* (ed. Rosenberg, R.N.), pp. III: 1–33. Churchill Livingston, London (1983).

89. McLendon, R.E., Crain, B.J., Oakes, W.J., and Burger, P.C. Cerebral polygyria in the Chiari Type II (Arnold–Chiari) malformation. *Clinical Neuropathology*, **4**, 200–5 (1985).

90. Walker, A.E. Lissencephaly. *Archives of Neurology and Psychiatry,* **48**, 13–29 (1942).

91. Dambska, M., Wisniewski, K., and Sher, J.H. Lissencephaly: two distinct clinico-pathological types. *Brain and Development,* **5**, 302–10 (1983).

92. Dobyns, W.B., Pagon, R.A., Armstrong, D., Curry, C.J., Greenberg, F., Grix, A., Holmes, L.B., Laxova, R., Michels, V.V., Robinow, M., and Zimmerman, R.L. Diagnostic criteria for Walker–Warburg syndrome. *American Journal of Medical Genetics,* **32**, 145–210 (1989).

93. Bordarier, C., Aicardi, J., and Goutières, F. Congenital hydrocephalus and eye abnormalities with severe developmental brain defects: Warburg's syndrome. *Annals of Neurology*, **16**, 60–5 (1984).

94. Williams, R.S., Swisher, C.N., Jennings, M., Ambler, M., and Caviness, V.R. Cerebro-ocular dysgenesis (Walker–Warburg syndrome): Neuropathologic and etiologic analysis. *Neurology*, **34**, 1531–41 (1984).

95. Norman, M.G., Thurber, L.A., and Wooley, H.E. Abnormal leptomeninges and vessels causing fetal hydrocephalus. Diagnosis of hydrocephalus at 19 weeks' gestation by ultrasound. *Acta Neuropathologica*, **54**, 283–6 (1981).

96. Lake, B.D. Lysosomal and peroxysomal disorders. In *Greenfield's Neuro-pathology, (5th edn)*, (ed. Adams, J.H. and Duchen, L.W.), pp. 709–801. Edward Arnold, London (1992).

97. Gilles, F.H. and Davidson, R.I. Communicating hydrocephalus associated with deficient dysplastic parasagittal arachnoidal granulations. *Journal of Neurosurgery*, **35**, 421–6 (1971).

98. Gutierrez, Y., Friede, R.L., and Kaliney, W.J. Agenesis of arachnoid granulations and its relationship to communicating hydrocephalus. *Journal of Neurosurgery*, **43**, 553–8 (1975).

99. Fishman, M.A., Hogan, G.R., and Didge, P.R. The concurrence of hydrocephalus and craniosynostosis. *Journal of Neurosurgery*, **34**, 621–9 (1971).

100. Wise, B.L., Sondheimer, F., and Kaufman, S. Achondroplasia and hydrocephalus. *Neuropediatrics*, **3**, 106–13 (1971).

101. Hoffman, H.J. and Hendrick, E.B. Early neurosurgical repair in craniofacial dysmorphism. *Journal of Neurosurgery*, **51**, 769–803 (1979).

102. Collmann, H., Sörensen, N., Krauss, J., Mühling, J. Hydrocephalus in craniosynostosis. *Child's Nervous System*, **4**, 279–85 (1988).

103. Cohen, M.M.Jr and Kreiborg, S. The central nervous system in Apert syndrome. *American Journal of Medical Genetics*, **35**, 36–45 (1990).

104. Sainte-Rose, L.H., LaCombe, J., Pierre-Kahn, A., Renier, D., and Hirsch, J-F. Intracranial venous sinus hypertension: cause or consequence of hydrocephalus in infants. *Journal of Neurosurgery*, **60**, 727–36 (1984).

105. Pierre-Kahn, A., Hirsch, J-F., Renier, D., Mitzger, J., and Maroteaux, P. Hydrocephalus and achondroplasia. A study of 25 observations. *Child's Brain*, **7**, 205–19 (1981).

106. Hogan, G.R. and Bauman, M.L. Hydrocephalus in Apert's syndrome. *Journal of Pediatrics*, **79**, 782–7 (1971).

107. Vigouroux, A. Écoulement de liquide céphelo-rachidien. Hydrocéphalie papillome des plexus choroides du IVe ventricule. *Revue Neurologique (Paris)*, **16**, 281–5 (1908).

108. Davis, L.E. A physio-pathologic study of the choroid plexus with a report of a case of villous hypertrophy. *Journal of Medical Research*, **44**, 521–34 (1924).

109. Laurence, K.M. The biology of choroid plexus papilloma and carcinoma of the lateral ventricle. In *Tumours of the brain and skull, Part II, Handbook of Clinical Neurology, Vol. 17* (ed. Vinken, P.J. and Bruyn, G.W.), pp. 555–95. Elsevier, Amsterdam (1974).

110. Lippa, C., Abroms, I.F., Davidson, R., and De Girolami, U. Congenital choroid plexus papilloma of the fourth ventricle. *Journal of Childhood Neurology*, **4**, 127–30 (1989).

111. Lawrence, K.M. General discussion. In *Ciba Foundation Symposium on the Cerebrospinal Fluid*, (ed. Wolstenholme, G.E.N. and O'Connor, C.M.), pp. 310–14. J. and A. Churchill, London (1958).

112. Welch, K., Strand, R., Bresnan, M., and Cavazzuti, V. Congenital hydrocephalus due to villous hypertrophy of the telencephalic choroid plexuses. *Journal of Neurosurgery*, **59**, 172–5 (1983).

113. Milhorat, T.H., Hammock, M.K., Davis, D.A., and Fenstermacher, J.D. Choroid plexus papilloma — proof of cerebrospinal fluid overproduction. *Child's Brain*, **2**, 273–89 (1976).

114. Ray, B.S. and Peck, F.C. Jr. Papilloma of the choroid plexus of the lateral ventricles causing hydrocephalus in an infant. *Journal of Neurosurgery*, **13**, 405–40 (1956).

115. Kahn, E.A. and Luros, J.T. Hydrocephalus from overproduction of cerebrospinal fluid (and experiences with other papillomas of the choroid plexus). *Journal of Neurosurgery*, **9**, 59–67 (1952).

116. Matson, D.D. and Crofton, F.D.L. Papilloma of the choroid plexus in childhood. *Journal of Neurosurgery*, **17**, 1002–27 (1960).

117. McDonald, J.V. Persistent hydrocephalus following the removal of papillomas of the choroid plexus of the lateral ventricles. *Journal of Neurosurgery*, **30**, 736–40 (1969).

118. Laurence, K.M., Hoare, R.D., and Till, K. The diagnosis of the choroid plexus papilloma of the lateral ventricle. *Brain*, **84**, 628–41 (1961).

119. Casey, K.F. and Vries, J.K. Cerebral fluid overproduction in the absence of tumor or villous hypertrophy of the choroid plexus. *Child's Nervous System*, **5**, 332–4 (1989).

120. Worthington, W.C. and Cathcart, R.S. Ciliary currents on ependymal surfaces. *Annals of the New York Academy of Sciences*, **130**, 944–50 (1965).

121. Afzelius, B.A. The immotile cilia syndrome and other ciliary diseases. *International Review of Experimental Pathology*, **19**, 1–43 (1979).

122. Greenstone, M.A., Jones, R.W.A., Dewar, A., Neville, B.G.R., and Cole, P.J. Hydrocephalus and primary ciliary dyskinesia. *Archives of Disease in Childhood*, **59**, 481–2 (1984).

123. De Santi, M.M., Magni, A., Valletta, E.A., Gardi, C., and Lungarella, G. Hydrocephalus bronchiectasis and ciliary aplasia. *Archives of Disease in Childhood*, **65**, 543–4 (1990).

124. Salonen, R., Herva, R., and Norio, R. The hydrolethalus syndrome: delineation of a 'new' lethal malformation syndrome based on 28 patients. *Clinical Genetics*, **19**, 321–30 (1981).

125. Lowry, R.B. Variability in the Smith–Lemli–Opitz syndrome: overlap with the Meckel syndrome. *American Journal of Medical Genetics*, **14**, 429–33 (1983).

126. Baraitser, M. Syndrome of the month: the orofaciodigital syndromes. *Journal of Medical Genetics*, **23**, 116–19 (1986).

127. Harper, C. and Hockey, A. Proliferative vasculopathy and an hydranencephalic–hydrocephalic syndrome: a neuropathological study of two siblings. *Developmental Medicine and Child Neurology*, **25**, 232–9 (1983).

128. Fowler, M., Dow, R., White, T.A., and Greer, C.H. Congenital hydrocephalus–hydranencephaly in five siblings with autopsy studies: a new disease. *Developmental Medicine and Child Neurology*, **14**, 173–88 (1972).

129. Chow, C.H., Anderson, R.McD., and Kelly, G.C.T. Neuropathology in cerebral lactic acidosis. *Acta Neuropathologica*, **74**, 393–6 (1987).

130. Harding, B.N., Egger, J., Portmann, B., and Erdohazi, M. Progressive neuronal degeneration of childhood with liver disease. A pathological study. *Brain*, **109**, 181–206 (1986).

131. Erdohazi, M. and Marshall, P. Striatal degeneration in childhood. *Archives of Disease in Childhood*, **54**, 85–91 (1979).

132. Montpetit, V.J.A., Andermann, F., Carpenter, S., Fawcett, J.S., Zborowska-Sluis D., and Giberon, H.R. Subacute necrotizing encephalomyelopathy. A review and study of two families. *Brain*, **94**, 1–30 (1971).

133. Tien, R., Harsh, G.R., Dillon, W.P., and Wilson, C.B. Unilateral hydrocephalus caused by an intraventricular venous malformation obstructing the foramen of Monro. *Neurosurgery*, **26**, 664–6 (1990).

134. Venkataramana, N.K., Kolluri, V.R., Swamy, K.S., Arya, B.Y., Das, B.S., and Reddy, G.N. Progressive unilateral hydrocephalus in adults. *Neurosurgery*, **24**, 282–4 (1989).

135. Maurice-Williams, R.S. and Choksey, M. Entrapment of the temporal horn: a form of focal obstructive hydrocephalus. *Journal of Neurology, Neurosurgery and Psychiatry*, **49**, 238–42 (1986).

136. Russell, D.S. and Rubinstein, L.J. *Pathology of tumours of the nervous system*, (5th edn), (ed. Rubinstein, L.J.). Arnold, London (1989).

137. Von Deimling, A., Janzer, R., Kleihues, P., and Wiestler, O.D. Patterns of differentiation in central neurocytoma. An immunohistochemical study of eleven biopsies. *Acta Neuropathologica*, **79**, 473–9 (1990).

138. Yagishita, S., Itoh, Y., Shiozawa, T., and Tanaka, T. Ultrastructural observation on a colloid cyst of the third ventricle. A contribution to its pathogenesis. *Acta Neuropathologica (Berlin)*, **65**, 41–5 (1984).

139. Kovacs, J. and Horvath, E. *Tumors of the pituitary gland. 2nd series. Fascicle 21*. Armed Forces Institute of Pathology, Washington DC (1986).

140. Gelabert, M., Bollar, A., Paseiro, M.J., and Allut, A.G. Hydrocephalus and intraspinal tumor in childhood. *Child's Nervous System*, **6**, 110–12 (1990).

141. Isaacman, D.J. Otitic hydrocephalus: an uncommon complication of a common condition. *Annals of Emergncy Medicine*, **18**, 684–7 (1989).

142. Butler, E.G. and Gilligan, B.S. Obstructive hydrocephalus caused by multiple sclerosis. *Clinical Experimental Neurology*, **26**, 219–23 (1989).

143. Hutchings, M. and Weller, R.O. Anatomical relationships of pia mater to cerebral blood vessels in man. *Journal of Neurosurgery*, **65**, 316–25 (1986).

144. Alcolado, R., Weller, R.O., Parrish, E.P., and Garrod, D. The cranial arachnoid and pia mater in man: Anatomical and ultrastructural observations. *Neuropathology and Applied Neurobiology*, **14**, 1–17 (1988).

145. Nicholas, D.S. and Weller, R.O. The fine structure of the spinal meninges in man. *Journal of Neurosurgery*, **69**, 276–82 (1988).

146. Zhang, E.T., Richards, H.K., Kida, S., and Weller, R.O. Directional and compartmentalised pathways for the drainage of interstitial fluid and cerebrospinal fluid from the rat brain. *Acta Neuropathologica*, **83**, 233–9 (1992).

147. Upton, M.L. and Weller, R.O. The morphology of cerebrospinal fluid drainage pathways in human arachnoid granulations. *Journal of Neurosurgery*, **63**, 867–75 (1985).

148. Kida, S., Yamashima, T., Kubota, T. *et al.* A light and electron microscopic and immunohistochemical study of human arachnoid villi. *Journal of Neurosurgery*, **69**, 429–35 (1988).

149. Pantazis, A. and Weller, R.O. CSF drainage by direct connections between the subarachnoid space and nasal lymphatics in the rat. (1992) (In preparation).

150. Pentland, B., Douglas Mitchell, J., Cull, R.E., and Ford, M.J. Central nervous system sarcoidosis. *Quarterly Journal of Medicine*, **56**, 457–65 (1985).

151. Tang Lok-Ming. Ventriculoperitoneal shunt in cryptococcal meningitis with hydrocephalus. *Surgical Neurology*, **33**, 314–19 (1990).

152. Torvik, A., Bhatia, R., and Murthy, V.S. Transient block of the arachnoid granulations following subarachnoid hemorrhage. *Acta Neurochirugica (Wien)*, **41**, 137–46 (1978).

153. Tomlinson, B.E. and Corsellis, J.A.N. Ageing and the dementias. In *Greenfield's neuropathology, (4th edn)*, (ed. Adams, J.H., Corsellis, J.A.N., and Duchen, L.W.), p. 951. Edward Arnold, London (1984).

154. Lantos, P.L. Ageing and dementias. In *Systemic pathology*, (3rd edn), *Nervous system, muscle and eyes*, (ed. Weller, R.O.) pp. 360–96. Churchill Livingstone, Edinburgh (1990).

155. De la Monte, S.M. Quantitation of cerebral atrophy in preclinical and end-stage Alzheimer's disease. *Annals of Neurology*, **25**, 450–9 (1989).

156. Graham, D.I. Trauma. In *Systemic pathology*, (3rd edn), *Nervous system, muscle and eyes*, (ed. Weller, R.O.), pp. 125–50. Churchill Livingstone, Edinburgh (1990).

157. Weller, R.O. *Colour atlas of neuropathology*. Harvey Miller and Oxford University Press, Oxford (1984).

158. Weller, R.O., Steart, P.V., and Powell-Jackson, J.D. Pathology of Creutzfeldt–Jakob disease associated with pituitary-derived human growth hormone administration. *Neuropathology and Applied Neurobiology*, **12**, 117–30 (1986).

159. Hakim, S. and Adams, R.D. The special clinical problem of symptomatic hydrocephalus with normal cerebrospinal fluid pressure. Observations on cerebrospinal fluid hydrodynamics. *Journal of Neurological Science*, **2**, 307–27 (1965).

160. Dauch, W.A. and Zimmerman, R. Normal pressure hydrocephalus. An evaluation 25 years following the initial description. *Fortschrift für Neurologie und Psychiatrie*, **58**, 178–90 (1990).

161. Leader article. Normal-pressure hydrocephalus. *Lancet*, **6**, 335, 22 (1990).

162. Akai, K., Uchigasaki, S., Tanaka. U., and Komatsu, A. Normal pressure hydrocephalus. Neuropathological study. *Acta Pathologica Japan*, **37**, 97–110 (1987).

163. Wikkelso, C., Andersson, H., Blomstrand, C., Matousek, M., and Svendsen, P. Computed tomography of the brain in the diagnosis of and prognosis in normal pressure hydrocephalus. *Neuroradiology*, **31**, 160–5 (1989).

164. De, S.N. A study of the changes in the brain in experimental internal hydrocephalus. *Journal of Pathology and Bacteriology*, **62**, 197–208 (1950).

165. Schurr, P.H., McLaurin, R.L., and Ingraham, F.D. Experimental studies on the circulation of the cerebrospinal fluid and methods of producing communicating hydrocephalus in the dog. *Journal of Neurosurgery*, **10**, 515–25 (1953).

166. Weller, R.O., Mitchell, J., Griffin, R.L., and Gardner, M.J. The effects of hydrocephalus upon the developing brain. Histological and quantitative studies on the ependyma and subependyma in hydrocephalic rats. *Journal of Neurological Science*, **36**, 383–402 (1978).

167. Takeuchi, I.K. and Takeuchi, Y.K. Congenital hydrocephalus following X-irradiation of pregnant rats on an early gestational day. *Neurobehav. Toxicol. Teratol.*, **8**, 143–50 (1986).

168. Stempak, G.J. Etiology of trypan blue induced antenatal hydrocephalus in the albino rat. *Anatomical Record*, **148**, 561–71 (1964).

169. Inouye, M. and Kajiwara, Y. Strain difference of the mouse in manifestation of hydrocephalus following prenatal methylmercury exposure. *Teratology*, **41**, 205–10 (1990).

170. Garro, F. and Pentschew, A. Neonatal hydrocephalus in the offspring of rats fed during pregnancy non-toxic amounts of tellurium. *Arch. Psychiat. Nervkrankh.*, **206**, 272–80 (1964).

171. Aikawa, H., Kobayashi, S., and Suzuki, K. Aqueductal lesions in 6-aminonicotinamide-treated suckling mice. *Acta Neuropathologica (Berlin)*, **71**, 243–50 (1986).

172. Carton, C.A., Pascal, R.R., and Tennyson, V.M. Hydrocephalus and vitamin-A deficiency in the rabbit. General considerations. In *Disorders of the developing nervous system*, (ed. Fields, W.S. and Desmond, M.M.), pp. 214–66. C.C. Thomas, Springfield, Illinois (1961).

173. Kanno, T., Nakamura, T., Jain, V.K., and Sugimoto, T. An experimental model of communicating hydrocephalus in C57 black mouse. *Acta Neurochirugica (Wien)*, **86**, 111–14 (1987).

174. Johnson, R.T., Johnson, K.P., and Edmonds, C.J. Virus-induced hydrocephalus: development of aqueduct stenosis in hamsters after mumps injection. *Science, NY*, **157**, 1066–7 (1967).

175. Margolis, G. and Kilham, L. Hydrocephalus in hamsters, ferrets, rats and mice following inoculations with Rheovirus Type I. II. pathologic studies. *Laboratory Investigation*, **21**, 189–98 (1969).

176. Weller, R.O., Mitchell, J., and Griffin, R.L. Cerebral ventriculitis in the hydrocephalic mouse: a histological and scanning electron microscope study. *Acta Neuropathologica (Berlin)*, Suppl VIII, 160–1 (1981).

177. Jones, H.C., Dack, S., and Ellis, C. Morphological aspects of the development of hydrocephalus in a mouse mutant (SUMS/NP). *Acta Neuropathologica (Berlin)*, **72**, 268–76 (1987).

178. Bronson, R.T. and Lane, P.W. Hydrocephalus with hop gait (hyh): a new mutation on chromosome 7 in the mouse. *Brain Res. Dev. Brain Res.*, **54**, 131–6 (1990).

179. Koto, M., Miwa, M., Shimizu, A., Tsuji, K., Okamoto. M., and Adach, J. Inherited hydrocephalus in Csk: Wistar–Imamichi rats; Hyd strain: a new disease model for hydrocephalus. *Jikken Dobutsu.*, **36**, 157–62 (1987).

180. D'Amato, C.J., O'Shea, K.S., Hicks, S.P., Glover, R.A., and Annesley, T.M. Genetic prenatal aqueductal stenosis with hydrocephalus in rat. *Journal of Neuropathology and Experimental Neurology.*, **45**, 665–82 (1986).

181. Yoshida, Y., Koya, G., Tamayama, K., Kumanishi, T., and Abe, S. Histopathology of cystic cavities in the cerebral white matter of HTX rats with inherited hydrocephalus. *Neurol. Med. Chir. (Tokyo)*, **30**, 229–33 (1990).

182. Raimondi, A.J., Soare, P., and Chicago, M.A. Intellectual development in shunted hydrocephalic children. *American Journal of Diseases of Children*, **127**, 664–71 (1974).

183. Hammer, R. Hydrocephalus in infancy. Normal cerebrospinal fluid dynamics, hydrocephalus — causes — therapy — lethality — prognosis. *Z. Geburtshilfe Perinatol.*, **190**, 233–42 (1986).

184. Hiratsuka, H., Tabata, H., Tsuruoka, S., Aoyagi, M., Okada, K., and Inaba, Y. Evaluation of periventricular hypodensity in experimental hydrocephalus by metrizamide CT ventriculography. *Journal of Neurosurgery*, **56**, 235–40 (1982).

185. Diggs, J., Price, A.C., Burt, A.M., Flor, W.J., McKanna, J.A., Novak, G.R., and James, A.E. Jr. Early changes in experimental hydrocephalus. *Invest. Radiol.*, **21**, 118–21 (1986).

186. Drake, J.M., Potts, D.G., and Lemaire, C. Magnetic resonance imaging of silastic-induced canine hydrocephalus. *Surgical Neurology*, **31**, 28–40 (1989).

187. Takei, F., Shapiro, K., Hirano, A., and Kohn, I. Influence of the rate of ventricular enlargement on the ultrastructural morphology of the white matter in experimental hydrocephalus. *Neurosurgery*, **21**, 645–50 (1987).

188. Higashi, K., Asahisa, H., Ueda, N., Kobayashi, K., Hara, K., and Noda, Y. Cerebral blood flow and metabolism in experimental hydrocephalus. *Neurological Research*, **8**, 169–76 (1986).

189. Okuyama, T., Hashi, K., Sasaki, S., Sudo, K., and Kurokawa Y. Changes in cerebral microvasculature in congenital hydrocephalus of the inbred rat LEW/Jms: light and electron microscopic examination. *Surgical Neurology*, **27**, 338–42 (1987).

190. Ogawa, H., Tsubokawa, T., Katayama, Y., Miyazaki, S., Iwasaki, M., Shibanoki, S., and Ishikawa, K. Facilitated growth of transplanted raphe cells in hydrocephalic interstitial edema. *Brain Research Bulletin*, **24**, 769–74 (1990).

191. Wisniewski, H., Weller, R.O., and Terry, R.D. Experimental hydrocephalus produced by the subarachnoid infusion of silicone oil. *Journal of Neurosurgery*, **31**, 10–14 (1969).

192. Collins, P. and Fairman, S. Repair of the ependyma in hydrocephalic brains. *Neuropathology and Applied Neurobiology*, **16**, 45–56 (1990).

193. Tamaki, N., Yamashita, H., Kimura, M., Ehara, K., Asada, M., Nagashima, T., Matsumoto, S., and, Hashimoto, M. Changes in the components and content of biological water in the brain of experimental hydrocephalic rabbits. *Journal of Neurosurgery*, **73**, 274–8 (1990).

194. Oi, S., Ijich, A., and Matsumoto, S. Immunohistochemical evaluation of neuronal maturation in untreated fetal hydrocephalus. *Neurologica Medica Chirurgica (Tokyo)*, **29**, 989–94 (1989).

195. Bruni, J.E. and Del Bigio, M.R. Reaction of periventricular tissue in the rat fourth ventricle to chronically placed shunt tubing implants. *Neurosurgery*, **19**, 337–45 (1986).

196. Oi, S. and Matsumoto, S. Morphological findings of postshunt slit-ventricle in experimental canine hydrocephalus. Aspects of causative factors of isolated ventricles and slit-ventricle syndrome. *Child's Nervous System*, **2**, 179–84 (1986).

197. Griebel, R.W., Black, P.M., Pile-Se-Spellman, J., and Strauss, H.W. The importance of 'accessory' outflow pathways in hydrocephalus after experimental subarachnoid hemorrhage. *Neurosurgery*, **24**, 187–92 (1989).

198. Ohata, K., Marmarou, A., and Povlishock, J.T. An immunocytochemical study of protein clearance in brain infusion edema. *Acta Neuropathologica*, **81**, 162–77 (1990).

199. Sahar, A., Hochwald, G.M., Sadik, A.R., and Ransohoff, J. Cerebrospinal fluid absorption in animals with experimental obstructive hydrocephalus. *Archives of Neurology*, **21**, 638–44 (1969).
200. Takei, F., Shapiro, K., and Kohn, I. Influence of the rate of ventricular enlargement on the white matter water content in progressive feline hydrocephalus. *Journal of Neurosurgery*, **66**, 577–83 (1987).

4 Clinical features of hydrocephalus in childhood and infancy

B.G.R. Neville

INTRODUCTION

Hydrocephalus in childhood has a significant mortality and morbidity. The disability syndrome that may be associated with hydrocephalus combines learning, central motor, and visual deficits, and tends to occur irrespective of the cause of the hydrocephalus or the age of the child. An important aim of the clinical approach to hydrocephalus is early identification and treatment, with the hope of minimizing that part of the disability which is directly attributable to distension of the CSF spaces and raised intracranial pressure. The pathologies underlying a congenital or acquired disturbance of CSF pathways and parenchymal brain lesions commonly coexist. Therefore not all of the disability, and sometimes none of it, can be prevented by early intervention. Many reported series of patients with hydrocephalus indicate delays of months up to several years from the likely onset to the time of diagnosis and treatment. There will inevitably be some delay in diagnosis unless there is a pre-existing strong suspicion of hydrocephalus occurring for example, in the presence of open spina bifida or when it is discovered by routine ultrasound. This clinical account assumes that an early diagnosis is desirable. This does not mean, however, that a later diagnosis is necessarily harmful or that all or the majority of the child's disability could have been prevented by early detection.

The detailed clinical aims, therefore, are as follows:

(1)   the identification of children with hydrocephalus arising as a primary condition or complicating other diseases or treatments;

(2)   the use of clinical assessment techniques to assist in decisions about treatment;

(3)   the identification of symptomatic hydrocephalus, for example tumours, and to treat both disorders effectively;

(4)   the provision of comprehensive management for those children with neurological disability;

(5)   to increase understanding of the natural history of hydrocephalus and to improve its management;

(6)   to give genetic counselling;

(7) and perhaps to give advice on what is the expected level of clinical competence.

The particular problems of hydrocephalus in premature babies and in the child who is acutely sick, for example with meningitis, are considered separately.

The clinical problem of distinguishing between ventriculomegaly, mild but acceptable hydrocephalus, i.e. with raised intracranial pressure, and significant hydrocephalus requiring treatment is difficult and the clinical problem can be best illustrated by a general example:

1. A child has ventriculomegaly without symptoms of raised intracranial pressure. Pressure monitoring would be required to decide if there is a significant rise in ventricular pressure.

2. The child has learning and motor problems, but the history and examination do not clearly indicate if these are static or progressive.

3. Since both pressure monitoring and shunt insertion are invasive and the latter is subject to possible complications, the question is asked 'Is this hydrocephalus significant enough to justify such a management plan?'

It is important that these three questions should be clearly separated in the analysis of the data. In this chapter, we are particularly concerned with problem 2, but cannot escape reference to the other questions.

GENERAL CLINICAL FEATURES IN INFANCY AND CHILDHOOD

The clinical setting of initial presentation

The primary presentation will usually be to a non-neurologist, who needs to decide which children should be referred to a paediatrician, neurologist or neurosurgeon. The history of babies with hydrocephalus is often not strongly suggestive of raised intracranial pressure. The commonest complaints are irritability, failure to feed, and vomiting. Lack of weight gain may be less obvious because of the increasing weight of the head. This group of symptoms, particularly feeding difficulties, are among the commonest in paediatric practice and can indicate a wide range of problems, most of them not neurological. These symptoms can also be a presenting problem in children with neurological disability who do not have hydrocephalus. However, in children with long-standing hydrocephalus such symptoms have often been regarded as due to oesophageal reflux. This problem should be regarded as a symptom of a wide range of disorders, including metabolic disease, severe neurological disability, and raised intracranial pressure. Since ultrasound through the fontanelle is such a simple investigation, it should be performed on those babies with anorexia, failure to thrive, and vomiting who do not respond rapidly to simple measures. Ultrasound may not reveal subdural collections which are the other common cause of raised intracranial pressure in babies.

The commonest neurological problems in the presentation of hydrocephalus are motor and general delay and failure to make appropriate visual and social contact. There may be a history of relative or absolute normality followed by increasing concern about development, but this is not alway easy to separate from realization of the extent of a fixed deficit. Babies and young children with such a history deserve urgent investigation, looking for hydrocephalus and a number of other treatable diseases which may present as developmental delay.

In a consecutive series of 107 patients from Edinburgh, a third showed evidence of failure to thrive. The frequency of symptoms were as follows: vomiting 33 per cent; behaviour change 33 per cent; drowsiness 28 per cent; headache 28 per cent; anorexia 14 per cent; stiff neck or backache 7 per cent; and 28 per cent were asymptomatic.[1]

The same Edinburgh series gave incidences of signs in the presentation of hydrocephalus: an excessive rate of head growth 40 per cent; fullness of the fontanelle 41 per cent; splayed sutures 21 per cent; scalp vein dilatation 15 per cent; sunsetting of the eyes and loss of upward gaze 14 per cent; reduced conscious level 12 per cent; neck retraction 10 per cent; acute strabismus 8 per cent; abnormalities of the pupils and papilloedema 7 per cent. Thirteen per cent had no symptoms. These clinical features need discussion in the context of clinical history taking and the examination of children.

History taking and neurological examination in young children

A history of the pregnancy, birth, neonatal period, and any significant illness should be taken. A developmental history is important and at its simplest should include:

1. An account of social responsiveness in the first few weeks of life.

2. The age of walking which may vary in normal children from under one year to more than two years, and being particularly delayed in some children who adopt a non-prone, including bottom shuffling, mode of locomotion between sitting and walking. However, it is more important to discover the degree of stability in walking after one to two months and the progress made to being able to run. A child with a gait disorder will usually be slow to walk independently and will walk round furniture or with support for some months before letting go, and will remain unsteady for several months afterwards.

3. The age at which the child puts words together into sentences, and thus the ability to communicate verbally.

4. For older children, the initial social and educational progress made at school.

5. The history of hand-function is obtained by early abilities with finger, spoon, and cup feeding. After this the range of skills involved in dressing and building games are helpful.

It is important to try to separate general delay, which is usually caused by a global cognitive deficit, from selective motor deficits, in which the movements are attempted but poorly performed. Hand preference is not usually obvious during the first two years of life and if clearly developed during that time is usually pathological.

The neurological examination of babies and young children requires specific training. The main principles are:

1. As much of the examination should be done by observation, with the gradual introduction of play material appropriate to the child's developmental age. The setting should be domestic with chairs and tables of paediatric scale in a simple, friendly, domestic atmosphere. Hospital uniforms do not help in this process.

2. The child's security is best maintained by starting the examination on their parent's lap and allowing the physical and emotional relationship to continue until they show themselves willing to separate. Between the developmental ages of 8 months and 18 months to 2 years children are often very apprehensive of strangers.

3. The examiner should have a scheme of developmental assessment with which he is familiar, for example Egan 1990.[2]

Because the child's co-operation is essential for the assessment of fine motor skills and visual acuity, certain physical contact aspects of the assessment, particularly measuring the head circumference and examination of the optic fundi should be delayed until the end. The traditional order of neurological examination, working down from the cranial nerves, is probably best more-or-less reversed.

Abnormalities of tone and relatively brisk reflexes may be difficult to judge if they are generalized. The best guide to their significance is whether or not they are accompanied by a functional deficit. In any paediatric neurological examination, it is the simple description, in non-medical language, of a child's performance that is most useful in judging later deterioration or improvement.

A full fontanelle means that with the head upright the fontanelle completes the dome of the skull, does not sink below it, and feels tense. With high pressures the normal pulsation is lost. This sign is not always reliable. The tension in normal babies increases with crying, initially, and may go down if the P_{CO_2} drops during prolonged crying, or if the baby is dehydrated. Dilated scalp veins and a full fontanelle are also seen in heart failure and venous obstruction, but such babies still require urgent investigation.

An excessive rate of head growth is probably the most important sign of hydrocephalus which has its onset in the first year of life. The head circumference is defined as the maximum that can be measured in a fronto–occipital direction. If the head circumference growth curve has crossed more than one standard deviation, this should be regarded as suspicious, and if two standard deviations then it is virtually diagnostic of expanding intracranial pathology. A head circumference which is more than two standard deviations above the mean also deserves investigation. It is very important that the head circumference is measured at birth and at one month to six weeks as a routine, and whenever the baby is seen for a medical problem. These figures and head circumference charts that cover at least two standard deviations above and below the mean and include figures for premature babies are essential and are shown in the Appendix. Many babies with a large head or one standard deviation rise in the rate of head growth will not have hydrocephalus on ultrasound, but many later CT scans could be avoided if these early criteria were used for referral for ultrasound.

Irritability and neck retraction are very common in acute rises in intracranial pressure, but may be entirely absent in slowly progressive hydrocephalus. It would seem that the relative laxity of the skull is associated with less direct symptoms.

The 'setting sun' sign indicates upper lid retraction with some depression of the globes and is usually combined with a defect of up-gaze. Mild degrees of lid retraction may occur in normal babies. The assessment of vision is important, since visual failure appears to be the least recoverable consequence of raised intracranial pressure. Babies under the age of six months have to be assessed by their ability to follow near objects. The ability to follow a suspended spinning ball within 2–6 feet is the standard test and if there is difficulty with this a face, a light-reflecting object, or a bright light are used, but there should be concern if these are required. A baby should be expected to follow both horizontally and vertically unless upper or lower motor neurone defects of eye movements interfere with these tests. Any baby of six weeks or more who is unable to visually follow should be urgently referred for further assessment. The testing of vision in children over the age of six months is an essential part of the assessment of a child with possible raised intracranial pressure, and should be available to the paediatrician, neurologist, and neurosurgeon at referral and follow-up of such patients. The limitations of such tests are important. A baby who can maintain visual following of a face at about two feet, may have quite severe visual disability in later life, and could be slipping from near normal to severe visual disability without any change in the response to this crude visual test. If pupil reactions to light are sluggish or unreactive, and there is no visual response, it is worth urgent investigation and treatment since it may be possible to retrieve a small amount of functional vision. The presence of roving eye movements suggests a poor visual outcome. A careful examination of the retina is important as a retinopathy can give a strong suggestion of either intrauterine infection or a dysplastic process affecting the retina and brain. While the fontanelle is open, the only change in the optic nerve is usually progressive atrophy. Papilloedema is usually only seen after closure of the anterior fontanelle, which occures somewhere between the age of six months and eighteen months but may be delayed in hydrocephalus. It is not, however, consistently seen even after that age, particularly if there is already a degree of optic atrophy. A unilateral or bilateral sixth nerve palsy is common in hydro-cephalus, and is often partial with the abducting eye drifting back or showing a slow paretic nystagmus.

The motor assessment in babies and young children suspected of having hydrocephalus has a number of specific features. Firstly, if the head is big, and therefore heavy, this can have the profound effect of delaying motor develop-ment. High intracranial pressure can produce transient pyramidal signs with usually flexed upper limbs and extended lower limbs, increased tone, and pathologically brisk tendon reflexes. Part of this may be the mass pattern that often accompanies neck retraction of any cause, including respiratory failure and upper airways obstruction as well as raised intracranial pressure. The clue that this is not a true spastic quadriplegia may come from the relative preservation of bulbar and intellectual functions and of the normal repertoire of spontaneous finger and toe movements which tend to be lost in pyramidal disease.

Intellectual function may be difficult or impossible to assess, particularly if the child is irritable or drowsy or otherwise disturbed by raised intracranial pressure. The assessment should be attempted but should not, of course, be regarded as an accurate predictor of future development. However, it is important to have a good clinical baseline assessment to compare with follow-up assessments of treated children. Therefore, perhaps one to two months after recovery from surgical treatment, a detailed physical, including visual, and developmental or psychological assessment, depending on age, should be performed. Whatever else the follow-up entails, there should be a similar annual review, and at a later age school progress may replace the need for psycholo-gical assessment.

The clinical follow-up for children with a degree of hydrocephalus which is not initially treated, for example in children with spina bifida and stable mild ventricular enlargement, is a similar developmental exercise. Children gain motor and intellectual skills throughout childhood, and assessments have to allow for this shifting baseline. One should be concerned that intellectual skills have been acquired at a slower rate than predicted even if they have not been lost.

An initial presentation with deepening coma and fading respiration is unusual in pure hydrocephalus unless it is very advanced, but is more commonly seen in an episode of acute shunt failure or in the presentation of symptomatic hydro-cephalus with, for example, a posterior fossa tumour.

Headache in childhood

Headache is a common symptom, particularly in older children;[3] 60–70 per cent of children have a headache at some time, 7 per cent have frequent non-migrainous headache, and 4 per cent have migraine. Migraine is relatively more common in older girls. It is important, therefore, to have some clinical guide to the separation of those children who may have a serious pathology, including hydrocephalus, and those who can be managed conservatively. The important features of a headache include the site, periodicity, and accompanying symptoms, including the child's behaviour. Headaches caused by raised intracranial pressure tend to be present early in the morning or even wake the child from sleep, to occur daily, and to be made worse on effort and coughing. The indications for further investigation of a child with headache include the following:

(1) the presence of neurological signs;

(2) a large head;

(3) nocturnal or early morning headaches;

(4) persistent vomiting or anorexia;

(5) failure to attend school or make progress there;

(6) a change in behaviour;

(7) epilepsy;

(8) the presence of insistent focal pain;

(9) complex 'migraine' with hemiplegia;

(10) inability to relieve headaches which are presumed to be migrainous or of psychogenic cause.

Clinical studies of consecutive patients have shown that over 90 per cent of children with raised intracranial pressure have neurological signs or an abnormal skull X-ray within a short time of the onset of symptoms.[4] Therefore, children who present with headache should undergo a clinical assessment at the first visit, including looking for infection and measuring blood pressure. A skull X-ray is usually performed at the second visit and CT scanning is used for the above more serious indications.

Migraine is quite common and, in general, the symptoms are similar to those in adults. However, there are some important features in childhood. The pain may not be of obviously throbbing character and only a minority report a hemicranial distribution. Twenty per cent of children complain of dizziness and light-headedness. The common provoking factors in childhood include upper respiratory infection, family stress, hypoglycaemia, certain specific foods, minor head trauma, menarche, flickering lights, and sleep deprivation. The 'periodic syndrome' in younger children of cyclical vomiting, abdominal pain, headache, dizziness, fever, and malaise lasting for one to three days seems to be a definite variant of migraine that is mainly seen in younger children. In childhood, as in adults, it is important that the symptoms are paroxysmal lasting usually up to one day with normal functioning between attacks.

Psychogenic headache caused by stress and unhappiness are common in older children. Such headaches are often continuous and occur daily. They tend to be less definite in character and localization. A detailed history usually reveals a loss of drive, interest, and ability to cope with life. These problems may be discovered through taking the history of a normal day's activity including eating, sleeping, play and communication. Increasing difficulty in attending school for reasons of minor illness is a common complaint. Headache is an important presenting symptom of depression, of covert abuse, and major family psychopathology. The elimination of organic disease is, therefore, only part of the doctor's role.

The presentation of simple hydrocephalus in older children

Hydrocephalus may present in older children without any obvious antecedents. The history may give hints of early episodes of headache and vomiting, or neurological dysfunction with ataxia and drowsiness, to which a variety of diagnoses may have been ascribed. There may also be evidence of a mild long-standing disability of learning, gait, or vision. Very often the only clue to the long-standing nature of the pathology is a large head. The commonest presentation in this group is of slowly progressive dementia and gait disorder, very often over months or even years, with visual loss as a late feature. Dementia in children is an uncommon clinical problem and may not be recognized, particularly if it starts before the child enters full-time education. Parents, however, are usually quite clear that their child's recent memory, ability and interest in constructive play, communication and care of their possessions and of themselves have deteriorated. The school performance will usually have deteriorated, but the signifance of this may not have been realized. The motor disorder begins as mild clumsiness of walking and hand function but progresses to a gross ataxia with signs of mild spasticity, usually worse in the legs, and a coarse intention tremor in all limbs. There is usually relative sparing of bulbar muscles. The motor signs are bilateral but not necessarily symmetrical. The visual assessment usually shows chronic papilloedema and reduced visual acuity. It is interesting how a child's vision can be deteriorating without it being recognized. Because of the occurrence of rapid visual loss in raised intracranial pressure it is very important that children with reduced vision are seen quickly. Sixth nerve palsies and some difficulty with up-gaze may be present. A cracked pot note (a high pitched sound) may be present on tapping the skull: the examiner applies one ear to the side of the head and gently taps the other side, providing he has practised this test on a large number of children! Many children will have had some symptoms of raised intracranial pressure with headache and vomiting, but the important point is that these symptoms may be mild, episodic, or totally absent. The motor signs can also show an episodic course. It is very interesting how good the motor, intellectual, and even visual recovery can be after adequate treatment, sometimes with the loss of all motor problems over a few weeks and a rapid rise in intellectual functioning over several months. Occasionally late onset hydrocephalus can present acutely, particularly after mild head trauma or a systemic, usually infective, illness with deepening coma, a third nerve palsy, extensor rigidity, and shallow or intermittent respiration. A respiratory arrest in the context of impaired cortical perfusion is better anticipated than treated after the event.

In a study of 250 cases of non-tumoural hydrocephalus, 32 children between the ages of two and fifteen had such a late presentation.[5] The clinical features in this study were a large head in 60 per cent, pyramidal signs in 40 per cent, psychomotor retardation and visual disturbance in 37 per cent, gait disturbance in 35 per cent, epilepsy in 22 per cent, nausea and vomiting in 20 per cent, endocrine disturbances in 20 per cent, headache in 15 per cent and incontinence, progressive mental deterioration, deafness, and scoliosis all occurring in less than 10 per cent. In a third, there was a possible cause, which included perinatal haemorrhage, leucomeningitis, neurofibromatosis, and an aneurysm of the great vein of Galen. This mode of presentation is very similar to that seen in adults. The commonest site of CSF obstruction is aqueduct stenosis. It needs to be emphasized that a number of such patients may have very slow-growing or static tumours of glial origin which do not behave like the more common fast-growing brainstem gliomas. They are often clinically inapparent except for hydrocephalus and can be missed on initial CT. MRI is probably a better method of finding such lesions. However, the management of the patients as isolated aqueduct stenosis is usually quite appropriate.

Occasionally, unusual clinical features are seen in the acute presentation of hydrocephalus. A syndrome of neurogenic pulmonary oedema may occur and persist, despite adequate ventricular drainage, and other acute measures, including atropine and positive pressure ventilation, used in an attempt to relieve it. Other unusual features include profuse sweating, a macular rash, abdominal pain, and palor. Although cranial nerve palsies, particularly causing stridor, are commoner with a Chiari malformation, they may occur without. Occasionally a pseudobulbar palsy can occur and sometimes these localized brainstem manifestations may appear following decompression.

Chronic communicating hydrocephalus

This condition is not always easily recognized, and the differential diagnosis from idiopathic or familial megalencephaly and cerebral atrophy may not always be clear. One presentation is with a baby in the first year of life with an excessive rate of head growth, or just a rather large head with few or no symptoms. The CT scan shows moderate enlargement of the ventricles and sometimes even greater enlargement of the extracerebral spaces. In the first year of life, it is not possible to identify mild learning difficulties and a mild degree of ataxia. The intellectual functioning of such children is clearly much better than would be expected in the setting of cerebral atrophy which could produce similar radiological findings, but in which one would expect the head to be small. This presentation in some children appears to resolve into a neurologically normal child with a discrepantly large head but with persistence of the CT appearances. Monitoring of intracranial pressure and shunt insertion would be hard to justify if the prognosis is known to be good and if all one is doing is producing some reduction in the eventual adult head circumference. It seems reasonable in such patients to measure the lumbar CSF pressure in a relaxed and usually, therefore, sedated child, and if it is clearly raised (more than 20 cm CSF) to treat with isosorbide and later confirm the reduction in pressure. During the second year, clinical assessment can be more definite in excluding disability or finding it on withdrawal of such treatment. If the child has symptoms which could indicate raised intracranial pressure, or has a neurological disability, then it seems reasonable to manage in the usual fashion for progressive hydrocephalus. It would appear that the CT appearances do not necessarily distinguish between subarachnoid and subdural fluid, since the protein content of fluid removed from what was confidently predicted to be the subarachnoid space may be very high. Some very handicapped children, not always with large heads, in fact sometimes with microcephaly, show deterioration in motor function and attention and similar CT scan appearances. It is certainly worth measuring the lumbar CSF pressure in such circumstances. Where a child is maximally handicapped with lissencephaly, this situation can arise, presumably as a result of under-development of arachnoid granulations, hydrocephalus may be missed for a long time and the episodes of anorexia, vomiting, and drowsiness misinterpreted.

CLINICAL FEATURES OF HYDROCEPHALUS IN PARTICULAR SYNDROMES

Hydrocephalus in the presentation of children with intracranial tumours

Hydrocephalus is a significant part of the presentation of many children with tumours and often requires separate management. It occurs in both benign and malignant posterior fossa tumours but is usually either absent or late in brainstem gliomas. In such patients, the presentation is usually that of focal symptoms and signs and rapidly progressive hydrocephalus. An acute presentation with reduced conscious level is much commoner in this situation than in simple hydrocephalus, presumably because of the greater posterior fossa pressure and displacement problems. It is worth noting that, in children treated for benign posterior fossa tumours, there is a significant incidence of intellectual and visual disability following treatment, and it is very likely that most of this is attributable to hydrocephalus before and during the acute management. Therefore a careful watch for hydrocephalus is an essential part of the management, particularly when it is not going smoothly. Tumours in the third ventricle often present with pure, rapidly progressive hydrocephalus. Tumours in the region of the foramen of Monro may present with unilateral hydrocephalus. This may give evidence of a general rise in intracranial pressure with hemiplegia and a contralateral fixed dilated pupil.

Epilepsy is not a common feature of hydrocephalus as such, unless the pathology involves the cerebral cortex, either acutely as in meningitis or head injury, or chronically. The incidence of epilepsy in children with hydrocephalus is increased over what one would expect for the degree of mental disability, presumably because of additional pathology. A rise in intracranial pressure may increase the frequency of epileptic attacks. However, most of the paroxysmal events that occur in hydrocephalus are non-epileptic episodes of vertical eye movements and extensor spasms which are attributable to coning.

Hydrocephalus in meningitis

Hydrocephalus is common in pyogenic meningitis and is particularly frequent in more chronic meningeal infections, for example tuberculosis, listeria, and yeasts. It usually does not require specific management, but in some acute situations, and many more chronic ones, deterioration or lack of improvement is directly attributable to untreated hydrocephalus. The common problems include persistent vomiting, drowsiness, and reduced visual acuity with loss of pupil responses. Such deterioration is usually reversible by insertion of a ventricular drain. It now seems clear that obsessional care of hydrocephalus in this setting can significantly reduce the morbidity of this aspect of meningitis.[6] The other major cause of cerebral damage is vasculitis and that, of course, requires different management. If the child is receiving intensive care for meningitis, monitoring of intracranial pressure or ventricular drainage is usually required because of the lack of physical signs in sedated ventilated patients. The intracranial pressure problems are often aggravated by inappropriate antidiuretic hormone secretion which is common in meningeal disease.

Hydrocephalus in premature babies

The epidemiological studies of B. and G. Hagberg, from Gothenberg, have helped in our understanding of the changes in clinical patterns of presentation of hydrocephalus in childhood over the past 40 years.[7] Their earlier studies show that infantile hydrocephalus and cerebral palsy were the two major neurological diagnoses which could be associated with a normal perinatal period, but that the risk of both increased sharply with decreasing gestational age. The brain insult appears to be perinatal, usually early postnatal, and both disorders can be used as measures of perinatal care. The survival of children with hydrocephalus has increased from around 50 per cent 40 years ago in mostly term babies to 85 per cent in the 1960s and 1970s, which included many more preterm infants. In the pre-shunting era, a syndrome of chronic brain dysfunction consisting of a large head, a diplegic distribution of motor disorder with hypotonia and marked motor delay, with or without pyramidal and cerebellar signs, and what was described as a 'dysplastic' body build of hypothalamic type, sometimes with precocious puberty was recognized. This was commonly combined with the expected visual problems and a cognitive dissociation with speech which was better than other intellectual abilities. In the Gothenberg series from 1967–1982, the birth prevalence of infantile hydrocephalus rose from 0.48 to 0.67 per 1000 live births. There were 201 children in their series of which 63 were preterm. Of these preterm babies with hydrocephalus, 26 died before the age of two years. At follow-up at the age of four and a half, about half had cerebral palsy, half had mental retardation, and a third had epilepsy. The extremely premature babies with hydrocephalus, that is a gestational age of less than 28 weeks, were all severely multiply disabled. This group of very premature babies with hydrocephalus were a new phenomenon resulting from the survival of such babies following modern intensive care.

Ventriculomegaly in sick premature babies is one of the most difficult areas of paediatric management.[9] The sequence of events is usually of a germinal matrix haemorrhage with spread to the ventricles and their subsequent enlargement. It is mostly seen in babies born before 35 weeks' gestation, and is usually a postnatal occurrence, but ventricular haemorrhage and hydrocephalus can occur before birth. In the vast majority, there is communication between the ventricles and subarachnoid space. The babies are often very sick, requiring ventilation, intravenous nutrition, and treatment of infection, including treatment of meningitis to which they are particularly prone. A mortality of 15 per cent and a morbidity of cerebral palsy, visual and hearing problems, and learning disorders has currently to be accepted in this group. In one recent series, only 15 per cent of such patients with ventriculomegaly were free of neuromotor signs at one year and further problems, particularly of educational and social functioning may be revealed later.

The ischaemic lesions of prematurity, periventricular leucomalacia, are the main cause of disability in this group, but the contribution of hydrocephalus, although not easily separable, seems likely to be a major adverse factor. The argument that children with pure hydrocephalus have a much better prognosis than this group of babies with hydrocephalus and the cerebral lesions of prematurity has been used to suggest that the hydrocephalus is not an important contributor to further damage. The situations are, however quite different.

Obvious signs and symptoms of hydrocephalus are often absent because of immaturity and the degree of illness of the babies. The CSF pressure is often not appreciably raised above its normal level of up to 6 cm.[8] Hence the use of the term ventriculomegaly. In many such babies with mild to moderate enlargement there is resolution or stability of ventricular size. There is no general agreement about the management of progressive ventriculomegaly in this group and attempts at drainage and shunting are often the start of a sequence of treatment complications, particularly infective. This can lead to a predicament of not knowing whether to withdraw treatment or to persist in the hope of minimizing an already established major neurological disability.

Approximately 25 per cent of the premature babies receiving intensive care have been reported to have ventricular dilatation, and of those who had parenchymal brain disease (periventricular leucomalacia and/or haemorrhage) 50–60 per cent develop ventricular dilatation at 14 days of age. However, a minority of such patients eventually come to ventricular shunting.[10]

Congenital expanding porencephaly

This condition arises from a focal destructive hemisphere lesion in which the subsequent cavity is in communication with the lateral ventricle. The typical presentation is of a child with a congenital hemiplegia who suffers an increase in the motor deficit and may develop symptoms secondary to pressure and midline shift of the upper brainstem. A related condition of unilateral expanding hydrocephalus consists of global dilatation of one lateral ventricle in which pressure symptoms are more common. This may arise from a background of ischaemic damage to one hemisphere, for example in periventricular leucomalacia or infarction within a vascular malformation, or the cause may be unknown. There has been a lot of discussion about the pressure relationships and causes of this dilatation, but it behaves as a localized form of hydrocephalus and usually responds to shunting of the expanding cavity. The presentation with deterioration of what was previously regarded as a fixed motor deficit, i.e. cerebral palsy, can cause confusion.

It is obviously important that diagnostic labels, such as mental retardation and cerebral palsy, are not assigned to children in a way which precludes the possibility of their having a progressive condition, particularly hydrocephalus, unless this has been positively excluded.

The Dandy–Walker syndrome

This condition of congenital outflow obstruction and cystic dilatation of the fourth ventricle with hypoplasia of the cerebellum usually presents as hydrocephalus. This may be at a late age, and there is rarely anything to suggest direct effects of raised pressure in the posterior fossa. The breathing abnormalities that are sometimes associated with cerebellar vermis dysgenesis, particularly in Joubert syndrome, are probably associated with primary brainstem defects. The skull shape is abnormal with a bulging posterior fossa. The Dandy–Walker syndrome is usually associated with relatively little disability.

Arachnoid cysts

Arachnoid cysts are sometimes found in children being investigated for hydrocephalus, one of the commonest sites being in the suprasellar region. In general the clinical presentation is similar to that of other children with hydrocephalus, but occasionally focal, usually brainstem, signs are seen as a direct consequence of the cyst. They are mainly important as they sometimes require separate surgical treatment in addition to the hydrocephalus.

The 'bobble–headed doll' syndrome

This rare presentation of hydrocephalus consists of regular nodding movements of the head in the sagittal plane. It seems to be particularly associated with lesions of the third ventricle and aqueduct. The distinction from head movements associated with congenital ocular nystagmus is made by the absence of such nystagmus and the fact that the movements that are associated with nystagmus are usually horizontal or rotatory.

Hydranencephaly

This condition may present in a similar clinical fashion to hydrocephalus. Pathologically it consists of subtotal or complete absence of the cerebral hemispheres with optic nerve atrophy or hypoplasia and no intellectual development. The head is often large and the fontanelle may be full. It results from severe global ischaemia to the cerebral hemispheres in the last trimester of gestation.

Hydrocephalus in open spina bifida

This is due to a Chiari malformation in which the brainstem is more inferiorly placed so that part of the medulla is in the upper cervical cord. The possibility of hydrocephalus developing is known from the time the diagnosis is made. The only unusual thing about the presentation of this condition is the relatively early involvement of cranial nerves, particularly causing stridor but also sometimes facial palsy or other cranial nerve lesions. They usually resolve rapidly after shunting. Presumably the longer route taken by the cranial nerves because of caudal displacement of the medulla and pons explains this phenomenon. This also occurs in some children with persistently raised CSF protein in which one presumes that there is arachnoiditis within the posterior fossa.

Prenatal hydrocephalus

With the increasing use of modern ultrasound, enlargement of the ventricles and of the head can often be detected in pregnancy and, therefore, the fetus can be examined in detail by an experienced ultrasonographer. This examination may reveal additional problems, for example an encephalocele or open spina bifida, and this may allow the offer of termination of the pregnancy, if such detection occurs sufficiently early. Ventriculomegaly may be detected at a later stage, but at the moment attempts at intrauterine treatment of hydrocephalus have not been successful. The warning, however, that a large head is present is helpful in planning the delivery. Occasionally, the process of cerebral infarction with ventricular dilatation and eventually hydranencephaly can be documented. Intraventricular haemorrhage and subsequent hydrocephalus has also been observed.

The developmental outcome of mild ventriculomegaly in pregnancy is not certain, therefore the obstetrician's and the parent's wish for a clear prognosis on which to base their management cannot, as yet, be met.

Stiff ventricles

Occasionally, one sees a child with severe symptoms of raised intracranial pressure, particularly pain, with ventricles that may be barely enlarged and the suspicion may arise that the symptoms are not organic. Sometimes, the ventricles do not appear to be particularly distensible but yet the pressure may be very high. It seems important, therefore, to initially regard such symptoms as being likely to be organic.

Migraine in children with hydrocephalus (see also pp. 105–6)

An important clinical phenomenon has been described in children with treated hydrocephalus, and regarded as migrainous.[11] It consists of episodes of headache, nausea, vomiting, sometimes with lateralized ischaemic phenomena, and usually drowsiness and sometimes coma. For obvious reasons, shunt dysfunction is suspected and surgically treated. In the five reported patients, however, because of the lack of response to such treatment, the intermittent nature of the symptoms, and the presence of a strong family history of migraine, they were treated with propranolol with good result. The reduction in conscious level makes it very difficult to exclude shunt dysfunction without appropriate investigation on the first occasion, but this phenomenon should be borne in mind for children with recurrent unexplained episodes.

Achondroplasia

A large head and ventriculomegaly is common in achondroplasia but progressive hydrocephalus, although uncommon, can also occur. It is usually accompanied by normal intellectual functioning and is treated in the usual fashion.

Meningeal infiltration

There are a wide variety of inflammatory and malignant infiltrations of the meninges, including a condition which occurs in association particularly with the X-linked variety of immune deficiency. In this situation, although the ventricles become somewhat enlarged, the subarachnoid space superficially becomes widely dilated and loculated. Meningeal inflammation may be accompanied by a degree of atrophy and pressure symptoms are not always present.

Mucopolysaccharidoses (MPS)[12]

Hydrocephalus caused by meningeal involvement is reported in MPS1H (Hurler syndrome) and MPSII (Hunter syndrome). In the latter, papilloedema can be caused by hydrocephalus or direct involvement of the optic nerve sheath. It can be difficult to decide on the main cause of visual failure in this condition in which retinal deterioration and corneal clouding also occur.

In MPS1H/S (Hurler/Scheie), a rather specific group of problems secondary to suprasellar arachnoid cysts occur. These include destruction of the sella and cribriform plate with rhinorrhoea and visual loss. Hydrocephalus has also been reported in MPSVI, the Maroteaux–Lamy syndrome. As well as having difficulty in deciding on the relative importance of hydrocephalus in the clinical picture of this group of children, the additional problems of these children include an underlying progressive neurological disorder, albeit slowly progressive in some, chronic upper airways obstruction, instability of the cervical spine, and a very thick skull vault. They may, therefore, constitute quite a difficult surgical problem.

Ciliary dysfunction

A syndrome of primary ciliary dysfunction producing hydrocephalus and bronchiectasis with mild bony dysmorphic features has been described.[13] It is of interest from the point of view of functional embryological mechanisms. Secondary loss of ventricular cilia in hydrocephalus is well described but of uncertain clinical significance.[14]

Syndromes associated with hydrocephalus

More than 100 syndromes associated with hydrocephalus have been described and some have already been mentioned. They include both genetic and sporadic conditions, and no attempt will be made to list them all. The important clinical conclusions of reviewing this large number of conditions is as follows:

1. Any child with hydrocephalus, particularly with other congenital defects, should be investigated in detail, including chromosomes, skeletal X-rays, echocardiography and ultrasound of the abdominal viscera.

2. The child's problem list should be checked against these conditions, preferably through a regularly updated computer database of these syndromes.[15]

3. There is a genetic issue for families who have a child with unexplained hydrocephalus and they require counselling. Simple hydrocephalus carries a similar recurrence risk of neural tube defects to that of open spina bifida and, therefore, a detailed discussion about methods of detection, obstetric management, and the range of disability which could be expected is required.

4. All still-births and neonatal deaths and, if possible, spontaneous abortions should undergo autopsy by an experienced paediatric pathologist. A number of conditions that cause hydrocephalus are obligatorily or optionally lethal. This information can be crucial to future genetic counselling. The reasons given for a neonatal death are often quite misleading unless records are examined.

5. Hydrocephalus is relatively common in association with brain defects (holoprosencephaly) and with abnormalities of development of the corpus callosum.

6. The X-linked recessively inherited condition of aqueduct stenosis with adducted thumbs which is quoted in many texts is a good example of Mendelian inheritance in hydrocephalus, but should perhaps not be given the prominence which might imply that most other cases of hydrocephalus are not genetically determined.

7. Hydrocephalus can occur in the two commonest genetically determined neurocutaneous syndromes. Ventricular dilatation occurs in about one-third

of cases of tuberous sclerosis.[16] It is associated with calcified subependymal nodules and is usually evidence of cerebral atrophy. True hydrocephalus is caused by a subependymal giant-cell astrocytoma developing in association with one of these nodules in the region of the foramen of Munro. These tumours can cause either unilateral or bilateral dilatation of the lateral ventricle and sometimes discrete enlargement of the third ventricle.

In neurofibromatosis at least three mechanisms of hydrocephalus have been described. These are the indolent glial tumours in the region of the aqueduct mentioned previously, a diffuse plexiform neurofibroma in the posterior fossa, and simple communicating hydrocephalus. The commonest neurological manifestation of neurofibromatosis is a combination of a rather large head and mild to moderate learning difficulties. Active hydrocephalus is, relatively, much less common.

Arteriovenous malformations with aneurysmal dilation of the great vein of Galen

In the situation where an arteriovenous malformation drains into the great vein of Galen the latter may dilate and produce secondary aqueduct stenosis and hydrocephalus. The condition may present with heart failure in the neonatal period, a very high venous return through the head and neck, and very widely dilated veins. At a later stage it may present with acute or chronic hemisphere ischaemia or progressive hydrocephalus. It is important that this rare cause of hydrocephalus is recognized before surgery. The clinical signs of not just widely dilated scalp veins but of large jugulars and the presence of a loud bruit will usually suggest this possibility. An enhanced CT scan is virtually diagnostic. The morbidity and mortality in the early presenting group is very high, but useful treatment of the malformation and hydrocephalus are available in those presenting later.

Benign intracranial hypertension

Benign intracranial hypertension is not usually regarded as a form of hydrocephalus but is an important differential diagnosis. The presentation is of raised intracranial pressure without disturbance of consciousness. In babies, there is usually irritability and vomiting, and a full fontanelle, and very commonly lateral rectus weakness. In older children there may be some symptoms of raised intracranial pressure, but the presentation may be purely ocular with diplopia caused by lateral rectus weakness and surprisingly gross papilloedema discovered on examination. In a minority of people with this condition, usually quoted as less than 10 per cent, there may be progressive visual loss. The CSF pressure is often very high but its constituents are normal. The advent of CT scanning has made the diagnosis much easier. The scan appearances may show widening of the subarachnoidal space over the cortex but the ventricular size is usually normal or reduced.

The pathophysiology is uncertain but the condition behaves as a peripheral absorption block to CSF flow and, therefore, perhaps quite closely related to communicating hydrocephalus except that it usually has a more acute onset. The original description of the condition was in association with severe otitis media and extensive intracranial venous thrombosis, which presumably interfered with the function of the arachnoid granulations. Other causes of this condition include:

(1) a sudden reduction in corticosteroid drug dosage;

(2) a number of drugs, including tetracycline and nalidixic acid;

(3) hypocalcaemia;

(4) vitamin A poisoning.

Many cases, however, do not have an obvious cause.

Psychiatric disorders in children with hydrocephalus

Psychiatric disorders are very common in children with neurological disability. The precise diagnosis of such problems is important since they may be totally unrelated to hydrocephalus, for example Tourette syndrome, obsessive compulusive disorder, or autism which would require quite separate management. The commonest reactive problems to neurological disability are depression and conduct disorders, and these often coexist. If the child has epilepsy, then the problems of hyperactivity, irritability, and aggression which may accompany epilepsy may also be present. Therefore, although deterioration in behaviour and social functioning in children with hydrocephalus may be due to raised intracranial pressure, it is important that psychiatric problems are both expected in this group of children and that the clinical team includes a paediatric neuropsychiatrist. Although we hope that the hydrocephalus part of a syndrome complex is the most remediable, there is a case for suggesting that the psychiatric problems are the most commonly overlooked.

CONCLUSIONS

Hydrocephalus in childhood is, therefore, a condition which can arise in a wide range of clinical situations, including the sick premature neonate, the child with life-threatening meningitis, in children who are found to have relatively mild developmental problems at surveillance, or whose parents just have the suspicion that something is not right. The condition can masquerade as gastrointestinal or ocular disease or be misinterpreted as an emotional disorder in a child who is failing at school. It is an important aspect of the management of many children with brain tumours. The decisions about whether the hydrocephalus is active or not are often very difficult. The manifestations have a regular pattern of disabilities but vary according to the selective vulnerability of the nervous system at different ages. There would appear to be a very large number of primary disorders which can lead to hydrocephalus. The clinical skills required in the detection and management of hydrocephalus are many and varied, and include those of neurosurgeons, paediatricians and paediatric neurologists, psychologists, psychiatrists with experience of complex handicap, and therapists who can both assess such patients and provide programmes of advice and intervention for their multiple problems.

REFERENCES

1. Kirkpatrick, M., Engleman, H., and Minns, R.A. Symptoms and signs of progressive hydrocephalus. *Archives of Disease in Childhood*, **64**, 124–8 (1989).
2. Egan, D.F. *Developmental examination of infants and pre-school children*, MacKeith Press, London (1990).
3. Barlow, C.F. *Headaches and migraine in childhood*. Clinics in Developmental Medicine No. 91. Spastics International Medical Publications Oxford (1984).
4. Honig, P.T. and Charney, E.B. Children with brain tumour headaches. *American Journal of Diseases of Children*, **136**, 121–4 (1982).
5. Rocco, C.D., Caldarelli, M., and Ceddia, A. 'Occult' hydrocephalus in children. *Child's Nervous System*, **5**, 71–5 (1989).
6. Visudiphan, P. and Chiemchanya, S. Hydrocephalus in tuberculous meningitis in children: Treatment with acetazolamide and repeated lumbar puncture. *Journal of Paediatrics*, **95**, 657–60 (1979).
7. Hagberg, B. and Hagberg, G. The changing panorama of infantile hydrocephalus and cerebral palsy over forty years — A Swedish survey. *Brain Development*, **11**, 368–73 (1989).
8. De Vries, L-S., Larroche, J.C., and Levine, M.I. 'Intracranial Sequelae' In *Fetal and neonatal neurology and neurosurgery*. (ed. Levene, M.I., Bennett, M.J., and Punt, J.), 346–53. Churchill Livingstone, Edinburgh (1988).
9. Volpe, J.J. and Hill, A.H. Normal pressure hydrocephalus in the newborn. *Paediatrics*, **68**, 623–9 (1981).
10. Whitelaw, A. Randomised trial of early tapping in neonatal posthaemorrhagic ventricular dilatation. *Archives of Disease in Childhood*, **65**, 3–10 (1990).
11. Nowak, T.P. and James, H.E. Migraine headaches in hydrocephalic children: a diagnostic dilemma. *Child's Nervous System*, **5**, 310–14 (1989).
12. Neufeld, E.F. and Muenzer, J. The Mucopolysaccharidoses. In *The metabolic basis of inherited disease*, pp. 1565–88. McGraw-Hill, (1989)
13. Greenstone, M.A., Jones, R.W.A., Dewer, A., Neville, B.G.R., and Cole, P.J. Hydrocephalus and primary ciliary dyskinesia. *Archives of Disease in Childhood*, **59**, 481–2 (1984).
14. Bannister, C.M. and Chapman, S.A. Ventricular ependyma of normal and hydrocephalic subjects: a scanning electromicroscopic study. *Developmental Medicine and Child Neurology*, **22**, 725–35 (1980).
15. Baraitser, M. *London Neurology Database*. Institute of Child Health, University of London (1990).
16. Gomez, M.R. *Tuberous sclerosis*, 2nd edn., Raven Press, New York (1988).

5 Radiological and other investigative techniques

R.O. Robinson

INTRODUCTION

The investigation of childhood hydrocephalus is directed towards

1. An architectural description of ventricular size (and by inference volume), associated obstruction to CSF flow, and associated brain anomalies — if any;
2. Measurement of CSF pressure;
3. Evaluation of the effects of hydrocephalus on brain function.

These will be considered in turn.

IMAGING

The advent of non-invasive imaging techniques have made pneumoencephalography and arteriography redundant in the investigation of hydrocephalus. Therefore these techniques will not be considered further.

Ultrasound imaging

Prenatal assessment

Prenatal assessment has recently been well reviewed.[1,2] Ultrasound, which should now be taken to mean real-time scanning, is currently the only method of assessment of fetal ventricular size. This technique uses the properties of tissues in altering ultrasound to generate an image. A source of ultrasound, the transducer, creates a beam of ultrasound waves. When the wave front strikes an interface between tissues which differ in their acoustical impedance an echo is reflected back to the transducer. By measuring the time taken for the echo to be received, the distance between the transducer and the interface can be calculated.

Using the reflected sound energy with the time interval data, an image can be generated which is displayed on a television monitor. If successive images are placed on the monitor at short intervals an image is produced in 'real time'. This allows movement within organs, vascular pulsation for example, to be displayed. Since major enlargement of the ventricles takes place before an increase in the biparietal diameter there is no substitute for the direct assessment of ventricular size. As the term hydrocephalus usually subsumes a clinical description, the situation of enlarged ventricles in fetal life is usually described as fetal ventriculomegaly. (Fig. 5.1). Because routine antenatal scanning is widely practised, this is now frequently a serendipitous finding, but the obstetric sonographer will pay particular attention to ventricular size where there is a family history of neurological defects or chromosomal anomalies, or where the maternal serum alpha fetoprotein is elevated. Ratios comparing ventricular to head size have been used, perhaps most widely the ratio of ventricular body width to head width. Since unaltered ratios can disguise real increases in size, actual measurements of ventricular size are preferred. Normal ranges by gestational age for different sites in the ventricles have been published. Of these, measurement of the atria is perhaps the single most useful measurement as this usually dilates earliest. This is particularly useful as, despite brain growth, from 13 to 38 post-menstrual weeks atrial size remains relatively constant at 7.6 ± 0.6 cm ($\pm$ SD).[3]

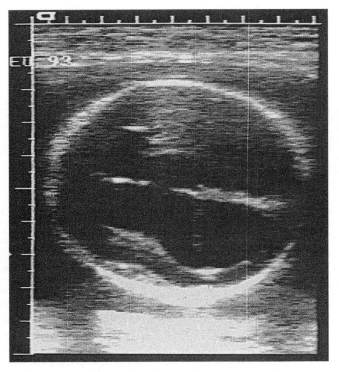

Fig. 5.1 Fetal ultrasound scan showing moderate ventriculomegaly at 23 weeks' gestation.

During the first trimester, and up to 16 weeks, gestation, the choroid plexuses almost entirely fill the lateral ventricles. Separation of the ventricular wall from the choroid plexus by more than a few millimetres has been taken by some as an additional useful sign of ventriculomegaly.

The early and accurate diagnosis of fetal ventriculomegaly is not merely an academic exercise. Approximately 80 per cent of those with enlarged ventricles will have associated anomalies either within or without the central nervous system, or both. (Figs 5.2 and 5.3). The majority of these anomalies can be correctly identified by careful ultrasound scanning which is therefore mandatory. Multiple associated anomalies outside the central nervous system are almost invariably associated with fetal mortality.[4] Survivors with severe anomalies outside the central nervous system also have a high mortality rate in the neonatal period. Rapidly progressive ventriculomegaly carries a poor prognosis. Additional items of information which need to be sought urgently in these cases are the fetal karyotype and evidence of intrauterine infection.

Most instances of fetal ventriculomegaly become apparent during the first trimester at a time when informed decisions about the course and termination of pregnancy can be made. Slight and questionable ventriculomegaly needs frequent subsequent ultrasound assessment as massive dilatation can take place within a fortnight,[5] become stable, or resolve.[6] As might be expected the outcome in the latter group may be good, if no additional anomalies are found.

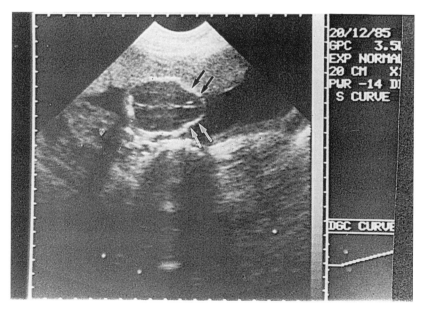

Fig. 5.2 Fetal ultrasound scan showing frontal scalloping ('lemon') deformity.

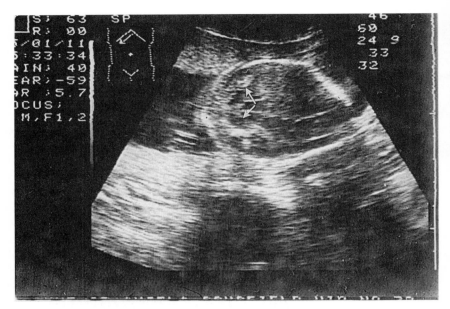

Fig. 5.3 Fetal ultrasound scan showing frontal scalloping ('lemon' deformity), and a curvilinear echodensity ('banana' deformity) — arrowed — a characteristic of the Arnold–Chiari malformation.

Neonatal assessment

This has also been well reviewed recently.[7] In the preterm infant post-haemorrhagic hydrocephalus is a frequent and difficult problem. Intraventricular haemorrhage occurs in approximately half those babies with a birthweight of less than 1500 g. Of these a quarter to a half will develop hydrocephalus. (Fig. 5.4). Ultrasound is the preferred investigation in this situation, being safer and more sensitive than computerized tomography (CT) for the detection of small haemorrhagic clots within the ventricles and for the identification of haematomas that are isodense on CT scanning.

The great majority of intraventricular haemorrhages occur during the first week after birth. Ventricular dilatation takes place at any stage during the next three months. Early and rapidly progressive hydrocephalus accompanied by raised intracranial pressure will almost certainly be evident by the end of the second week.[8] More occult increase in ventricular size, initially without a detectable rise in intracranial pressure, can take place at varying intervals thereafter; sometimes with an intervening period of stability lasting up to three months.[6] During this period ventricular dilatation may arrest without further change or ventricular size may diminish. These various changes, with the management decisions based upon them, can be followed without difficulty by serial ultrasound scans because the anterior fontanelle will remain sufficiently

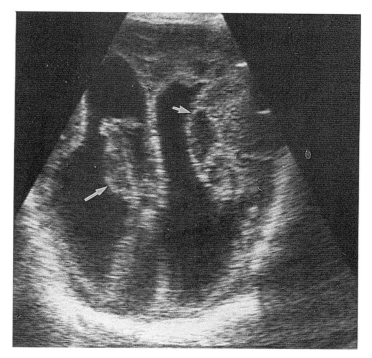

Fig. 5.4 Longitudinal ultrasound scan showing hydrocephalus and intra-ventricular haemorrhage — arrowed.

patent for at least this period of time. Routine scanning to detect ventricular dilatation will be most effectively carried out halfway through the first week and at the end of the first week, at the end of the second week, and at three months.

In both neonatal and fetal assessment, an actual measurement of ventricular size is to be preferred.[9] Using ultrasound techniques we can also assess the efficacy of shunt placement in respect of subsequent changes in ventricular size and also the width of the cortical mantle (Fig. 5.5), as well as detecting complications of shunting such as ventriculitis.[10]

Computerized tomography

By contrast when the aetiology of neonatal hydrocephalus is not clear, that is to say that it is not post-haemorrhagic, then better definition of intracranial structures is required than can be provided by ultrasound in the neonatal period (Figs 5.6 and 5.7). Similarly ultrasound is precluded as the fontanelle closes. Most experience at the present time has been acquired with US or CT (Figs 5.8–13), but where magnetic resonance imaging (MRI) is available it will undoubtedly be preferred because of its improved ability to delineate periaqueductal and posterior fossa structures. With both techniques acceptable images can only be

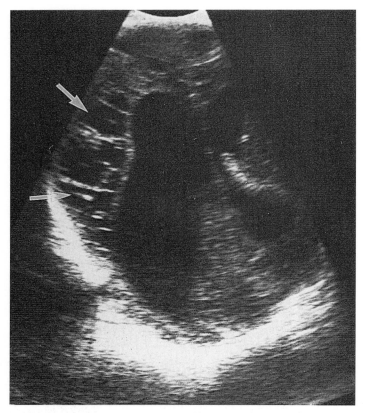

Fig. 5.5 Longitudinal ultrasound scan showing cystic periventricular leucomalacia — arrowed.

produced if the child is still. This may require a brief general anaesthetic which, in the case of MRI, has to be administered using special equipment in which only non-ferrous metal is used.

A host of normal values for the size of different ventricular structures and the ratios between them are available, and have been reviewed by Naidich et al.[11] However, experienced radiologists and clinicians rely not only on the proportion of the intracranial area occupied by the ventricles, but also on other features, such as the dilatation of the temporal horns, rounding of the superolateral angles of the frontal horns, and compression and inferior displacement of the thalami. Ventricular enlargement due to atrophy (hydrocephalus *ex vacuo*) can be distinguished from obstructive hydrocephalus, as in the former the frontal horns, although enlarged, retain their shape and, in addition, sulci are more evident.[12]

Attempts to gauge the site of the obstruction to CSF flow by evaluation of dilatation of some parts of the ventricular system as compared with others can

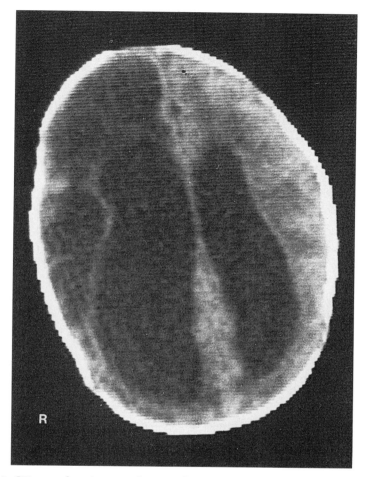

Fig. 5.6 CT scan showing post-haemorrhagic hydrocephalus and extensive hypoxic ischaemic damage.

be misleading, as only approximately one third of cases of communicating hydrocephalus will have a dilated IVth ventricle.

Indications for computerized tomography may be summarized as follows:

1. Any child with symptoms or signs of raised intracranial pressure (see Chapter 4).

2. Any child with an increased rate of head growth. This has to be assessed by plotting successive head measurements of the child against the normal trajectories of head size and postnatal age. Previous measurements from health clinic charts may be very valuable here.

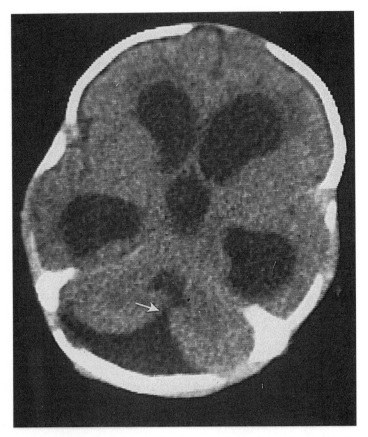

Fig. 5.7 CT scan showing hydrocephalus together with a Dandy–Walker malformation and agenesis of the vermis — arrowed.

3. Commonly previous measurements are not available. If the child is developmentally appropriate for its age, neurologically normal, asymptomatic, and the head size is not greater than three standard deviations above the mean, it is reasonable to temporize whilst establishing the rate of head growth, particularly if one or both of the parents have large heads. Conversely, if one or more of these does not apply, CT is indicated.

Conventional X-rays

It may seem odd to mention plain skull films only at this stage. Raised intracranial pressure may separate cranial sutures in children and, if prolonged, may accentuate the gyral patterning on the inner calvarium, erode the posterior clinoid processes, and expand the pituitary fossa (Fig. 5.14). However, it should be clear by now that skull X-rays cannot reliably exclude raised intracranial

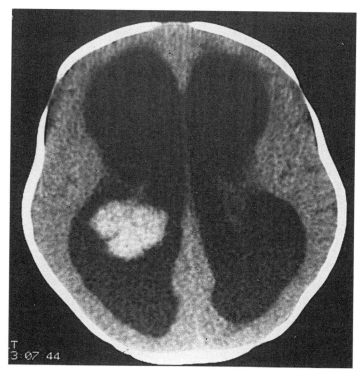

Fig. 5.8 CT scan showing a choroid plexus papilloma causing hydrocephalus.

pressure let alone assess ventricular size. Nevertheless, they can occasionally provide useful information such as in complete cranial synostosis, a rare cause of raised intracranial pressure with little or no ventricular dilatation, the volume of the posterior fossa, or by showing scattered cerebral calcification where toxoplasmosis has caused hydrocephalus. They are also indispensable of course in assessing shunt continuity in cases of suspected shunt malfunction.

Magnetic resonance imaging

As mentioned above, where available, this investigation is likely to displace CT. Small periaqueductal tumours, easily missed on CT, are readily seen on sagittal MRI views, particularly on T2 images.[13] The ability to reformat sagittal images easily may show additional changes less easily appreciated on CT, such as thinning and smooth elevation of the corpus callosum, helpfully distinguishing hydrocephalus from atrophy.[14] Improved visualization of the posterior fossa, and particularly foramen magnum relationships, can be helpful when assessing Chiari malformations, associated syringomyelia, and Dandy–Walker malformations.[15] CSF volume may be derived from MRI. Being highly reproducible this may prove a sensitive index of change of ventricular size.[16]

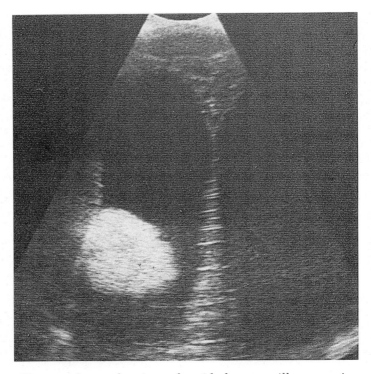

Fig. 5.9 Ultrasound scan showing a choroid plexus papilloma causing hydrocephalus.

Attention has recently been directed to the dynamics of CSF flow. A variety of MRI techniques will show fast laminar flow as a low signal ('flow void' sign) (Fig. 5.15). This is usually present in narrow CSF spaces, such as the aqueduct and basal cisterns. Therefore, when a flow void is seen aqueduct stenosis can be excluded. 'Gating' data collection to the cardiac cycle can demonstrate to and fro CSF flow during systole and diastole. More specialized techniques can demonstrate turbulent CSF flow, for example in the IVth ventricle[17](which means that the relationship between flow and pressure has become non-linear). Whilst these developments are not as yet clinically applicable, it is possible that they may become so if, for example, CSF pulse amplitude can be measured.

PRESSURE MEASUREMENTS

Clinicians tend to associate symptoms with elevated intracranial CSF pressure, although this is not always the case.[18] Single pressure measurements using the manometer or fluid-filled transducer attached to a lumbar puncture needle, are of

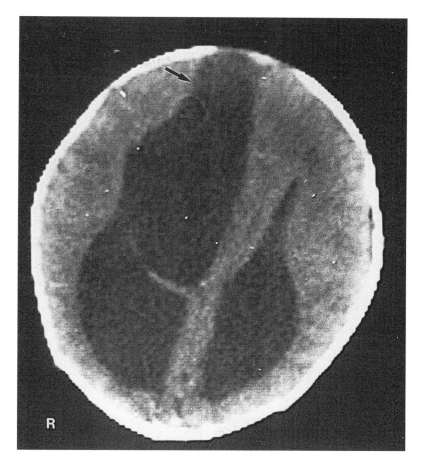

Fig. 5.10 CT scan showing hydrocephalus accompanying an arachnoid cyst and agenesis of the corpus callosum.

limited value. The child must be tranquil (not crying) and relaxed (which implies some spinal and hip extension from the traditional flexed position used for lumbar CSF puncture). An unequivocally raised pressure measurement when this situation is achieved, if necessary with the help of sedation, is very helpful. However, a normal single reading does not exclude periods of significantly raised intracranial pressure. Continuous CSF pressure monitoring in doubtful or difficult cases is, therefore, frequently regarded as the 'gold standard'. This may be achieved by passing a soft catheter through a lumbar puncture needle into the subarachnoid space, removing the needle and after securing the catheter to the skin attaching a fluid-filled transducer. This will allow the child a reasonable degree of mobility.

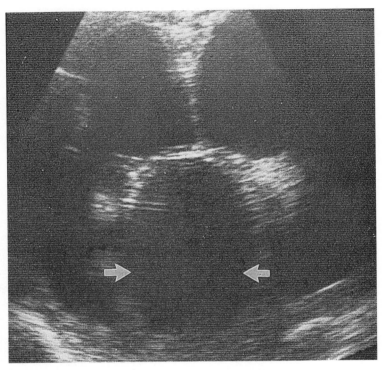

Fig. 5.11 Ultrasound scan of an aneurysm of the vein of Galen — arrowed.

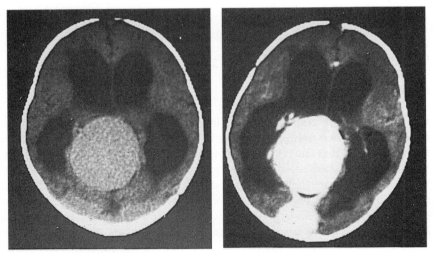

Fig. 5.12 CT scan showing hydrocephalus caused by an aneurysm of the vein of Galen. Left, scan unenhanced; Right, scan enhanced.

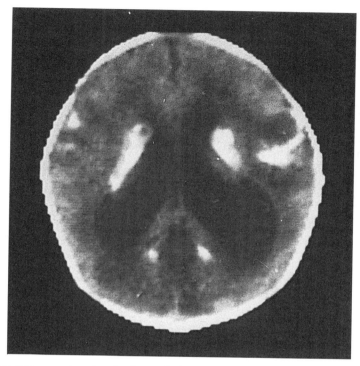

Fig. 5.13 CT scan showing hydrocephalus and intracerebral calcification due to toxoplasmosis.

Over-drained ventricles can lead to a system with reduced compliance which is very volume sensitive. In this situation symptoms caused by transient rises in CSF pressure or occult increases during sleep, may be relieved by subtemporal decompression. Similarly, intracranial pressure monitoring may be helpful in assessing the need for shunt revision or the need for CSF diversion in older children with tumours.[19] McCullough[19] found continuous CSF pressure monitoring less predictive in younger children. This may be partly because the period of normal pressure hydrocephalus in some infants had not at that time been appreciated,[6] but possibly also because less attention than it deserves has been given to the CSF pressure amplitude.[20] Di Rocco convincingly demonstrated that ventricles may be dilated rapidly by an increased pulse pressure amplitude even when the mean CSF pressure remains normal.[21] Whether this can produce symptoms is as yet unclear. Partly because of these difficulties, partly to obviate the need for diurnal recording and partly to improve our ability to detect 'latent' hydrocephalus, various workers have assessed the place of pressure/volume relationships in children with hydrocephalus. From the pressure response to rapid volume changes (either bolus addition or withdrawal)

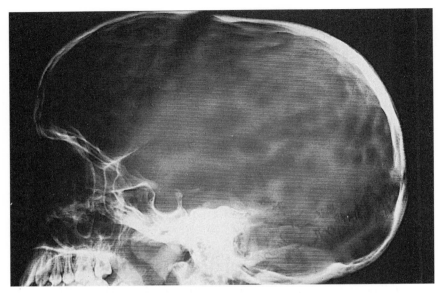

Fig. 5.14 Plain X-ray showing suture diastasis, enlargement and thinning of the skull due to hydrocephalus.

inferences about the compliance of the system can be made. Additionally, lumbar infusions either at a steady rate or to maintain a steady pressure, may allow inferences about the rate of and threshold for CSF absorption. Di Rocco *et al.* studied 18 children with apparently arrested hydrocephalus using this steady lumbar infusion technique. They found that although the resting pressure in all children was normal, CSF pressure stabilized in six children at an abnormally high value during this procedure. Five of these six children had shunt revisions, all five apparently showed clinical improvement.[22]

Caldarelli *et al.*[23] successfully distinguished hydrocephalus from atrophy using this technique. In the hydrocephalic group CSF pressure plateaued at more than 300 mm of water, whereas in the atrophic group plateauing occurred at less than 300 mm of water, usually around 200 mm. Shapiro and Fried[24] showed, in 20 children with acute shunt malfunction, that individual children had a specific point on the pressure/volume curve, usually between 20 and 30 mm Hg, beyond which acute deterioration occurred. The same workers showed that unlike adults, children with more subtle signs of shunt malfunction had abnormally compliant ventricles, which they equated with continuing shunt dependency.[25]

This work, based on sound physiological principles has been quoted at some length because it appears to take a logical approach to improving our understanding of the problems of hydrocephalus. Although these techniques have been described for up to 20 years they have not, however, found wider clinical application, partly because the information they provide can usually be derived

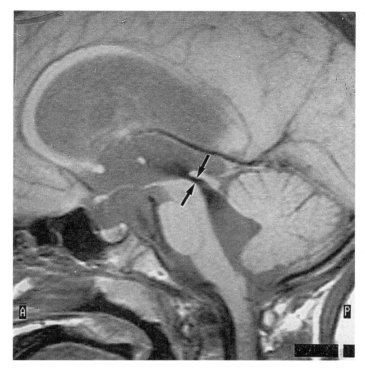

Fig. 5.15 Sagittal MRI scan showing a 'flow void' throughout the aqueduct — arrowed.

from serial non-invasive imaging, with the resort to simple pressure recording in difficult cases.

CSF dynamics have also been studied by imaging the radio-isotope diethylenetriaminepentaacetic acid (DTPA) injected into the lumbar space of 34 infants with ventricular enlargement.[26] All but six showed some degree of ventricular filling with varying rates of 'clearance' of isotope from within the ventricles. There did seem to be some correlation between signs of raised intracranial pressure and clearance rate but this was not clear cut. This technique does not recommend itself to many because of the concern about local radiation dosage.

EFFECTS OF HYDROCEPHALUS

The direct measurement of aspects of cellular metabolism in hydrocephalus whilst now technically feasible using positron emission tomography, infra-red or magnetic resonance spectroscopy has not yet been undertaken in children. Our evaluation of the effects of hydrocephalus must be necessarily indirect. Not surprisingly there is little recent literature on the effect of raised intracranial pressure on the electroencephalograph (EEG) in untreated hydrocephalus. In one study findings in 17 such children were reported.[27] EEG abnormalities were found in 16. Nine had generalized polymorphic delta activity, five had multifocal 'epileptiform' activity, and four had generalized abnormalities such as 'paroxysmal' 4/s rhythms. There was EEG evidence, therefore, of both white and grey matter involvement, with the former perhaps predominating.

Ines *et al.* provided good EEG evidence of cortical dysfunction with shunt insertion.[28] These authors studied 92 patients in the paediatric age range retrospectively. Eighty one had one or more ventriculo–atrial shunts inserted and eleven had not. Fifty three (65.4 per cent) of the shunted group had fits as compared with two (18.2 per cent) of the unshunted group. Whilst it might be argued that this represented the effects of less extreme hydrocephalus in the unshunted group (which was the case in all but two) EEG findings were against this. EEG abnormalities were largely focal, but more particularly showed slow wave predominance over the shunted hemisphere. In more than half of these the abnormality was localized to the shunt site itself. A useful clinical point that emerged from this work was that of the 53 children in the shunted group who had fits, 42 developed them within four months of shunt insertion.

Evoked potentials

As hydrocephalus is a condition the brunt of which falls on the white matter, it is logical to examine the effect on evoked potentials.

Visual evoked potentials

Several studies suggest increased latency of early components of the visual evoked response which appears to depend on raised intracranial pressure rather than increased ventricular size.[29,30] CSF diversionary procedures will restore latencies to normal within one week, again irrespective of a change in ventricular size.[31] It is not clear whether these effects are caused by chiasmal and anterior pathway compression or by pressure on post-chiasmatic pathways, or their blood supply.

Auditory evoked potentials

Auditory evoked potentials (AEPs) have been less extensively studied. Whilst in cats, an increase in acute intracranial pressure had no apparent effect on AEPs,[32] 16 babies with hydrocephalus showed changes compared with age-matched controls.[33] Although there was a lower mean latency and lower mean amplitude of waves I and IV, only one hydrocephalic baby had a latency of more than 2 standard deviations above the normal mean. A lower amplitude of wave V was the most consistent finding. In addition, all hydrocephalic babies had an elevated auditory threshold in one or both ears which was thought to be central in origin, rather than representing peripheral hearing loss. However, it is not known whether the cochlear aqueduct will transmit pressure increases sufficient to affect middle ear function. An interesting technique which deserves further study is the possibility of non-invasive evaluation of changes of CSF pressure. The oval window is, via the perilymph and cochlear aqueduct, in communication with the subarachnoid space. Displacement of the oval window with a rise in intracranial pressure alters the movement of the middle ear ossicles and hence the tympanic membranes. This can be appreciated by the acoustical stimulation of the stapedial reflex.[34]

Other studies

Apart from effects of pressure on neurones, pressure and distortion may affect intracranial arteries, raising the possibility of secondary ischaemic damage. This has been studied by using pulsed Doppler ultrasound to measure blood flow velocity. Comparison of flow velocities in systole and diastole, the 'pulsatility index,' gives an indirect assessment of peripheral resistance. Hill and Volpe studied anterior cerebral artery flow in 11 untreated hydrocephalic infants. Impaired flow was demonstrated in all cases, and improved with shunting or ventriculostomy.[35] Interestingly, the intracranial pressure measured non-invasively was normal in two, suggesting that the impaired flow was due to dislocated vascular architecture rather than the increased pressure. An increased pulsatility index has been confirmed by others, such as Anderson and Mawk[36] and Alvisi *et al.*[37] The latter authors emphasized that their findings were not sufficiently consistent to form a basis for management decisions. Most recently the finding has been replicated *in utero* where an inverse relationship was found between ventricular size and pulsatile flow, flow during diastole being better with smaller ventricles.[38]

Support for a measure of brain ischaemia comes from the study of xanthine and hypoxanthine levels in CSF. During tissue hypoxia there is increased catabolism of adenosine nucleotides, and hence an increase in the concentrations of hypoxanthine and xanthine. Levin *et al.* were able to show a convincing linear correlation between maximum intracranial pressure and oxypurine levels.[39] These levels fall with shunting.[40] Further work needs to be done to ·assess the place for this information in the management of doubtful and difficult cases.

CONCLUSIONS

Non-invasive imaging represents a major advance in the investigation of hydrocephalus. It is of course far more comfortable for the patient than the now outmoded pneumoencephalogram. Both CT and MRI can show cerebral anatomy very clearly and these frequently demonstrate in elegant detail the cause of the hydrocephalus.

Patients, however, continue to puzzle clinicians with unexpected responses (beneficial or otherwise) to shunting procedures. Some of these difficulties may be resolved by an improved understanding of CSF flow and pressure dynamics. It is to be hoped that in the future, perhaps with further development of MRI, we will be able to study them less invasively than at present. This, coupled with information about regional brain metabolism, should greatly improve our understanding of the processes of hydrocephalus as well as our ability to manage these patients more effectively.

REFERENCES

1. Birnholz, J.C. Ultrasound evaluation of fetal neurology. In *Fetal and neonatal neurology and neurosurgery*, (ed. Levine, M.I., Bennett, M.J., and Punt, J.), pp. 91–107. Churchill Livingstone, Edinburgh (1988).

2. Pilu, G. and Hobbins, J.C. The ultrasound appearances of normal and abnormal anatomy of the fetal central nervous system. In *Fetal and neonatal neurology and neurosurgery*, (ed. Levine, M.I., Bennett, M.J., and Punt, J.), pp. 108–21. Churchill Livingstone, Edinburgh (1988).

3. Cardoza, J.D., Goldstein, R.B., and Filly, R.A. Exclusion of fetal ventriculomegaly with a single measurement: the width of the lateral ventricular atrium. Radiology, **169**, 711–14 (1988).

4. Nyberg, D.A., Mack, L.A., Hursch, J., Payon, R.O., and Shepard, T.H. Fetal hydrocephalus: sonographic detection and clinical significance of associated anomalies. *Radiology*, **163**, 187–91 (1987).

5. Chervenak, F.A., Berkowitz, R.L., Tortora, M., Chitkara, U., and Hobbins, J.C. Diagnosis of ventriculomegaly before fetal viability. *Obstetrics and Gynecology*, **64**, 652–6 (1984).

6. Hill, A. and Volpe, J.J. Normal pressure hydrocephalus in the newborn. *Pediatrics*, **68**, 623–9 (1981).

7. Levene, M.I., Williams, J.L., and Fawer, C.L. Ultrasound of the infant brain. Clinics in Developmental Medicine, No. 92. SIMP Blackwell Scientific Publications Limited, Oxford (1985).

8. Partridge, J.C., Babcock, D.S., Steichen, J.J., and Han, B.K. Optimal timing for diagnostic cranial ultrasound in low birthweight infants. *Journal of Pediatrics*, **102**, 281–7 (1983).

9. Levene, M.I. Measurement of the growth of the lateral ventricles in preterm infants with real time ultrasound. *Archives of Disease in Childhood*, **56**, 900–4 (1981).

10. Reeder, J.D and Sanders, R.C. Ventriculitis in the neonate: recognition by sonography. *American Journal of Neuroradiology*, **4**, 37–41 (1983).

11. Naidich, T.P., Schott, L.H., and Baron, R.L. Computed tomography in evaluation of hydrocephalus. *Radiological Clinics of North America*, **20**, 143–67 (1982).

12. Heinz, E.R., Ward, A., Drayer, B.P., and du Bois, P.J. Distinction between obstructive and atrophic dilatation of ventricles in children. *Journal of Computer Assisted Tomography*, **4**, 320–5 (1980).

13. Lee, B.C.P. Magnetic resonance imaging of periaqueductal lesions. *Clinical Radiology*, **38**, 527–33 (1987).

14. El-Gammel, T., Allen, M.B., Brooks, B.S., and Mark, E.K. Magnetic resonance evaluation of hydrocephalus. *American Journal of Radiology*, **149**, 807–13 (1987).

15. Hanigan, W.C., Wright, R., and Wright, S. Magnetic resonance imaging of the Dandy–Walker malformation. *Paediatric Neuroscience*, **12**, 151–6 (1985–6).

16. Condon, V., Patterson, J., Wyper, D., Hadley, D., Grant, R., Teasdale, G., and Rowan, J. Use of magnetic resonance imaging to measure intracranial cerebrospinal fluid volume. *Lancet*, **i**, 1355–7 (1986).

17. Joleiz, F.A., Patz, S., Hawkes, R.C., and Lopez, I. Fast imaging of cerebro-spinal fluid flow/motion patterns using steady state free precession (SSFP). *Investigative Radiology*, **22**, 761–71 (1987).

18. Kirkpatrick, M., Engleman, H., and Minns, R.A. Symptoms and signs of progressive hydrocephalus. *Archives of Disease in Childhood*, **64**, 124–8 (1989).

19. McCullough, D.C. A critical evaluation of continuous intracranial monitoring in paediatric hydrocephalus. *Child's Brain*, **6**, 225–41 (1980).

20. Foltz, E.L. Hydrocephalus and cerebro-spinal fluid pulsatility: clinical and laboratory studies. In *Hydrocephalus*, (ed. Shapiro, K., Marmarou, A., and Portnoy, H.), pp. 337–62. Raven Press, New York (1984).

21. Di Rocco, C., Di Tripani, G., Pettovorsi, U.E., and Caldarelli, M. On the pathology of experimental hydrocephalus introduced by artificial increase in endoventricular cerebro-spinal fluid pulse pressure. *Child's Brain*, **5**, 81–95 (1975).

22. Di Rocco, C., Caldarelli, M., Maira, G., and Rossi, G.F. The study of cerebro-spinal fluid pressure dynamics in apparently arrested hydrocephalus in children. Child's Brain, **3**, 359–74 (1977).

23. Caldarelli, M., Di Rocco, C., and Rossi, G.F. Lumbar subarachnoid infusion test in paediatric neurosurgery. *Developmental Medicine and Child Neurology*, **21**, 71–82 (1974).

24. Shapiro, K. and Fried, A. Pressure volume relationships in shunt dependent childhood hydrocephalus. The zone of pressure instability in children with acute deterioration. *Journal of Neurosurgery*, **64**, 390–6 (1986).

25. Fried, A. and Shapiro, K. Subtle deterioration in shunted childhood hydro-cephalus. A biomechanical and clinical profile. *Journal of Neurosurgery*, **65**, 211–6 (1986).

26. Velardi, F., Hoffman, H.J., Ash, J.M., Hendrick, E.B., and Humphreys, R.P. The value of cerebro-spinal fluid flow studies in infants with communicating hydro-cephalus. *Children's Nervous System*, **2**, 139–43 (1986).

27. Bogacz, J. and Rebollo, M.A. Electroencephalographic abnormalities in non tumour hydrocephalus. *Electroencephalography and Clinical Neurophysiology*, **14**, 123–5 (1962).

28. Ines, D.F. and Markand, E.N. Epileptic seizures and abnormal electroencephalo-graphic findings in hydrocephalus and their relation to shunting procedures. *Electroencephalography and Clinical Neurophysiology*, **42**, 761–8 (1977).

29. Coupland, S.G. and Cochrane, D.D. Visual evoked potentials, intracranial pressure and ventricular size in hydrocephalus. *Doc. Ophthalmol.*, **66**, 321–30 (1987).

30. York, D.H., Pulham, M.W., Rosenfeld, J.G., and Watts, C. Relationship between visual evoked potentials and intracranial pressure. *Journal of Neurosurgery*, **55**, 909–16 (1981).

31. Ehle, A. and Sclar, F. Visual evoked potentials in infants with hydrocephalus. *Neurology*, **29**, 1541–4 (1979).

32. Sutton, L.N., Cho, B., Jaggi, J., Joseph, P.M., and Bruce, D.A. Effects of hydrocephalus and increased intracranial pressure in auditory and somato-sensory responses. *Neurosurgery*, **18**, 756–61 (1986).

33. Edwards, C.G., Durieux-Smith, A., and Picton, T.W. Auditory brain stem response audiometry in neonatal hydrocephalus. *Journal of Otolaryngology*, **14** (Suppl. 14), 40–6 (1985).

34. Marchbanks, R.J., Reid, A., Martin, A.M., Brightwell, A.P., and Bateman, D. The effect of raised intracranial pressure on intracochlear fluid pressure: three case studies. *British Journal of Audiology*, **21**, 127–30 (1987).

35. Hill, A. and Volpe, J.J. Decrease in pulsatile flow in the anterior cerebral arteries in infantile hydrocephalus. *Pediatrics*, **69**, 4–7 (1982).

36. Anderson, J.C. and Mawk, J.R. Intracranial arterial duplex Doppler wave form analysis in infants. *Child's Nervous System*, **4**, 144–8 (1988).

37. Alvisi, C., Cerisoli, M., Giulioni, M., Moneri, P., Salvioli, G.P., Sandri, F., Lippi, C., Bovicelli, L., and Pilu, G. Evaluation of cerebral blood flow changes by transfontanelle Doppler ultrasound in infantile hydrocephalus. *Child's Nervous System*, **1**, 244–7 (1985).

38. Degani, S., Lewinsky, R., Shapiro. I., and Sharf, M. Decrease in pulsatile flow in the internal carotid artery in fetal hydrocephalus. *British Journal of Obstetrics and Gynaecology*, **95**, 138–41 (1988).

39. Levin, S.D., Brown, J.K., and Harkness, R.A. Cerebrospinal fluid hypoxanthine and xanthine concentrations as indicators of metabolic damage due to raised intracranial pressure in hydrocephalic children. *Journal of Neurology, Neurosurgery and Psychiatry*, **47**, 730–3 (1984).

40. Castro-Gago, M., Logo, S., Del Rao, R., Rodriguez, A., Novo, I., and Rodriguez-Segade, S. The concentrations of xanthine and hypoxanthine in cerebro-spinal fluid as therapeutic guides in hydrocephalus. *Child's Nervous System*, **2**, 109–11 (1986).

6 Principles of CSF diversion and alternative treatments

J. Punt

INTRODUCTION

There are few conditions in neurosurgical practice more frustrating to manage than hydrocephalus. It is a disturbance whose capricious nature has it origins in an incomplete understanding of the pathophysiology; where diagnostic difficulties abound despite sophisticated aids to investigation; and for which apparently straightforward operative procedures may have devastatingly disastrous consequences.

The modern era of active intervention has followed a sequence of developments commencing with the more accurate anatomical descriptions given by various writers from the 16th to the 19th centuries;[1-5] complimented by the later physiological studies of Key and Retzius[6] and Dandy and Blackfan;[7] rationalized by the pathological observations of Russell;[8] and culminating in the invention of valved shunt systems by Holter and their application by Nulsen and Spitz.[9] Finally, there have been the major advances in diagnostic imaging of the central nervous system afforded by computerized tomographic scanning (CT), magnetic resonance imaging (MRI) and real-time ultrasound (US). Despite this apparently satisfactory evolution imperfections in understanding exist at almost all levels, ranging from the dynamics of production and absorption of cerebrospinal fluid (CSF), to the interpretation of diagnostic images in given clinical contexts, as exemplified by such conditions as benign intracranial hypertension and normal pressure hydrocephalus.[10] The more ancient and historic methods of treatment have been well catalogued elsewhere,[11,12] and this chapter will concentrate on more recent, modern and current practices, their short falls, and their complications.

MEDICAL TREATMENT

Compressive head wrapping

Blane[13] first mentioned success in treating infantile hydrocephalus by compressive head wrapping, and further encouraging reports appeared from Girdlestone and Costerton[14] and Barnard:[15] moist muslin bandages firmly applied, adhesive plaster or, preferably, rubber bandages were used to support the fragile neonatal calvarium. Epstein *et al.*[16,17] resurrected the technique following observations on the effects of radical craniectomy on the ventricular size in cats; massive ventriculomegaly ensued which could be stabilized by reconstitution of the calvarium. The hypothesis was that wrapping would overcome the expansile skull and that the resultant rise in intracranial pressure (ICP) would increase transependymal reabsorption of CSF and might also force open compromised pathways. Certainly very high ICP was obtained and 8 out of 11 babies treated appeared to benefit; when reviewed between 12–24 months of age they showed normal development and had not required other treatment for hydrocephalus. Meyer *et al.*[18] were less successful, finding the procedure ill-tolerated. Porter[19] reported a single success. Despite the initial enthusiasms of Epstein *et al.*[16,17] and Porter[19] larger series never materialized and the procedure has again been relegated to history.

Drug treatment

An ideal pharmacological treatment for hydrocephalus would be one that reduced the imbalance of CSF secretion over absorption, allowing ventricular pressure and size to stabilize without producing unacceptable side effects. Sadly such a perfect agent does not exist, but a number of drugs have been found useful in the management of selected cases, especially in infancy.

Isosorbide is a derivative of mannitol; it is osmotically active and probably works by creating an osmotic gradient between serum and ventricular CSF[20] thus removing intracerebral fluid and possibly reducing CSF formation.[21–23] Concerned by very high rates of complications following ventricular shunting procedures Lorber[24] introduced isosorbide as a possible drug treatment for neonatal and infantile hydrocephalus. The dose was 2 g/kg bodyweight 6-hourly, increasing to 3 g/kg 6-hourly for maintenance. Treatment was continued for up to 18 months. The major complications, occurring in about a quarter of those babies treated, were diarrhoea, vomiting, and hypernatraemia. In a series of 101 children a shunt was avoided in 36 cases and a worthwhile delay in shunting was achieved in a further 39 cases. Babies with congenital hydrocephalus, especially associated with myelomeningocele, more frequently benefited than those with post-haemorrhagic or post-meningitic hydrocephalus.[25] Although overall head size was larger in children who were not shunted there was no apparent intellectual handicap correlating with the macrocephaly. Isosorbide has been used elsewhere with success but has generally fallen out of favour, being supplanted by acetazolamide. Isosorbide has not proved of value in the treatment of hydrocephalus in older children or adults. It has to be acknowledged that enthusiasm for its use waned in proportion to distance from Sheffield, England!

Acetazolamide is a carbonic anhydrase inhibitor which has been shown to reduce CSF production by the choroid plexus by as much as 70 per cent in animals.[26,27] Although ineffective in infants with hydrocephalus in association with myelomeningocele,[28] acetazolamide has found a very definite role in the management of premature infants with post-haemorrhagic hydrocephalus. In a study with admirably strict entry requirements, Shinnar *et al.*[29] demonstrated success in terms of avoiding a ventricular shunt in more than 50 per cent of babies in whom hydrocephalus was not associated with myelomeningocele; in the latter only 26 per cent benefited. An initial dose of 25 mg/kg bodyweight/24 hours, in divided doses two or three times per day, is recommended. The principal complication is metabolic acidosis which can be prevented by the administration of citrate, usually as the potassium salt, using a divided dose of 3–20 mEq/kg bodyweight/day. Of particular value in very small premature babies with post-haemorrhagic hydrocephalus is the ability of acetazolamide to control the condition until the child is a few weeks or months older and, therefore, more resilient, hopefully discharged from the neonatal intensive care unit, and even out of the hospital; such a worthwhile delay in shunt insertion does seem to reduce complications from shunting, especially infection. Finally, acetazolamide can be of value in treating post-operative CSF fistulae, cranial and spinal, both in children and adults, in circumstances such as following repair of lipomyelomeningocele and trans-sphenoidal hypophysectomy. The combination of acetazolamide and serial lumbar punctures is additive. It does also have a role in the treatment of benign intracranial hypertension.

Lumbar puncture

When Quincke[30] introduced lumbar puncture as a treatment for hydrocephalus, he recognized the importance of making a relatively large puncture in the spinal dura and arachnoid so as to encourage leakage of CSF. This technique has currently returned to favour in the management of post-haemorrhagic ventriculomegaly,[31–33] and when combined with acetazolamide it is highly effective in reducing the need for shunt insertion and also for delaying the time before a shunt is needed.[34] Lumbar puncture is also of value in treating disturbances of CSF circulation after intracranial surgery, particularly operations for intracranial aneurysm and procedures in the posterior cranial fossa; with patience and repeated therapeutic lumbar puncture taps withdrawing generous volumes of CSF through large needles (18 gauge), the normal CSF circulation can often be re-established and a shunt avoided. Lumbar puncture taps are also useful in the treatment of post-operative CSF fistulae, especially when combined with acetazolamide, and in the management of benign intracranial hypertension. Lastly, some authors have described an improvement in the clinical condition of patients with normal pressure hydrocephalus after drainage of CSF by lumbar puncture, and felt that such improvement was a good way to predict which patients would benefit from subsequent shunting.[35,36]

SURGICAL TREATMENT

Choroid plexectomy

Attempts to relieve hydrocephalus by destruction of the choroid plexus date back to Lespinasse in 1910 (quoted by Davis in 1936[37]) who used an endoscopic technique to coagulate the choroid plexus. Subsequent surgeons have used either extirpation at open operation[38,39] or endoscopic coagulation,[40] and although each new generation of endoscopes brings a resurgence of minority interest in this approach it has never gained anything more than transient acceptance because of the relatively high morbidity and mortality, and its fundamental ineffectiveness due to extrachoroidal CSF production.[39]

As all forms of hydrocephalus in humans are essentially obstructive in nature, the ideal surgical treatment would be the removal of the obstructing lesion. Clearly there are many cases in which excision of a tumour or cyst from an intraventricular or paraventricular site achieves that ideal. However, for the most part it is a matter of bypassing the obstruction by a drainage procedure. In addition, a number of patients with tumoral hydrocephalus will present in such a severely ill condition that some form of ventricular drainage is urgently required to save life or vision, and to render them fit for definitive excision of the causative lesion.

External ventricular drainage

Following the pioneering manoeuvres of Wernicke,[41] Keen,[42] and Broca[43] external drainage of CSF, either by intermittent ventricular taps via the anterior fontanelle in babies or a surgical burrhole in older children and adults, or by an inserted drainage tube, has been an important method of relieving hydrocephalus. Although such measures are essentially temporary solutions they remain of real value in dire emergencies when life or vision are threatened by severe hydrocephalus. They are also useful when it is felt that hydrocephalus may be a transient phenomenon, as in some cases of intraventricular haemorrhage or infection, and also when the CSF is unsuitable for insertion of an implanted shunt, because of the presence of blood, pus, debris, or very high protein content. The major hazards of repeated ventricular punctures are haemorrhage, infection and, in infants, the development of a focal porencephalic cyst; a late complication is epilepsy. Haemorrhage and infection can mostly be avoided by an immaculate technique. The principal concern with external ventricular catheter drainage is infection; even with the modern closed drainage systems and tunnelled ventricular catheters the risk is significant. Indeed the present writer senses an increased incidence in recent years despite apparently better equipment compared to the not too distant past when, prior to the introduction of CT scanning and MRI, a diagnosis was principally made by ventriculography, and external ventricular drainage was a very frequent event. For this reason many practitioners prefer to insert a definitive internal ventricular shunt even in dire emergencies rather than risk the perils of an infected external drain. The disadvantage with this policy is that one cannot then observe whether the CSF is in fact draining and the patient is also probably committed to a permanent shunt which in itself may have distant complications. The author's policy is, therefore, to employ external ventricular drainage for very sick patients if there is a reasonable prospect of relieving the primary cause of the hydrocephalus within 24–48 hours, and to use an internal shunt if no such prospect exists or if any such attempt cannot follow very promptly. Numerous commercially produced external ventricular drainage kits exist, most of them exorbitantly expensive and indistinguishable in their indifferent qualities. The vital requirements are simplicity with a minimum of connections, stopcocks, measuring devices, and bags; a relatively wide-bore ventricular catheter that is capable of draining blood, pus, and debris, and that can be tunnelled several centimetres away from the site of insertion.[44] If employed, external ventricular drains demand fastidious attention by experienced medical and nursing staff, with a maximum working life of any drain of about 7 days if infection is to be avoided. Daily microbiological examination of the CSF is essential: prophylactic antibodies are not, unless drainage is contemplated for more than 72 hours.[45]

Intracranial shunts

If the subarachnoid space around the brain and in the basal cisterns is patent then it is theoretically possible to employ an intracranial shunt. Only two routes, third ventriculostomy and ventriculocisternostomy, have ever gained much popularity.

Third ventriculostomy

This procedure was introduced by Dandy[46,47] as an open transcranial technique, but it carried a high mortality.[48] Subsequent percutaneous techniques using either an endoscope[49] or a leucotome[50,51] to create a fistula between the third ventricle and the interpeduncular cistern have reduced morbidity and mortality substantially, but these methods have never gained widespread popularity. Suitable cases are relatively scarce and most surgeons have preferred to use extracranial shunts. It is possible that a new generation of fine fibre-optic endoscopes may bring about a resurgence of interest and improved results in an attempt to avoid implanted shunt material, the major advantage of the procedure.

Ventriculocisternostomy

This operation was devised by Torkildsen[52] to treat hydrocephalus resulting from congenital aqueduct stenosis or other obstructions at the level of the posterior third ventricle and midbrain, such as pineal tumours and midbrain gliomas. Operative mortality was not inconsequential (25–40 per cent) and successful initial arrest of hydrocephalus was unpredictable (20–77 per cent).[48] Although now an obsolete technique, it is of some continuing interest as some patients are still alive and in a good condition who were treated in this way and who have eventually come to extracranial shunt insertion many years after the initial Torkildsen operation.

Extracranial shunts

The ingenuity of surgeons in diverting CSF into almost every other body cavity and endothelial lined tube is well documented elsewhere.[11,12,48] The only routes that remain in current use are ventriculoperitoneal (VP), ventriculoatrial (VA), ventriculopleural (VPL), and thecoperitoneal (TP). The modern era of ventricular shunting was ushered in by the invention of valved shunting systems by Nulsen and Spitz[9] working in conjunction with Holter, and by Pudenz *et al.*[53] Interestingly, early reviews of these methods of treatment were not always favourable. Scarff,[48] for example, reported operative mortalities equal to that of the open operation of up to 18 per cent, and an overall rate of late complications of 35–100 per cent, some 10–20-fold greater than that of third ventriculostomy or of endoscopic cauterization of the choroid plexus; he, therefore, strongly advocated a return to the open procedures.

Ventriculoatrial and ventriculoperitoneal shunts

These pioneering valved shunt systems were all used to divert CSF to the intravascular compartment, and for the first two decades of valved devices the VA shunt was the preferred option. However, the serious nature of the complications of this route led to a trend towards the VP shunt which is now firmly established as the standard treatment. Several reports attested to the serious hazards of VA shunts,[54–56] in particular superior and inferior vena cava thrombosis, pulmonary embolism, fatal cor pulmonale, and perforation of the heart.[57] Furthermore, infection of VA shunts carries much more serious consequences than infection of VP shunts, for example chronic bacteraemia, septicaemia, and shunt nephritis.[58] Comparative studies of VA and VP shunts have concluded[59] that the peritoneal route is far preferable, especially for children in whom the need to revise the shunt because of growth of the trunk can be avoided by use of a peritoneal catheter of a suitable length: also the overall rate of late complications is less with VP shunts and their nature is less serious than with VA shunts. It must be concluded that the hazards of the VA shunt no longer justify its use except in the very exceptional circumstance of neither the peritoneal nor the pleural cavities being available.

Whereas there may be universal acceptance of the diversionary route there are very differing opinions as to which hardware to employ to get there. Despite very detailed investigation of the hydrodynamic properties of shunts[60] the choice that a particular surgeon makes from the wide variety of devices commercially available is essentially a personal one. Claims of benefits accruing from the use of very complex, programmable shunts remain to be justified. One-piece systems are free from the risk of disconnection but are necessarily less easy to revise.[61] Price is also a significant factor in making a choice. This author personally favours a multicomponent system with separate ventricular and peritoneal catheters and a ventricular reservoir, accepting its imperfections but learning to live with them. Each surgeon is well advised to find the device that suits him or her and to stick with it, resisting the sales pitch of the manufacturers to change to the latest modifications or the newest model. The anti-siphon valve[62] is a theoretically useful addition, utilizing the influence of atmospheric pressure through the scalp to eliminate any tendency towards a siphoning effect when the head is higher than the peritoneal cavity; by preventing this effect the incidence of shunt dependence with small ventricles in infants and of chronic subdural haematoma in the elderly might hopefully be reduced. Although employed by some surgeons it has failed to achieve universal popularity. All other 'add-ons' are best avoided.

Each surgeon will naturally develop their own personal technique of insertion, some preferring to operate alone, others with an assistant in a simultaneous combined procedure which can reduce operating time to a matter of 20 minutes or so. What matters is attention to detail and a rapid unencumbered technique. Preoperative inspection of the skin is crucial, especially in babies and in the elderly; any napkin rash or other sore must be eliminated and any infective lesion dealt with, especially perineal candidiasis. Babies in the neonatal intensive care unit must have the operative sites liberated from stick-on monitoring devices several days before surgery so as to permit the skin to recover. Scalp vein needles must be prohibited. Any source of infection, such as chest or urinary tract must be purged. Preoperative cleaning of the skin with antiseptic baths may be helpful. During the operation an uninterrupted passage for the patient through a closed operating room with prohibition of unnecessary staff movement is advisable. Isolation of the operative site with adhesive drapes is useful and obviously minimal handling of the implanted device is essential. The avoidance of intermediate skin incisions by employing a catheter passer of suitable length is important, not least cosmetically.

The site of ventricular catheter insertion is crucial. Interestingly for many years the posterior temporal region was chosen; perhaps a legacy from Broca[43] who claimed it to be the best place for ventricular puncture. This site has nothing to recommend it: it is not the easiest route for obtaining a good position of the ventricular catheter; it traverses eloquent brain; it leaves the shunt, sandwiched between the bony prominence and the rather poor skin of the mastoid region, a sure candidate for erosion. The best sites are either frontal or on the lambdoid suture. The former has the advantage of easy placement in the frontal horn and the latter the possibility in infants of opening an already diastased suture. However, frontal shunts may have a significantly higher risk of producing epilepsy.[63] Precise placement of the ventricular catheter is crucial as a poor position is the commonest cause of early shunt failure. Flanged catheters carry no proven advantage. The peritoneal catheter should be long enough to be placed well within the peritoneal cavity, and in infants and children it should be of a length to entertain the child's future growth into adult height: there is little logic in placing short catheters in children, condemning them to certain revision at a later age. The modern silastic catheters are virtually free of any risk of erosion or perforation of the viscera. Wounds should be closed meticulously in layers using absorbable suture materials. Postoperatively, babies, especially premature ones, must not be allowed to lie for long periods on the ventricular reservoir because of the danger of decubitus ulceration. Some surgeons select 'mini' systems for their premature babies for this reason, but the author has found them to be unnecessary as long as a generous craniectomy is made at the lambdoid suture and a slightly larger scalp flap is employed to eliminate any tension on the skin, and if the nurses and parents are suitably instructed to prevent decubitus.

Complications

The complications of ventricular shunts are truly legion and include blockage, infection, disconnection and fracture of components, ulceration of overlying skin, erosion and perforation of abdominal and pelvic viscera, subdural effusions, intraperitoneal cyst formation, slit-ventricle syndrome, secondary craniosynostosis, tumour metastasis, epilepsy, and more. The most commonly encountered, frequently misunderstood and therefore mismanaged complications, will be dealt with here in relationship to VP shunts.

Shunt blockage   With VP shunts the problem is principally one of obstruction of the ventricular catheter; early postoperative blockage is usually due to poor placement or occasionally to intraventricular bleeding if ventricular cannulation has been difficult or clumsy. Later the catheter may be obstructed by the choroid plexus or may embed in the ventricular wall or become plugged with ependymal tissue; placement of the tip of the ventricular catheter anterior to the Foramen of Monro reduces the incidence of plugging from choroid plexus but increases blockage by ependyma.[64] Sterile shunt blockage may be associated with the finding of inflammatory cells within shunts employing proximally placed valves,[65] although it is unclear whether this is cause or effect. Early blockage of the peritoneal catheter is invariably due to malpositioning in an extraperitoneal site; this can be avoided by careful surgical technique and by the use of a long peritoneal catheter which is virtually impossible to place outside the peritoneal cavity. Late blockage of the peritoneal catheter may be due to growth if a short catheter has been inserted early in childhood or to the formation of a loculated intraperitoneal CSF collection.[66] It is very important to recall that intraperitoneal CSF loculation is most frequently due to shunt colonization.[67] This can be detected by simple imaging: the tip of a peritoneal catheter is usually freely mobile within the abdominal cavity and if it appears constantly in one place on serial plain radiography then US examination of the region should be performed to seek a loculus of CSF around the tip; if such is found then shunt colonization should be strongly suspected.

The patient with a blocked VP shunt will usually present with a recurrence of symptoms of raised ICP; some patients will however develop other symptoms, such as deteriorating mental state, eye movement disorder, or gait disturbance. Loss of upgaze is a very useful sign, more so than papilloedema, and it is wise to keep a written record of the completeness, or otherwise, of upgaze in health, for future reference. Some patients with myelomeningocele will develop clinical features relating to their Chiari malformation at times of shunt obstruction, such as neck and upper limb girdle pain. Chronic shunt malformation in patients with myelomeningocele may manifest itself as frank hydromyelia with deteriorating limb function or disproportionate spinal deformity. The occasional patient will develop a unique pattern of disturbance and it is wise to take the experience of the patient and his or her family into consideration in this regard; for example one of the author's patients develops very small pupils when shunt malfunction is brewing. Epileptic seizures are, on the other hand, virtually never due to shunt blockage; a clear distinction does, however, need to be made between epileptic fits and the hydrocephalic attacks of severely raised ICP; many physicians have never encountered the latter and will mistake them for epilepsy, with a potentially disastrous outcome, especially if diazepam is foolishly given thereby precipitating respiratory depression.[68] The rate at which deterioration may take place is very variable, ranging from many months to a few hours; fortunately few patients decline at an alarmingly rapid pace but they are also notoriously unpredictable, so those caring for patients with shunted hydrocephalus must never be complacent or tardy in attendance or in seeking neurosurgical advice. Certain patients, especially those with aqueductal stenosis, seem to be particularly brittle. Mismanagement of blocked shunts features large in medicolegal practice. If shunt malfunction is diagnosed clinically then plain radiographs of the skull, chest, and abdomen are required to identify any malposition or disconnection of the shunt components. According to age, US or CT scanning is needed to show ventricular size and to exclude other possibilities, such as subdural effusions, loculated ventricles, or progression of any primary disease either suspected previously or occult. Indeed when confronted with a patient with recurrent symptoms and suspected shunt malfunction it is a useful discipline to briefly review the supposed aetiology of the original hydrocephalus and to consider critically whether the symptoms are indeed those of shunt malfunction or whether they represent recurrence of the primary disease or progression of a hitherto unsuspected condition, in particular tumour. It should be emphasized that the radiological examination does not make the diagnosis of shunt malfunction; this is principally and almost exclusively a clinical diagnosis regardless of ventricular size. Some radiological features may, however, be helpful: sutural diastasis on plain radiographs clearly indicates the presence of raised ICP, and the finding of a ventricular catheter in a poor position or of a peritoneal catheter in an extraperitoneal location will raise suspicions. On US and on CT the shunted lateral ventricle is often smaller than its fellow if the shunt is functioning. CSF may extravasate along the track of a blocked ventricular catheter producing a focal interstitial CSF oedema on CT. Obliteration of the perimesencephalic cistern on CT correlates with a very real danger of sudden and life-threatening deterioration.[69] The best quality real-time US will now display changes in cerebral vascular resistance in the presence of raised ICP, and may even demonstrate CSF flow from catheter tips. Digital compression of the shunt cannot be relied upon as a test of patency.[70] Various techniques for testing shunt patency have been devised, these include the injection of radio-opaque contrast medium,[71] or radioisotopes,[72,73] and the use of thermistors to detect CSF flow in the shunt:[74] the present author has not found the need to resort to these methods. Exceptionally it has proved necessary to measure ICP either transiently, by needle puncture of the reservoir, or over a longer period, by a subarachnoid screw inserted at a safe distance from the shunt: this can usefully be coupled with simultaneous electroencephalography when looking for evidence of seizure activity or raised ICP (Henderson and Punt. 1992, unpublished data). Neurosurgeons, especially those specializing in paediatrics, should be aware of the tendency to attribute all symptoms in shunted patients to a complication of the shunt and they should remember to review the whole patient for alternative diagnoses. At special hazard are children unfortunate enough to be admitted to adult services. Some children with shunted hydrocephalus will regularly become quite drowsy and lethargic with upper respiratory and middle ear infections. This may represent a measure of marginal shunt malfunction brought to light by altered CSF dynamics due to the infection or associated fever. Occasionally such children will develop frank shunt malfunction shortly after a well-documented and undisputed infection of this type.

Disconnection of shunt components   This is a risk inherent to multi-piece systems, it may occur spontaneously or after local trauma and usually affects the peritoneal catheter. It is more likely to occur if both ends of the peritoneal catheter are anchored at the time of insertion. Frequently it is due to fracture of the peritoneal catheter just distal to the connector on the outlet of the reservoir or proximal valve. Presentation is usually with features of raised ICP but may be preceded by discomfort over the course of the peritoneal catheter. CSF may extravasate along the path of the disconnected catheter giving the impression on palpation that the peritoneal catheter is still present even after it has distracted and migrated into the peritoneal cavity. The diagnosis is confirmed radiologically, and operation should proceed without delay as the catheter may migrate over a few hours and then be difficult to retrieve short of laparotomy. Occasionally a ventricular catheter may disconnect or fracture through the inlet to the shunt and then there is a particular hazard of losing the ventricular catheter at the time of revision. The fractured catheter may be identified on CT by a break in continuity highlighted by an intracerebral collection of CSF just below the cortical surfaces.

Migration of shunt tubing   Such migration is principally a complication of disconnection or fracture, but certain older types of one-piece system are notorious for migrating into the peritoneal cavity or even cranially into the ventricle despite the use of anchoring devices.

Infection   This is the single most serious complication of VP shunts; serious because of the need for lengthy in-patient treatment and because of the potentially deleterious effects on cerebral function. In children shunt infection correlates with poor intellectual development, even in the absence of ventriculitis.[75] Infection rates in the order of 7–10 per cent are the sorry norm[76] and anything under 5 per cent is deemed excellent, only usually being attained by specialist paediatric neurosurgeons.[77] Age is an important aetiological factor;

under six months old carrying a 2.5-toldrisk compared to over one year of age,[76] premature babies being at particular hazard. The elderly are also more susceptible.[78] Other factors include poor skin condition; intercurrent infections at other sites in the body and post-operative wound breakdown. Reinsertions following treatment for shunt infection are twice as likely to become infected as primary procedures. Revisions are least likely to become infected, but within that context ventricular catheters are at a 3-fold risk over distal catheters.[76] The experience and technique of the individual surgeon may carry a 25-fold variance in infection rate[79] and emergency procedures are more often followed by infection than elective operations. The source of the infection may be the operating room environment, including personnel, but in the majority of cases it is from the patient's own skin.[80] Up to 90 per cent of infections are with staphylococci, *Staphylococcus epidermidis* being much commoner than *Staphylococcus aureus*. Occasional infections with diphtheroids and Gram-negative bacilli are encountered.[81] Rarely, infection of the shunt with *Haemophilus influenzae*, *Streptococcus pneumoniae*, or *Neisseria meningitidis* may follow on from an incidental primary meningitis in a shunted patient. Occasionally the soft tissues around the shunt track may become acutely inflamed in the early post-operative period giving rise to a rapidly spreading erythema. This is invariably due to streptococcus infection and the shunt must be removed very rapidly to prevent disastrous intracranial infection: bruising around the shunt track is acceptable, erythema spells infection. The majority of infected VP shunts present within one month of insertion.[79] The commonest presentation is with symptoms of shunt malfunction, but faced with this the surgeon must always consider the possibility of infection, especially if the shunt is well positioned, and in the light of any known risk factors such as prematurity or old age. Systemic symptoms of infection are relatively unusual with VP shunts and blood cultures are typically negative, except very occasionally in premature babies. A more chronic presentation is of recurrent transient niggling abdominal pains with slight fever; such episodes, suggestive of chronic colonization of the shunt, may continue for many years. Indeed it must be remembered that a VP shunt may remain colonized for very long periods of time and the possibility of any blocked shunt being infected must be borne in mind; clues may lie in the circumstances of the original procedure or in events such as early revision operations and wound dehiscence. The presence of an encysted peritoneal CSF collection usually indicates colonization, as does repeated unexplained shunt failures. It is often not appreciated that in up to 50 per cent of colonized shunts microorganisms cannot be cultured from CSF aspirated from the shunt and that the diagnosis will only be made on examination of removed hardware: it follows that components changed at operation must always be examined microbiologically as well as CSF. Examination of CSF obtained at lumbar puncture is pointless and occasionally dangerous, but is still occasionally pursued by uninitiated physicians. Treatment is traditionally by shunt removal, with or without interval drainage, followed by appropriate antibiotics and then re-insertion through fresh incisions. Accurate microbiological diagnosis is essential, and the wise surgeon works closely with the microbiologist in selecting the appropriate antibacterial chemotherapy and in deciding the route and duration of therapy. More than one agent is usually chosen, especially if staphylococcus is the target. In the case of functioning, but colonized, shunts it is occasionally possible to treat with antibiotics alone as long as the appropriate agents are given in high doses by intravenous and intrashunt injections and bactericidal levels achieved in the CSF.[82,83] However, this treatment is prolonged and most have found the 50 per cent failure rate unacceptable.[84] This medical treatment will only work if the shunt is fully functional and if there are no stray shunt components. It has a value in the occasional patient in whom further surgery would be particularly unwelcome: for example the patient with a malignant brain tumour awaiting radiation therapy. Prevention of shunt infection is clearly the ideal to be worked towards. Some have found prophylactic antibiotics useful[85] but there has been no universal acceptance of their employment; careful skin preparation is very important[86] and the use of a surgical isolator may contribute.[87] By far the most important consideration is an immaculate operative technique.

Abdominal complications   Although the catalogue of recorded catastrophes is horrendous when assembled,[88] intra-abdominal and pelvic complications of VP shunts are, in reality, unusual with modern silastic catheters. Events reported include perforation of the abdominal wall, intra-abdominal viscera, and the vagina; volvulus, intussusception, and torsion; sterile and infected CSF cysts; umbilical CSF fistula; inguinal hernia and hydrocele. The latter are particularly common in premature babies because of the patent processus vaginalis.

Subdural haematoma (SDH)   Subdural haematoma is a particularly tiresome complication of any shunting procedure, be it VA, VP, or TP. It is especially likely to occur in patients with very large heads and relatively chronic hydrocephalus, in whom the cerebral mantle cannot reconstitute sufficiently to obliterate the space remaining when the ventricular CSF is drained out. SDH is usually bilateral and may remain asymptomatic. Alternatively, they may produce recrudescence of symptoms of raised ICP; deterioration in mental function; disturbance of eye movement; or return of focal neurological signs relating to the site of the primary pathology, for example ataxia after removal of a cerebellar tumour. The groups most at risk are macrocephalic infants and those adults with normal-pressure hydrocephalus. In the latter, the incidence reaches 20 per cent or more.[89] Anti-siphon devices do not apparently reduce the risk of SDH,[90] neither do high-pressure shunt systems.[91] If asymptomatic then no intervention is required beyond careful observation. Often simple burr-hole drainage will suffice, but in refractory cases ligation of the shunt or upgrading of its pressure rating may be needed; the latter procedure is usually promptly followed by a recurrence of the symptoms of raised ICP. In some patients, including most children, a subdural–peritoneal or subdural–pleural shunt is needed. A particular diagnostic difficulty arises in elderly patients with alleged normal-pressure hydrocephalus who fail to improve following shunting and who are found to have SDH on CT or MRI; it may be impossible to decide whether they have not improved because of the SDH or because they were fundamentally incapable of improvement. A variant of post-shunting SDH is seen as a particular complication in children who have undergone craniotomy to relieve the primary pathology in the presence of a previously placed VP shunt, especially if chronic intracranial hypertension has produced macrocephaly; these children develop chronic subdural CSF effusions, quite different in character to SDH. Subdural–pleural or subdural–peritoneal shunting is the correct line of management. It is ironic that the most unpredictable and unrewarding group of patients, namely the elderly demented with dubious normal-pressure hydrocephalus, are those most prone to develop SDH and this complication adds significantly to the 33–51 per cent morbidity.[10]

Slit-ventricle syndrome   This arises as a medium-term to late complication of ventricular shunting which principally afflicts those shunted from early childhood. The pathology is not straightforward; although simple mechanical 'overdrainage' of the ventricles is the seductively simple answer.[92] However, this does not explain why only 5 per cent of children develop the condition, neither does it elucidate why some patients may have very small ventricles while the shunt is working and yet effortlessly develop ventriculomegaly when the shunt blocks, while apparently identical peers do not. Other factors clearly operate to prevent the ventricles dilating and they presumably relate to changes in the ventricular walls and periventricular tissues. It may be of considerable relevance that premature babies suffering post-haemorrhagic hydrocephalus seem particularly susceptible. These patients are very liable to repeat shunt malfunction due to obstruction of the ventricular catheter and at such times are likely to deteriorate very rapidly, a particularly hazardous circumstance since shunt revision may be very difficult, not least because of the rigid ventricular wall which may deflect the new ventricular catheter. A further trap for the uninitiated is that as the ventricles are small the CT may be taken erroneously to represent a functioning shunt. Often these patients suffer repeated episodes of transient shunt malfunction which may go misinterpreted and thus incorrectly treated. Occasionally in very difficult cases, ICP monitoring and electro-encephalography are of value in reaching a diagnosis. (Henderson and Punt — unpublished data) Those patients who present with acute deterioration require shunt revision urgently, and it may be easier to relocate the ventricular catheter to a frontal (coronal) location for ease of insertion in the small ventricle and to ensure frontal horn placement. For those who display a chronic, recurrent clinical picture, subtemporal decompression is the ideal treatment.[93,94] Not only is it a safe extracerebral procedure but it avoids any influence that overdrainage may have in aggravating the condition. In addition, the decompression is a useful practical guide to the interpretation of symptoms in the future, extremely helpful in the mentally handicapped, the polysymptomatic, the difficult adolescent, and also in managing patients at a geographical distance from their neurosurgeon. It can be repeated if necessary. The author's preference is to perform a wide decompression beneath temporalis on the same side as the ventricular catheter and to open the dura widely in cruciate fashion, closing the wound carefully in layers over a sheet of gelfoam. Interestingly, parents of children undergoing the procedure frequently comment on a general improvement in intellect, temperament, and behaviour; an observation made so often that it is hard to attribute it purely to a placebo effect. (Punt — unpublished data) Another useful application is in patients with infected shunts in whom the ventricles are small and who might be expected to have slit-ventricle syndrome; when the infected shunt is removed, a decompression is fashioned on the same side as the next shunt will be inserted.

Trapped ventricle   This term is used to describe isolated dilatation of a single ventricle, either a lateral or the fourth being affected. It typically occurs in circumstances predisposing towards ependymal scarring, such as post-haemorrhagic hydrocephalus;[95] neonatal meningitis, especially when there has been ventriculitis;[96] after intraventricular surgery, including frequent shunt revisions, notably for infection. It may also complicate hydrocephalus in association with myelomeningocele.[97] Symptoms include recurrence of raised ICP and focal neurological signs; when the fourth ventricle is involved a brainstem syndrome may result. Failure to appreciate the significance of the disproportionate ventriculomegaly may result in respiratory arrest. Treatment is usually by insertion of a shunt system from the dilated cavity to the peritoneal cavity. It is preferable to place an entirely separate device rather than to succumb to the temptation to create a shunt into the original system, such conjoined shunts give endless trouble in the author's experience, not least in assessing which limb is not working at times of malfunction.

Epilepsy   Epilepsy in patients with ventricular shunts is variously reported as occurring in 18 per cent[98] and in 48 per cent of cases,[99] although the only really substantial series[63] found a more reassuring figure of 9.4 per cent. Factors associated with the development of epilepsy include, under one year of age at the time of initial shunt insertion, frontal location of the ventricular catheter and multiple revisions of the ventricular catheter. The risk falls substantially with time, from 5 per cent in the first post-operative year to 1 per cent by the third. The pathology of the hydrocephalus must also be a significant factor, with conditions that produce cortical damage such as neonatal meningitis, head injury, and supratentorial surgery being of relevance. The substantially higher incidence with frontally placed shunts might provide justification for relocating the shunt if epilepsy were a major problem for an individual patient, or even removing it if it were not needed at all.

Tumour metastases   Tumour metastases via ventricular shunts was first described in cases of cerebral glioblastoma producing extraneural metastases in pleura, bone, and lymph nodes.[100,101] Medulloblastoma spreading widely via a ventriculovenous shunt was also recognized,[102] but was not thought to be a major hazard until Hoffman *et al.*[103] described 4 children out of 41 receiving routine preoperative VP shunts: in each case the presentation was with abdominal mass, ascites or abdominal pain, and widespread metastases were identified in bone marrow, skeleton, liver, and spleen, even though there was no evidence of residual or recurrent central nervous system disease. The outcome was uniformly fatal within 1–13 months despite chemotherapy. The insertion of a 3 μm porosity Millipore filter* along the shunt was advocated. Subsequent studies have failed to confirm any overall increase in the risk of systemic spread of medulloblastoma in children with shunts for other reasons. In any event it seems prudent to avoid shunts in patients with CNS malignancy if at all possible.

Shunt-independence   Although it is an unquestionable observation that some patients become independent of their shunt, it must be emphasized that there is no accurate or reliable test of this state of affairs, although various tests have been proposed from time to time.[104] It is a major error to assume that a particular patient no longer requires a CSF diversion because he or she has not undergone any shunt surgery for many years. Unfortunately it remains a widely held belief, especially among paediatricians, and occasionally with disastrous consequences.

Ventriculopleural shunts

This route, first described by Heile[105] and later developed by Ransohoff *et al.*,[106] has never achieved great popularity because of the tendency for the pleural cavity to lose its absorptive capacity, with the consequent formation of a frank and symptomatic pleural effusion. It is also unsuitable for use in the first 18 months of life for the same reason. Nevertheless, it is almost certainly under-rated and is a useful bypass if the peritoneal cavity is not available. The author would always prefer it to a VA shunt because of the very dangerous potential of the latter. It is of particular value in older patients with severe myelo-meningocele if deformity of the thoracic spine makes a free pass of the peritoneal catheter difficult. It has proved valuable in some older myelo-meningocele victims with abdominal wall stomas and urinary diversions. It may have advantages in patients with hydromyelia associated with hydrocephalus. It is a straightforward procedure with few complications and deserves wider use.

---

* Made by Holter Division of Extracorporeal Medical Specialties Inc. Royal and Ross Roads, King of Prussia, Pennsylvania 19406, USA

Thecoperitoneal shunts

Ferguson[107] was the first to devise a method of diverting CSF from the lumbar subarachnoid space to the peritoneal cavity, but his three patients did badly as did other early pioneering attempts. Shunts using polyethylene tubing were then introduced but were found to carry a very high incidence of subsequent arachnoiditis with spinal deformity and even major neurological deficit.[108] The later development of silastic shunts brought a resurgence of interest in the operation. Two types of shunt exist: either a simple silastic tube with distal slit valve introduced via a modified Tuohy needle[109] or a silastic T-tube, the crossbar of which is inserted into the lumbar subarachnoid space via an open interlaminar approach.[108] The latter has the advantage of being free of the major hazard of the former, namely migration, but is a more major procedure. Both types are obviously only of value in cases of communicating hydrocephalus. Although the TP shunt has not gained wide acceptance for use in infants and children, it is frequently of value in treating normal-pressure hydrocephalus, post-surgical and post-subarachnoid haemorrhage hydrocephalus. It is also of value in treating severe benign intracranial hypertension and CSF fistulae. Some have found a very low morbidity in treating normal-pressure hydrocephalus by this shunt.[110] Formation of subdural haematomas remains a risk, especially in the elderly. Slit-ventricle syndrome can develop. Those children with communicating hydrocephalus in association with a skull base anomaly are particularly prone to this complication and to deteriorate very rapidly at times of shunt malfunction because of the tight craniovertebral junction.

CONCLUSIONS

There remain many challenges and unanswered questions in the management of hydrocephalus. For example the 'ideal' ventricular size, if such exists, is yet to be determined as is a method of maintaining it. Shunt complications continue to blight many patients and their families, although by concentrating on technique many can be eliminated. The correct management of the hydrocephalic fetus is yet to be agreed upon; early forays into intrauterine ventricular drainage have not yielded many happy outcomes. Although not always perceived as the most glamorous end of the neurosurgical spectrum, the management of patients with hydrocephalus is eminently worthy of attention which will increasingly come from specialist neurosurgeons in order to maximize the potential for a good outcome.

REFERENCES

1. Vesalius, A. Opera omnia anatomica et chirurgica. *J du Vivie and J and H Verbeek, Batavorum*, Vol. 1, p. 572 and Vol. 2, pp. 577–1156 (1725).
2. Morgagni, J.B. *The seats and causes of diseases investigated by anatomy: in five books, containing a great variety of dissections, with remarks,*.Vol. 1, pp. xxxii &

868. (trans. by Alexander, B. Published by Millar, A. and Cadell, T., Johnson and Payne, London, (1769).

3. Whytt, R. Observations on the most frequent species of the hydrocephalus internus viz. The dropsy of the ventricles of the brain. In *The works of Robert Whytt, MD*, pp. 1X and 762. J. Balfour, Edinburgh (1768).

4. Magendie, F. *Recherches philosophiques et cliniques sur le liquide cephalo–rachidien ou cerebro–spinal*, pp. 40. Mequignon–Narvis, Paris (1842).

5. Luschka, H. *Die Struktur der serosen Häute des Menschen*. vi and pp. 98. Laupp and Siebeck, Tübingen. (1851).

6. Key, A. and Retzius, G. *Studier: nervsystemets anatomi*, pp. 68. P.A. Nerstedt & Sence, Stockholm (1872).

7. Dandy, W.E. and Blackfan, K.D. An experimental and clinical study of internal hydrocephalus. *Journal of the American Medical Association*, **61**, 2216–2217 (1913).

8. Russell, D.S. Observations on the pathology of hydrocephalus. *MRC Special Report Series No. 265*, pp. vi and 138. HMSO, London (1943)

9. Nulsen, F.E. and Spitz, E.B. Treatment of hydrocephalus by direct shunt from ventricle to jugular vein. *Surgical Forum*, **2**, 399–403 (1952).

10. Pickard, J.D. Normal pressure hydrocephalus – to shunt or not to shunt? In *Dilemmas in the management of the neurological patient*, (ed. Warlow, C, and Garfield, J.), pp. 207–14. Churchill Livingstone, Edinburgh (1984).

11. Fisher, R.G. Surgery of the Congenital Anomalies. In *A history of neurological surgery*, (ed. Walker, A.E.), pp. 334–47. Baillire, Tindall and Cox, London. (1951).

12. Pudenz, R.H. The surgical treatment of hydrocephalus — an historical review. *Surgical Neurology*, **15**, 15–26 (1980).

13. Blane, G. On the effect of mechanical compression of the head, as a preventive and cure in certain cases of hydrocephalus. *London Medical and Physical Journal*, **46**, 353–6 (1821).

14. Girdlestone, T. and Costerton, C. On the benefit arising from pressure applied to the head, in certain cases of hydrocephalus. *London Medical and Physical Journal*, **47**, 183 (1822).

15. Barnard, J.F. Case of hydrocephalus chronicus (chronic water of the brain) in which pressure proved most beneficial. *Lancet*, **i**, 360 (1823).

16. Epstein, F., Hochwald, G.M. and Ransohoff, J. Neonatal hydrocephalus treated by compressive head wrapping. *Lancet*, **i**, 634–636 (1973).

17. Epstein, F., Wald, A. and Hechwald, G.M. Intracranial pressure during compressive head wrapping in treatment of neonatal hydrocephalus. *Pediatrics* **54**, 786–90 (1974).

18. Meyer, H., Price, B.E. and Reubel, C.D. Complications arising from head wrapping for the treatment of hydrocephalus. *Pediatrics*, **52**, 867–72 (1973).

19. Porter, F.N. Hydrocephalus treated by compressive head wrapping. *Archives of Diseases of Childhood*, **50**, 816–18 (1975).

20. Hayden, P.W., Foltz, E.L. and Shurtleff, D.B. Effect of an oral osmotic agent on ventricular fluid pressure of hydrocephalic children. *Pediatrics*, 41, 955–67 (1968).

21. Heisey, S.R., Held, D. and Pappenheimer, J.R. Bulk flow and diffusion in the cerebrospinal fluid system of the goat. *American Journal of Physiology*, **203**, 775–81 (1962).

22. MacNab, G.H. The development of the knowledge and treatment of hydrocephalus. *Developmental Medicine and Child Neurology*, 7 (Suppl. 11), 1–9 (1965).

23. Wealthall, S.R., Hudson, J. and Sherriff, S. The effects of position, state of consciousness and drugs on cerebrospinal fluid absorption, estimated by I^{125} Hipparan resorption. *Developmental Medicine and Child Neurology*, **14**, (Suppl. 27), 140–145 (1972).

24. Lorber, J. Isosorbide in the treatment of infantile hydrocephalus. *Archives of Disease in Childhood*, **50**, 431–6 (1975).

25. Lorber, J., Salfield, S. and Lonton, T. Isosorbide in the management of infantile hydrocephalus. *Developmental Medicine and Child Neurology*, **25**, 502–11 (1983).

26. Tschirgi, R.D., Frost, R.W. and Taylor, J.L. Inhibition of cerebrospinal fluid formation by a carbonic anhydrase inhibitor, 2-acetylamino-1, 3, 4-thiadiazole-5-sulfonamide (Diamox). *Proceedings of the Society of Experimental Biology and Medicine*, **87**, 373–6 (1954).

27. Oppelt, W.W., Paclak, C.S. and Rall, D.P. Effect of certain drugs on cerebrospinal fluid production in the dog. *American Journal of Physiology*, **206**, 247–50 (1964).

28. Mealey, J. Jr. and Barker, D.T. Failure of oral acetazolamide to avert hydrocephalus in infants with myelomeningocele. *Journal of Pediatrics*, **72**, 257–9 (1968).

29. Shinnar, S., Gammon, K., Bergman, E.W., Epstein, M. and Freeman, J.M. Management of hydrocephalus in infancy: use of acetazolamide and furosemide to avoid cerebrospinal fluid shunts. *Journal of Pediatrics*, **107**, 31–7 (1985).

30. Quincke, H. Die Lumbalpunction des Hydrocephalus. *Berliner Klinische Wochenschrift*, **28**, 929–33 and 965–8 (1891).

31. Goldstein, G.W., Chaplin, E.R., Maitland, J. and Norman, D. Transient hydrocephalus in premature infants: treatment by lumbar punctures. *Lancet*, **i**, 512–14 (1976).

32. Papile, L., Burstein, J., Burstein, R., Koffler, H., Koops, B.L. and Johnson, J.D. Post-hemorrhagic hydrocephalus in low birth weight infants: Treatment by serial lumbar punctures. *Journal of Pediatrics*, **97**, 273–7 (1980).

33. Levene, M.I. and Starte, D.R. A longitudinal study of post-haemorrhagic ventricular dilatation in the newborn. *Archives of Disease in Childhood*, **56**, 905–10 (1981).

34. Kreusser, K.L., Tarby, T.J., Kovnar, E., taylor, D.A., Hill, A. and Volpe, J.J. Serial lumbar punctures for at least temporary amelioration of neonatal post-haemorrhagic hydrocephalus. *Pediatrics*, **75**, 719–24 (1985).

35. Fisher, C.M. Communicating hydrocephalus. *Lancet*, **i**, 37 (1978).

36. Wikkelso, C., Andersson, H., Blomstrand, C. and Lindquist, G. The clinical effect of lumbar puncture in normal pressure hydrocephalus. *Journal of Neurology, Neurosurgery and Psychiatry*, **45**, 64–9 (1982).

37. Davis, L. *Neurological Surgery*, p. 429. Lea and Febiger, Philadelphia (1936).

38. Dandy, W.E. Extirpation of the choroid plexus of the lateral ventricles in communicating hydrocephalus. *Annals of Surgery*, **68**, 5–11 (1918).

39. Milhorat, T. Failure of choroid plexectomy as treatment for hydrocephalus. *Surgery, Gynaecology and Obstetrics*, **139**, 505–8 (1974).

40. Scarff, J.E. The treatment of non-obstructive (communicating) hydrocephalus by endoscopic cauterisation of the choroid plexus. *Journal of Neurosurgery*, **33**, 1–18 (1970).

41. Wernicke, C. *Lehrbuch der Gehirnkrankheiten fur Aerzte und Studirende*, Vol. 3, 253–372 Fischer, Berlin (1881).

42. Keen, W.W. Exploratory trephining and puncture of the brain almost to the lateral ventricle, for intracranial pressure supposed to be due to an abscess in the

temporo–sphenoidal lobe. Temporary improvement; death on the fifth day; autopsy; meningitis with effusion into the ventricles, with a description of a proposed operation to tap and drain the ventricles as a definite surgical procedure. *Medical News*, **53**, 603–9 (1888).

43. Broca, A. Drainage des ventricules cerebraux pour hydrocephalic. *Revue de chirugie, Paris*, **11**, 37–52 (1891).

44. Friedman, W.A. and Vries, J.K. Percutaneous tunnel ventriculostomy. Summary of 100 procedures. *Journal of Neurosurgery*, **53**, 662–5 (1980).

45. Wyler, A.R. and Kelly, W. Use of antibiotics with external ventriculostomies. *Journal of Neurosurgery*, **37**, 185–7 (1972).

46. Dandy, W.E. The diagnosis and treatment of hydrocephalus due to occlusions of the foramina of Magendie and Luschka. *Surgery, Gynaecology and Obstetrics*, **32**, 112–24 (1921).

47. Dandy, W.E. An operative procedure for hydrocephalus. *Bulletin of Johns Hopkins Hospital*, **33**, 189–90 (1922).

48. Scarff, J.E. The treatment of hydrocephalus. A historical and critical review of methods and results. *Journal of Neurology, Neurosurgery and Psychiatry*, **26**, 1–26 (1963).

49. Sayers, M.P. and Kosnik, J. Percutaneous third ventriculostomy, experience and technique. *Child's Brain*, **2**, 24–30 (1976).

50. Hoffman, H.J. The advantages of percutaneous third ventriculostomy over other forms of surgical treatment for infantile obstructive hydrocephalus. In *Current controversies in neurosurgery*, (ed. Morley, T.), pp. 691–703. W.B. Saunders, Philadelphia (1974).

51. Hoffman, H.J., Harwood-Nash, D., Gilday, D.L. and Craven, M.A. Percutaneous third ventriculostomy in the management of non-communicating hydrocephalus. In *Concepts in pediatric neurosurgery*, Vol. 1 pp. 87–106. (American Society of Paediatric Neurosurgery), Karger, Basel (1981).

52. Torkildsen, A. A new palliative operation in cases of inoperable occlusion of the Sylvian aqueduct. *Acta Chirugica Scandinavica*, **82**, 117–24 (1939).

53. Pudenz, R.H., Russell, F.E., Hurd, A.H. and Sheldon, C.H. Ventriculo–auriculostomy. A technique for shunting cerebrospinal fluid into the right auricle. Preliminary report. *Journal of Neurosurgery*, **14**, 171–9 (1957).

54. Strenger, L. Complications of ventriculo–venous shunts. *Journal of Neurosurgery*, **20**, 219–24 (1963).

55. Nugent, G.R., Lucas, R., Judy, M., Bloor, B.M. and Warden, H. Thrombo-embolic complications of ventriculo–atrial shunts. Angiocardiographic and pathologic correlations. *Journal of Neurosurgery*, **24**, 34–42 (1966).

56. Forrest, D.M. and Cooper, D.G.W. Complications of ventriculo–atrial shunts. A review of 455 cases. *Journal of Neurosurgery*, **29**, 506–12 (1968).

57. Dzenitis, A.J., Mealey, J. Jr and Waddell, J.R. Myocardial perforation by ventricular shunt tubing. *Journal of the American Medical Association*, **194**, 1251–3 (1965).

58. Stauffer, U.G. 'Shunt nephritis': diffuse glomerulonephritis complicating ventriculo–atrial shunts. *Developmental Medicine and Child Neurology*, **12**, (Suppl. 22), 161–4 (1970).

59. Keucher, T.R. and Mealey, J. Jr. Long-term results after ventriculo–atrial and ventriculo–peritoneal shunting for infantile hydrocephalus. *Journal of Neurosurgery*, **50**, 179–86 (1979).

60. Portnoy, H.D. Hydrodynamics of shunts, In *Monographs in neural sciences*, (ed. Cohen, M.M.), Vol. 8, *Shunts and problems in shunts*, (ed. Choux, M.), pp. 179–183. S Karger, Basel (1982).

61. Raimondi, A.J., Robinson, J.S. and Kuwamura, K. Complications of ventriculo–peritoneal shunting and a critical comparison of the three-piece and one-piece systems. *Child's Brain*, **3**, 321–42 (1977).

62. Portnoy, H.D., Schulte, R.R., Fox, J.L., Croissant, P.D. and Tripp, L. Anti-siphon and reversible occlusion valves for shunting in hydrocephalus and preventing post-shunt subdural hematomas. *Journal of Neurosurgery*, **38**, 729–38 (1973).

63. Dan, N.S. and Wade, M.J. The incidence of epilepsy after ventricular shunting procedures. *Journal of Neurosurgery*, **65**, 19–21 (1986).

64. Collins, P., Hockley, A.D. and Woolam, D.H.M. Surface ultrastructure of tissues occluding ventricular catheters. *Journal of Neurosurgery*, **48**, 609–13 (1978).

65. Traynelis, V.C., Willison, C.D., Follett, K.A., Chambers, J., Schochet, S.S. Jr. and Kaufman, H.H. Millipore analysis of valvular fluid in sterile valve malfunctions. Neurosurgery, **28**, 848–52 (1991).

66. Parry, S.W., Schumacher, J.F. and Llewellyn. R.C. Abdominal pseudocysts and ascites formation after ventriculoperitoneal shunt procedures. Journal of Neuro-surgery, **43**, 476–80 (1975).

67. Grosfeld, J.L., Cooney, D.R., Smith, J. and Campbell, R.L. Intra-abdominal com-plications following ventriculo–peritoneal shunt procedures. *Pediatrics*, **514**, 791–6 (1974).

68. Eldridge, P.R, and Punt, J.A.G. Risks associated with giving benzodiazepines to patients with acute neurological inquiries. *British Medical Journal*, **300**, 1189–90 (1990).

69. Johnson, D.L., Fitz, C., McCullough, D.C. and Schwartz, S. Perimesencephalic cistern obliteration: a CT sign of life-threatening shunt failure. *Journal of Neuro-surgery*, **64**, 386–9 (1986).

70. Osaka, K., Yamasaki, S. and Hirayama, A. Correlation of the response of the flushing device to compression with the clinical picture in the evaluation of the functional status of the shunting system. *Child's Brain*, **3**, 25–30 (1977).

71. Evans, R.C., Thomas, M.D. and Williams, L.A. The use of the valvogram for the detection of shunt blockage in hydrocephalic children. *Developmental Medicine and Child Neurology* **17**, (Suppl. 35), 94–8 (1975).

72. Frick, R.M., Rosler, H. and Kinser, J. Functional evaluation of ventriculo–atrial and ventriculo–peritoneal shunts with 99m Tc-pertechnetate. *Neuroradiology*, **7**, 145–52 (1974).

73. Graham, P., Howman-Giles, R., Johnston, I and Besser, M. Evaluation of CSF shunt patency by means of technetium-99m DTPA. *Journal of Neurosurgery*, **57**, 262–6 (1982).

74. Chiba, Y. and Yuda, K. Thermosensitive determination of CSF shunt patency with a pair of small disc thermisters. *Journal of Neurosurgery*, 52, 700–4 (1980).

75. McLone, D., Czyzewski, D. and Raimondi, A.J. The effects of complications on intellectual function in 173 children with myelemeningocele. Cited by Reigel, D.J. Spina Bifida. In *Pediatric Neurosurgery: surgery of the developing nervous system*, pp. 23–47. Section of Pediatric Neurosurgery of the American Association of Neurological Surgeons, Grune and Stratton, New York (1982).

76. Renier, D., Lacombe, J., Pierre-Kahn, A., Sainte-Rose, C. and Hirsh, J-F. Factors causing acute shunt infection. Computer analysis of 1174 operations. *Journal of Neurosurgery*, **61**, 1072–78 (1984).

77. O'Brien, M., Parent, A. and Davis, B. Management of ventricular shunt infection. *Child's Brain*, **5**, 304–9 (1979).

78. Udvarhelyi, G.B., Wood, J.H. and James, A.E. Results and complications in 55 shunted patients with normal pressure hydrocephalus. *Surgical Neurology* **3**, 271–5 (1975).

79. George, R., Leibrock, L. and Epstein, M. Longterm analysis of cerebrospinal fluid shunt infections. A 25 year experience. *Journal of Neurosurgery*, **51**, 804–11 (1979).

80. Bayston, R. and Lar, J. A study of the sources of infection in colonised shunts. *Developmental Medicine and Child Neurology*, **16**, (Suppl. 32), 16–22 (1974).

81. Schoenbaum, S.C., Gardner, P. and Shillito, J. Infections of cerebrospinal fluid shunts: epidemiology, clinical manifestations and therapy. *Journal of Infectious Disease*, **131**, 543–52 (1975).

82. Wald, S.L. and McLaurin, R.L. Cerebrospinal fluid antibiotic levels during treatment of shunt infections. *Journal of Neurosurgery*, **32**, 41–6 (1980).

83. Frame, P.T. and McLaurin, R.L. Antibiotic therapy in central nervous system infections. In *Pediatric neurosurgery: surgery of the developing nervous system*, pp. 591–9. Section of Pediatric Neurosurgery of the American Association of Neurological Surgeons, Grune and Stratton, New York (1982).

84. Forward, K.R., Fewer, D. and Stiver, H.G. Cerebrospinal fluid shunt infections: a review of 35 infections in 32 patients. *Journal of Neurosurgery*, **59**, 389–94 (1983).

85. McCullough, D.C., Kane, J.G., Presper, J.H., and Wells, M. Antibiotic prophylaxis in ventricular shunt surgery. I: Reduction of operative infection rates with methicillin. *Child's Brain*, **7**, 182–9 (1980).

86. Venes, J.L. Control of shunt infection. Report of 150 consecutive cases. *Journal of Neurosurgery*, **45**, 311–14 (1976).

87. Hirsh, J.F., Renier, D., and Pierre-Kahn, A. Influence of the use of a surgical isolator on the rate of infection in the treatment of hydrocephalus. *Child's Brain*, **4**, 137–50 (1978).

88. Davidson, R.I. Peritoneal bypass in the treatment of hydrocephalus: historical review and abdominal complications. *Journal of Neurology, Neurosurgery and Psychiatry*, **39**, 640–6 (1976).

89. Samuelson, S., Long, D.M., and Chou, S.N. Subdural hematoma as a complication of shunting procedures for normal pressure hydrocephalus. *Journal of Neurosurgery*, 37, 548–51 (1972).

90. McCullough, D.C. and Fox, J.L. Negative intracranial pressure hydrocephalus in adults with shunts and its relationship to the production of subdural haematoma. *Journal of Neurosurgery*, **40**, 372–5 (1974).

91. Hughes, C.P., Siegel, B.A., and Coxe, W.S., Gado, M.H., Grubb, R.L., Coleman, R.E., and Berg, L. Adult idiopathic communicating hydrocephalus with and without shunting. *Journal of Neurology, Neurosurgery and Psychiatry*, **41**, 961–71 (1978).

92. Gruber, R., Jenny, P., and Herzog, B. Experiences with the anti-siphon device (ASD) in shunt therapy of pediatric hydrocephalus. *Journal of Neurosurgery*, **61**, 156–62 (1984).

93. Epstein, F.J., Fleischer, A.J., Hochwald, G.M., and Ransohoff, J. Subtemporal craniectomy for recurrent shunt obstruction secondary to small ventricles. *Journal of Neurosurgery*, **41**, 29–31 (1974).

94. Epstein, F., Marlin, A.E., and Wald, A. Chronic headache in the shunt-dependant adolescent with nearly normal ventricular volume: Diagnosis and treatment. *Neurosurgery*, **3**, 351–5 (1978).

95. Eller, T.W. and Pasternak, J.F. Isolated ventricles following intraventricular haemorrhage. *Journal of Neurosurgery*, **62**, 357–62 (1985).

96. Kalsbeck, J.E., DeSouza, A.L., Kleinman, M.B., Goodman, J.M., and Franken, E.A. Compartmentalization of the cerebral ventricles as a sequel of neonatal meningitis. *Journal of Neurosurgery*, **52**, 547–52 (1980).

97. Scotti, G., Musgrave, M.A., Fitz, C.R., and Harwood-Nash, D. The isolated fourth ventricle in children — CT and clinical review of 16 cases. *American Journal of Radiology*, **135**, 1233–8 (1980).

98. Marossero, F., Massarrotti, M., and Migliore, A. Anormalita EEG i idrocefali infantili dopo derivazione ventriculo–atriale. *Rivista di Neurologica*, **40**, 239–41 (1970).

99. Graebner, R.W. and Celesia, G.G. EEG findings in hydrocephalus and their relation to shunting procedures. *Electroencephalography and Clinical Neurophysiology*, **35**, 517–21 (1973).

100. Wolf, A., Cowen, D. and Stewart, W.B. Glioblastoma with extracranial metastasis by way of a ventriculopleural anastomosis. *Transactions of the American Neurological Association*, **79**, 140–2 (1934).

101. Wakamatsu, T., Matsuo, T., Kawano, S., Teramoto, S., and Matsamura, H. Glioblastoma with extracranial metastasis through ventriculopleural shunt. Case Report. *Journal of Neurosurgery*, **34**, 697–701 (1971).

102. Makeever, L.C. and King, J.D. Medulloblastoma with extracranial metastases through a ventriculovenous shunt. Report of a case and review of the literature. *American Journal of Clinical Pathology*, **46**, 245–9 (1966).

103. Hoffman, J.H., Hendrick, E.B., and Humphreys, R.P. Metastasis via ventriculo–peritoneal shunt in patients with medulloblastoma. *Journal of Neurosurgery*, **44**, 562–6 (1976).

104. Howman-Giles, R., McLaughlin, A., Johnston, I., and Whittle, I. A radionuclide method of evaluating shunt function and CSF circulation in hydrocephalus. Technical note. *Journal of Neurosurgery*, **61**, 604–5 (1984).

105. Heile, B. Zur chirurgischen Behandlung des Hydrocephalus internus durch Ableistung der Cerebrospinalflüssigkeit nach der Bauchhole und nach der Pleurakuppe. *Archive für klinike Chirurgie*, **105**, 507–16 (1914).

106. Ransohoff, J., Shulman, K., and Fishman, R. Hydrocephalus. A review of etiology and treatment. *Journal of Pediatrics*, **56**, 399–411 (1960).

107. Ferguson, A.H. Intraperitoneal diversion of the cerebrospinal fluid in cases of hydrocephalus. *New York Medical Journal*, **67**, 902 (1898).

108. Hoffman, J.H., Hendrick, E.B., and Humphreys, R.P. New lumbo–peritoneal shunt for communicating hydrocephalus. Technical note. *Journal of Neurosurgery*, **44**, 258–61 (1976).

109. Spetzler, R., Wilson, C.B., and Schulte, R. Simplified percutaneous lumboperitoneal shunting. *Surgical Neurology*, **7**, 25–9 (1977).

110. Selman, W.R., Spetzler, R.F., Wilson, C.B., and Grollmus, J.W. Percutaneous lumboperitoneal shunt; review of 130 cases. *Neurosurgery*, **6**, 255–7 (1980).

7 Results of treatment in infants and children

E. Bruce Hendrick

INTRODUCTION

The complications and consequences of the treatment of hydrocephalus can be divided into acute events, which may occur at any time during the patient's treatment such as shunt malfunction and infection, and the long-term effects on intellectual function, sexual activity, marriage, and pregnancy, as well as life expectancy.

SHUNT MALFUNCTION

Shunt obstruction

Proximal end

Ventricular catheter obstruction is said to be the most common cause of shunt problems.[1] In my experience, obstruction occurs with equal frequency at either end. Proximal obstruction is most often the result of inappropriate placement within the ventricle. The position of choice would appear to be in the frontal horn or the anterior third of the body of the ventricle, in order to avoid contact with, and subsequent obstruction by, the choroid plexus. This positioning may be achieved through a frontal or posterior occipital burr hole. In the latter insertion site, care must be taken to place the catheter tip anterior to the foramen of Monro. Positioning, however accurate, may be self-defeating. With adequate drainage the ventricular size diminishes and the catheter tip moves into contact with the ventricular ependyma and the plexus. Far too often, particularly in inexperienced hands, the ventricular catheter may be partially or completely inserted through the ventricular wall into cerebral tissue. Much has been made of the need for careful handling of shunt materials before and during placement in order to avoid contamination, but surely this is just a common-sense observation of surgical technique.[2] The removal of obstructed ventricular catheters, particularly those embedded or adherent to the ventricular wall, with or without choroid plexus attachment, is very often a hazardous manoeuvre. Tugging or abrupt withdrawal of the catheter may produce significant intraventricular haemorrhage with associated neurological deficits, and may lead to great difficulty in the establishment of free drainage from the ventricle. Slow withdrawal of the catheter from the point of cortical insertion, so that the adherent choroid plexus may be coagulated and separated, will prevent bleeding in most instances. If the catheter does not withdraw easily, the insertion of a metal catheter stylet into the full length of the plastic catheter and the application of a cutting current to the stylet for three to four seconds will free the catheter from the ventricular ependyma, in most instances. If the catheter, in spite of all efforts, remains adherent, then prudence dictates that the old tube be left in place and a new ventricular catheter be inserted, either parallel to it through the original burr hole or through a new burr hole.

Slit-ventricle syndrome

This term is used to describe a small but troublesome group of shunt-dependent individuals, with chronic or recurrent complaints of shunt obstruction and intermittent episodes of increased intracranial pressure, who show very small or slit ventricles on CT scanning.[3–6] There have been a number of mechanisms suggested as causes of this complicated and troublesome syndrome. These include overdrainage, subependymal periventricular gliosis with decreased intracranial compliance, intermittent ventricular obstruction, and even intracranial hypotension or 'low pressure syndrome'.[7,8] It would appear that there is no one consistent cause of 'slit-ventricle syndrome', and that treatment is successful only when appropriate to the underlying cause. The diagnosis is confirmed when the patient presents with headaches that are chronic, episodic, and recurrent. Minor viral infections, general or nasopharyngeal, may produce headache in a child whose hydrocephalus is marginally controlled. Chronic intracranial hypotension may produce headaches which only occur in the upright posture and relieved by recumbency. The shunt reservoir if present, usually empties rapidly and refills very slowly over a period of two to three minutes, the rate of refilling slowing proportionately to the number of times the pump is depressed. This usually indicates a limited ventricular volume. Papilloedema is unusual unless the symptoms are long standing and there is evidence of some degree of obstruction at either or both ends. The obvious signs of decompensated intracranial pressure, such as a decreasing level of consciousness, hypertension with or without accompanying bradycardia, require immediate treatment. CT scanning is readily performed and is diagnostic if done during the period of symptomatic headache. The ventricles may be minimally enlarged in comparison to previous studies carried out during an asymptomatic period. Radionucleide scanning for determination of shunt function should be carried out to exclude the presence of decreased flow in a partially obstructed system during an asymptomatic interval. Intracranial pressure monitoring is of value only when other methods fail to provide a diagnosis.[9]

Treatment should be kept as simple as possible, with the more complex and hazardous options reserved for circumstances where the less complicated procedures have proven unsatisfactory. Shunt revision, usually involving the ventricular catheter will often be sufficient to correct the problem. However, as one gains experience, it often seems sensible to replace the entire shunt rather than be faced with revision of the peritoneal end within three to four days after the initial procedure. One must decide at the time of complete replacement whether an increase in overall shunt-line resistance and opening pressure is necessary to prevent recurrence of symptoms, particularly in adolescent and adult patients. The placement of an antisyphon device, downstream from the upper end, during replacement of the ventricular catheter has been recommended. Personal experience with antisyphon devices has been disappointing. The devices function for intermittent and unpredictable intervals and have a tendency to become obstructed by debris, which would normally pass through the shunt system. Most devices must be removed or replaced within a period of a few months. One must agree with Wisoff and Epstein[9] that elective upgrading of shunt systems to a higher pressure, with or without an antisyphon device or the insertion of an antisyphon device during upper end revision, does not constitute a 'prudent therapeutic option'. There is nothing to suggest that enlarging the ventricular volume by increasing the latent intracranial pressure serves the patient's best interest, and it raises concerns about the possible deterioration of cognitive function as a result of chronically increased intracranial pressure. Replacement of the ventricular catheter or the complete system appears to be the safest and most reliable primary treatment. It has been noted that a partially obstructed ventricular catheter may fail to compensate for sudden, intermittent, and occasionally prolonged increases in intracranial pressure and may precipitate a sudden episode of clinical obstruction. In such a situation, replacement of the ventricular catheter solves the problem. If catheter or shunt replacement fails to alleviate the patient's symptoms, bony decompression may be the procedure of choice. In my experience, posterior calvariectomy[10] has not been necessary. An adequate subtemporal decompression on the side of the shunted ventricle has produced clinical improvement and adequate shunt function.[11]

Adequate subtemporal decompression means a large (5×6 cm) bony removal through a temporoparietal musculocutaneous flap based inferiorly and a wide dural opening with the dural flap based superiorly, to prevent unsightly bulging during intermittent episodes of increased intracranial pressure with associated ventricular dilatation.

Slit-ventricle syndrome should always be considered as a diagnosis in the shunted patient who presents with a history suggestive of intermittent obstruction, with or without progressive symptoms of increased intracranial pressure. Careful investigation and a logical sequential approach to surgical treatment will eliminate reckless and impulsive surgical intervention, but on the other hand, causes postponement of treatment to the detriment of the patient.

Distal end

In spite of the general impression that obstruction of the distal end of a shunt system as a single entity is rare, it is my impression that lower end obstruction, for whatever reason, occurs almost as frequently as does upper end obstruction. The causes of lower end failure are many, and vary from simple withdrawal with growth of the patient to perforation of a hollow viscus. Withdrawal of the peritoneal catheter with growth is usually the direct result of using an inadequate length of tubing at the time of the initial shunt insertion. Excluding small and premature infants, at least 60–70 cm of peritoneal catheter should be inserted. There is little or no problem with kinking, and adequate catheter length would appear to ensure constant mobility of the system within the peritoneum, preventing the formation of adhesions and local adherence to the omentum and the appendices epiploicae, thus decreasing the incidence of peritoneal loculation and the formation of cerebrospinal fluid pseudocysts.

Problems may arise during insertion of the peritoneal catheter if the neurosurgeon has little experience in abdominal surgery or can be due to the presence of intraperitoneal adhesions resulting from previous surgery or infection. At such times, it is wise to enlist the help of an abdominal surgeon to ensure correct placement of the peritoneal catheter within a free and adequate intraperitoneal space.

Peritoneal catheter shortening may be predicted by periodic X-ray films of the abdomen. Elective lengthening should be undertaken before the catheter tip has withdrawn close to the point of peritoneal insertion. In the young child, with a great deal of further growth to be compensated for, the revision should extend distally from the lower end of the pumping device. In the adolescent, or adult patient, revision may safely be carried out at the point of peritoneal insertion, making sure that the upper end of the original shunt and the new peritoneal end fit completely over the connector, allowing free movement within the fibrous sheath which has developed around the original shunt.

Shunt disconnection

Shunt disconnections may occur as a result of traction between components, usually at the point of connection between the ventricular catheter or pumping device and the distal end. Initially the problem may not be recognized by the patient, patient's family, or family physician, due to the ability of the fibrous sheath surrounding the tubing to maintain adequate flow between the separated ends for surprisingly long periods of time. The development of a soft fluctuant subcutaneous swelling along the course of the shunt, usually beginning at the point of discontinuity, may be the earliest sign. Occasionally, in more active patients, a blow or sudden stretching during rough play or participation in contact sports will produce a separation of the shunt with subsequent swelling and malfunction. Palpation along the subcutaneous length of the tubing will often identify the point of separation. If the shunt material is radiopaque, the discontinuity is readily confirmed by X-ray. Elective revision should be carried out before there is extensive migration of the separated ends and prior to the development of clinical signs of shunt obstruction.

Fibrous sheath effect

In older patients, the fibrous sheath, with associated shunt shortening, will produce a painful and unsightly 'checkrein or bowstring' effect subcutaneously in the posterior triangle of the neck or anterior upper thorax. This requires not only lengthening of the tubing, by insertion of an extension at the site of the disfigurement, but surgical excision of the fibrous sheath for a length of 6–10 cm.

Shunt migration

Shunt migration can occur with separation of the components or as a movement of the whole shunt system into the ventricle or peritoneal cavity. Total intraventricular migration can occur, but intraperitoneal lodgement is more common. Most often, it is the portion of the shunt distal to the pump or the ventricular catheter that migrates. One finds at operation that the lower end of the shunt has slipped off the connector due to inadequate fixation, or has fractured as a result of poor immobilization of the upper end, producing continuous movement of the catheter against the metal or plastic connector. These problems can be avoided by adequate anchoring of the upper components and careful fixation of all areas where the tubing is fastened to the appropriate connectors. The mixing of components from various manufacturers may result in a poor fit of the connecting segments or early material fatigue.

Bowel perforation

Perforation of the bowel during trochar insertion of the intraperitoneal end of the shunt can and does occur, with subsequent contamination of the shunt and peritoneal cavity. The use of a trochar is dangerous and offers no advantage over the insertion of the catheter into the peritoneal cavity under direct vision. With experience, there is little risk in direct transperitoneal insertion and correct placement of the tubing is assured. The abandonment of the use of the wire coil non-kinking catheter has all but eliminated the chance of bowel penetration. However, penetration of a hollow viscus by the modern soft catheter can and does occur. Protrusion of the catheter tip at the anal orifice is an obvious and alarming indication of bowel perforation. Less obvious, is a history of persistent watery stools, in the absence of any other sign of infection or gastroenteritis. Radionuclear studies will readily confirm this latter complication. Occasionally, during revision of the distal end of a ventriculoperitoneal shunt, the lower end of the withdrawn peritoneal catheter will show yellowish discoloration, which should be assumed to indicate that the catheter has been positioned within the bowel lumen for some time. The presence of loculated intraperitoneal pseudocysts, containing infected cerebrospinal fluid, should also suggest bowel penetration. Catheters presenting at the anus should be disconnected at the point of abdominal insertion and the protruding material withdrawn via the anus. Stained catheters and catheters from pseudocysts should be removed and cultured. The patient's intracranial pressure should be controlled by external ventricular drainage. Appropriate systemic and intraventricular antibiotics should be administered before shunt reinsertion, until confirmation of sterile cerebrospinal fluid is obtained. Pseudocysts disappear within 5–10 days after the removal of the abdominal catheter. Ultrasonography is useful in the initial determination of the presence of the pseudocyst and its subsequent reabsorption. There have been very few instances of generalized peritonitis arising from bowel penetration and subsequent catheter removal. This may be due to the very small penetration defect and the ability of the peritoneal cavity to wall off minor areas of contamination.

Subdural haematoma

The development of subdural haematomas in shunted hydrocephalic patients has been much less of a problem since the replacement of the open distal shunt by valve regulated systems. Treatment has been and always will be a frustrating and prolonged problem of drainage of the subdural spaces, while maintaining an intraventricular pressure high enough to re-expand the ventricles without producing further injury or signs of debilitating increases in intracranial pressure. The use of external ventricular drainage, following burr hole drainage of the subdural haematoma, allows for regulation and monitoring of the pressure required. Shunt re-insertion must wait upon the satisfactory resolution of the haematoma.

Iatrogenic synostosis

This clinical complication was most often seen in the grossly hydrocephalic infant who had been treated by the early unregulated shunt systems. It is a rare problem today because of earlier diagnosis and the use of appropriate pressures in the valve systems used. It still occurs, even with the best of clinical treatment. Early craniectomy is not advisable, but craniofacial reconstruction at a later date, if desired, appears to offer the most satisfactory solution.

INFECTION

Shunt infection is the single most controversial problem facing those who would treat hydrocephalus. The mortality from infection has been reported as ranging as high as 30 to 40 per cent.[12,13] Morbidity, in terms of intellectual deterioration and increased neurological deficits, is significant and increases with successive episodes of infection. Secondary problems of shunt obstruction, adhesive peritonitis, and septicaemia with multiple system involvement, take a further toll.[14,15]

Epidemiology

The literature dealing with shunt infections is voluminous and demonstrates significant differences in results. There are so many variables, controlled and uncontrolled, that any comparison of published results reveals inconsistencies and is misleading. Luthardt,[16] in a review of 17 articles, reported an average rate of infection of 13.5 per cent. This may be due to different patient population, age, patient selection, treatment modes, site of infection, the number of operative procedures, operative technique, the organism involved, and the duration of clinical observation. Early reports of post-operative infections produce rates of 10–15 per cent, but in the last 10–12 years the rates appear to have dropped to a range of 2 per cent to 5 per cent.[13,16–22] The reasons for the apparent improvement are not clear, but the increasing tendency toward the concentration of paediatric neurosurgical procedures in specialized units and the resultant consistency of treatment may be two factors. The majority of shunt infections occur within 2 months following surgery, although sporadic cases may occur up to 6 years later.[12,22,23] The method of shunting does not appear to be a major factor in the incidence of infection. The rates of infection for ventriculoperitoneal and ventriculoatrial shunts are not significantly different. Although, one might suspect that initial shunt procedures would have a lower infection rate than shunt revisions this is not so.[21,22,25]

Consistency of surgical treatment, i. e. the same surgeon, the same shunting mechanism, reduction in anaesthetic and operative times, avoidance of soft tissue trauma, meticulous haemostasis, and prophylactic antibiotics, are the most probable reasons for the reduction in shunt infection rates. One would expect higher rates of infection when the surgery is relegated to the resident staff with less experience, hence longer wound and shunt exposure time and less attention to haemostasis and tissue trauma. Several reviews have shown that there is no correlation between operative time, type of procedure, or shunt materials used.[20,21,26] George *et al.*[12] state that a surgeon's experience was the single most important factor in the reduction of infection. Infections following shunt procedures are most likely to occur in the very young or premature infant and in the very old. This is not surprising, as this group of patients are considered to be a high risk for almost any surgical procedure.[12,17,18,27]

Infecting organism

The majority of shunt infections are due to coagulase-negative *Staphylococcus epidermidis*.[28] This would suggest that subcutaneously placed shunts are easily contaminated by organisms from the patient's skin. Bayston and Lari[29] carried out preoperative skin and intraoperative wound cultures in 100 shunt procedures. Wound contamination was present in 58 per cent by the end of surgery, but only 55 per cent of this group showed the organism that had been present on the patient's skin prior to surgery. Shapiro, *et al.*[20] compared cultures from the operative sites in 413 paediatric shunt procedures with cultures taken from 20 subsequent shunt infections occurring in this group. Organisms, identical to those cultured from the skin of the same patient, occurred in only four (20 per cent) instances. It was suggested that the source of many shunt infections may be inoculation from the patient's nasopharynx, the operating room personnel or prior operating room contamination.

Perforation of the intestine, although less common with the use of flexible silastic tubing, is still a significant and potentially devastating source of infection in the shunted hydrocephalic patient.

Fluid flow through the shunt, itself, may produce contamination. Ventriculitis or intraperitoneal infection from a ruptured appendix can result in colonization of the tubing with bacteria, producing obstruction of the lumen or valve by inflammatory debris, by associated ventriculitis, or by omental adhesions. One might argue against retrograde bacterial migration in the shunt and valve systems, but clinically it does appear to occur. It must be assumed that if any part of the shunt system is proven to be infected, then the whole apparatus is involved.

The role of the materials from which the shunt is constructed, acting as a foreign body perpetuating infection, must be taken into consideration.[30] Plastic materials have physical properties which may promote bacterial propagation by making the organisms inaccessible to either the host defences or appropriate bactericidal drugs.[31] In addition, staphylococci have been shown to produce a mucoid substance which allows them to adhere to the shunt components.[32] When failure of the patient's host defence mechanism occurs due to the inability of phagocytes to clear bacteria from the shunt, and is included with the preceding factors, infection occurs.[33]

Clinical presentation of infection

The symptoms and signs of shunt infection vary widely from the overt to the insidious. They may appear as inflammatory changes in surrounding tissues, as a generalized systemic infection, as shunt obstruction, or as any combination of these. Walters et al.,[13] in a review of 267 infections in both peritoneal and cardiac shunts, found obvious meningeal or peritoneal signs in only 2 per cent of each group. Shunt obstruction and soft tissue infection were each seen in 23 per cent, and fever alone, acute or chronic in 18 per cent. Shunt obstruction, alone or with other signs, was most common. Pulmonary and cardiac involvement occurred in 18 per cent, or 8 out of 50, cardiac shunts. Chronic anaemia, failure to thrive, and symptoms of low-grade systemic infection were also presenting factors in a small group. The development of shunt nephritis in the patient with a ventriculocardiac shunt, leading to immune-mediated glomerulonephritis and progressive renal damage can be eliminated by aggressive treatment of the infection and replacement of the cardiac shunt by a peritoneal shunt.[34] Since the signs and symptoms are so often non-specific and treatment, either medical or surgical, carries significant risk, there must be proof of infection in the form of a positive culture. The clinician must be prepared to maintain a constant awareness about the possibility of infection and be willing to secure repeated cultures at the least suspicion, such as fever, persistent or intermittent pain, and tenderness or swelling along the shunt site. Such occurrences, during the immediate post-operative period, leave little doubt as to the diagnosis. However, similar complaints occurring at some time after surgery, require persistent and rigorous investigation. A positive diagnosis of infection may require repeated cultures over a period of 10–14 days to confirm the presence of organisms in an indolent infective process. Ready access to the shunt system for repeated cultures is necessary and certainly justifies the inclusion of some form of reservoir or pumping device in every shunt system. All cultures, whether from an external ventricular drain or from the shunt reservoir, must be carried out under a scrupulous aseptic technique so as to preclude the chance of a false-positive infection report which could lead to a progression of unwarranted surgical and antibiotic interventions. Schoenbaum *et al.*[35] compared the reliability of cultures from different areas in different shunt systems. Positive blood cultures were more frequently found in cardiac shunts (95 per cent) than in peritoneal (20 per cent) shunt infections. Fluid obtained for culture by ventricular or lumbar puncture, was a very poor source of positive culture (7–26 per cent). However, in all system types, culture of the cerebrospinal fluid obtained by direct aspiration of the shunt showed the presence of infection in 95 per cent of cases. Culture of the shunt material removed at operation, produced a positive result in 92 per cent of patients suspected of being infected. All shunt material, whether from partial or complete systems, should be cultured at the time of removal, whether or not infection is suspected.[13]

Treatment

There are almost as many treatment regimes as there are major centres concerned with the treatment of hydrocephalic patients. It is, however, generally agreed that the use of systemic antibiotics, with the addition of intraventricular therapy, preferably with the same antibiotic, is necessary in the treatment of shunt infections. Arguments exist as to whether the complete shunt must be removed with immediate replacement, or if subsequent replacement should take place after a period of external ventricular drainage with repeated negative cerebrospinal fluid cultures. Arguments appear to be based upon the judgment of the risks of treatment and are often tempered by the individual clinician's personal experience.

Immediate shunt replacement may require extensive and unduly prolonged surgery, involving the removal of the original shunt and insertion of a new system in a clean area. In many instances, all this being undertaken in a very ill patient. In a functioning shunt, there may be an additional hazard in the removal of an adherent ventricular catheter and the replacement of a new ventricular catheter in a slit-like ventricle. Immediate replacement may provide a rapid means of dissemination of infected material from the infected ventricle into the peritoneal cavity or heart, producing further problems and increasing the risk of distal obstruction.

Removal of the complete system necessitates the immediate insertion of an external ventricular drainage device, preferably in the frontal horn. This method is to be preferred to multiple ventricular punctures in order to obtain specimens for culture and to instil antibiotics. External ventricular drainage, unless treated with meticulous care, presents risks for secondary infection and overdrainage with excessive fluid loss and electrolyte imbalance, especially in small infants. External ventricular drainage, after complete removal of the infected system, would still appear to be the best approach to treatment.

It is now generally accepted that the treatment of infection should involve removal of the entire shunt apparatus, insertion of an external ventricular drain, and the administration of both systemic and intraventricular antibiotics. After three successive negative cerebrospinal fluid cultures, carried out at 2-day intervals, the drain may be removed and a new shunt inserted at a fresh site. Systemic antibiotics should be continued for a total period of 2–3 weeks from the time of initiation of therapy.

The treatment of infection by systemic antibiotics alone, without shunt removal, has been found to be unsatisfactory.[35,36] Although a small number of shunt infections may be treated successfully with systemic antibiotics alone, there are more negative than positive sides to this method. Walters et al.[13] showed that patients receiving only medical treatment initially, required, on average, more hospital days per infection (88 versus 71) and had twice the mortality (36 per cent versus 18 per cent), as compared with those initially treated by some form of shunt removal in addition to antibiotics.

Prevention of shunt infection

The use of prophylactic antibiotics as a routine in shunt surgery has been, and still is, a contentious issue. There has been a plethora of publications comparing infection rates in shunted patients who have or have not received antibiotics before, during, and after surgery. To date, no study has had sufficient case-related data to withstand scientific appraisal. The jury is still out!

In clean neurosurgical operations, Haines[22,37] suggested that an infection rate of 0.8 per cent–5.7 per cent might be expected. Young and Lawner[38] and Tenney et al.[39] have reported rates of infection of 3.6 per cent and 2.6 per cent, respectively, in neurosurgical procedures carried out with prophylactic antibiotic coverage. Current shunt infection rates vary from 2 per cent to 5 per cent. Burke[40] in a laboratory study using guinea-pigs, placed strong emphasis on the timing of the delivery of systemic antibiotic prophylaxis. Maximum suppression of infection occurred if the administration preceded invasive procedures. Subsequent administration became rapidly ineffectual, becoming useless if given 3 hours after the contamination. As a result of this study, it is apparent that to be effective, antibiotics must have saturated the tissues before inoculation occurs, and that antibiotics administered topically or post-operatively have little or no effect in the prevention of infection.

It has been my experience, that there are three groups of patients in whom it is wise to begin prophylactic antibiotic therapy 12–24 hours before surgery and to continue with such treatment for 4–5 days into the post-operative period. Premature infants with intraventricular haemorrhage, low weight infants under 6 months of age, and newborn infants with myelomeningoceles, previously repaired or not, constitute what I feel to be high risk-groups.

It must be continually emphasized that prophylactic antibiotics represent only one weapon in the constant battle against shunt infection. Careful preoperative evaluation to exclude other sources of infection, such as the skin or upper respiratory tract, meticulous preparation of the operative site, avoidance of undue tissue trauma during insertion of the shunt tubing, haemostasis, and the elimination of factors producing prolonged anaesthesia and surgery, all play equally important parts in the elimination of this major complication in the care of hydrocephalic patients.

QUALITY OF LIFE

Intellectual function

Predictive factors

It is very difficult to establish predictive or prospective criteria on the intellectual development of patients with infantile hydrocephalus with any degree of accuracy. Anyone, with a large experience in the treatment of these patients will realize that there are wide variations in function, with university graduates and competent business people at the upper end and severely retarded individuals at the other. The great majority of treated hydrocephalic patients fall into a vague but large group between these two aforementioned extremes. One of the difficulties is the method or form of testing used in an attempt to predict the developmental outcome of treated patients. One of the initial efforts was made by Young and co-workers.[41] This paper analysed 147 surgically treated hydrocephalic children older than 3 years of age. At that time, the thickness of the cerebral mantle was determined by 'bubble' ventriculography. The results suggested that in patients with pure hydrocephalus, a cerebral mantle thicker than 2.8 cm after shunting was consistent with normal development. If the cerebral mantle was thinner than 2.8 cm mental retardation was a foregone conclusion. They emphasized that the thickness of the mantle before shunting was not of predictive value. An adequate cerebral mantle (> 2.8 cm) was obtained in almost every child shunted before 6 months of age. This of course, was obviously inconclusive. In my experience there are a number of treated children in whom the cerebral mantle appears of normal thickness, as demonstrated either by ventriculography or by CT scanning, who are well below the average in terms of intelligence. On the other hand, there are individuals with persistent ventricular dilatation and thinning of the cerebral mantle who are of normal intelligence. Another early study, by Nulsen and Rekate,[42] indicated that patients in whom the mantle was thinner than 2.0 cm were barely educable or ineducable. Patients whose cerebral mantles were between 2.0 and 3.0 cm had IQ scores below 100. However, if a patient's mantle was thicker than 3.0 cm the probability was that they would have a normal IQ. This implied that successful intellectual development does not depend upon the restoration of the ventricle to normal size, which would be reflected by a mantle of 5 or 6 cm. They conclude that the failure to achieve a mantle consistent with normal development would appear to be related to delay in shunting during infancy. However, it was also suggested that as hydrocephalus progresses irreversible damage does not occur until a critical point is reached and that thereafter the damage would result in poor developmental performance.

A study using CT scanning was reported by Oberbauer.[43] In this investigation, a computer program was based on the differential densities of cerebrospinal fluid and brain tissue. The results were expressed as 'Brain–Ventricle Index' or BVI. The normal BVI is 35–40, but hydrocephalic children ranged from 0.5 to 12.5. There was little chance of predicted normal development in patients with an initial BVI of less than 1.5. Above that level it was difficult to establish a positive relationship, although if there was an improvement in the BVI on follow-up then there was a better relationship between ventricular index and intelligence. Dennis and associates[44] reviewed a group of 78 children in detail. These children were between the age of 5–15 years and had been shunted within the first year after the diagnosis of hydrocephalus. It was noted that uneven cognitive development had been reported previously, so that some studies had shown patients' language to be lacking in substantive content. Other studies had shown a selective loss of visual or perceptive skills. Dennis and her associates[45] found that the particular aetiology of the hydrocephalus affected the pattern of intelligence. Children with pure aqueduct stenosis demonstrated lower levels of non-verbal intelligence in relation to their verbal cognitive skills than did those with postnatal aetiologies. They also noted that the type and number of shunts performed did not affect intelligence. It was therefore concluded that cognitive defects were not related to hydrocephalus but to other developmental brain anomalies.

Although a hydrocephalic child is now less at risk for global mental retardation than would have previously been the case, the child is still vulnerable to cognitive impairments in language and non-language function, as reported by Fletcher and Levine.[46] In some domains of cognitive function, hydrocephalic children function as well as their age peers, while in other domains they perform less well. Some aspects of hydrocephalic medical history are associated with poor cognitive development, whereas other aspects appear unrelated.

Language function

It has been shown by many authors that disturbances of language function are not uncommon in early hydrocephalic conditions. The domains of speech and language that have been particularly studied in hydrocephalic children are: the ability to find names or substantive words; language fluency and automaticity; immediate verbal memory; the understanding of syntax or grammar, and metalinguistic awareness. In other words, the control function whereby children are able to monitor and judge the appropriateness of the language that they hear and reproduce. The language of hydrocephalic children is neither globally impaired nor globally proficient. It seems to involve well-maintained linguistic forms or structures that give rise to language output that, while acceptably fluent, is poor in substance and imperfectly monitored. Hydrocephalic speech has been described as lacking appropriate substance and content[47] and as containing a high proportion of inappropriate words in conversational and contextual frames.[47] In hydrocephalic children, verbal fluency may be high, with the speech seeming overautomatized and full of fluently pronounced but stereotype phrases.[48] Hydrocephalic children show poor metalinguistic awareness, being unable to explain, reflect upon, or monitor the language that they use.[49] Not all aspects of verbal function are poor, however; immediate sentence memory, the use of morphology, and the understanding of grammar have been described as adequately developed.[47,50–52] Tew and Laurence[52] have selected hydrocephalic subjects on the basis of a particular pattern of aberrant verbal and personality functioning, the 'Cocktail Party Syndrome', characterized by fluent and well-articulated speech, verbal perseveration, an excessive use of social phrases, irrelevant verbosity, and overfamiliarity of manner.

Generalizations concerning the incidence and characteristics of poor language in hydrocephalic children and adolescents have been difficult to abstract from the literature. This may be partly due to the fact that studies of children selected to approximate the original hydrocephalic case with 'Cocktail Party Syndrome' language,[49] cannot be readily related to empirical studies of verbal function in hydrocephalic children who have not been preselected to show abnormal speech and language.

An important and understudied question continues to be whether, and by what means, language function and language development can be predicted from the medical histories of hydrocephalic children. The literature on early hydrocephalus and language provides some suggestions about historical variables which may be indicative of a particular language syndrome or cognitive defect. How these factors operate within reach of the typical forms of hydrocephalus has not been studied to any great degree, either in detail or depth. It is not clear in published studies whether some degree of difficulty in speech or language function characterizes all forms of early hydrocephalus, or if instead it occurs only, or principally, in particular aetiologies, such as those patients with spina bifida.

As a result several issues critical to the identification of cognitive and educational difficulties of hydrocephalic children and adolescents are poorly understood. A recent study[45] explores whether hydrocephalic children and adolescents developed a more restricted language system, and/or acquired language skills more slowly than their non-hydrocephalic peers. This study had three aims: first, to compare the acquisition of five different language domains (word finding, fluency and automaticity, immediate sentence memory, understanding of grammar, and metalinguistic awareness) in 75 hydrocephalic children and 50 control children and adolescents over the age range during which core educational skills are mastered (6–14 years); second, to assess the extent to which differences in language skills were associated with differences in intelligence; and third, to relate each language function to the medical variables that code the signs, symptoms, and treatment procedures associated with early hydrocephalus.

Language skills improved with age in the hydrocephalics and in the controls, suggesting that the pathological reorganization of the brain, imposed by early hydrocephalus, produces a neural substrate that allows some degree of later language development to occur. Language and intelligence had only modest amounts of shared common variance, showing that language testing tapped functions substantially different from those involved in intelligence.

For several language functions, the trend towards improved language performance with age was one that occurred similarly in both groups; for other functions, however, the rate of improvement with age was significantly less for the hydrocephalics, such that, with increasing age, hydrocephalics were less able than the controls to maintain age-appropriate increments in language performance. These interactions between age and the presence of hydrocephalus have important implications. They suggest that some effects of the hydrocephalus on later language or cognitive functioning may become more, rather than less, apparent as the child develops. It was predicted, on the basis of language tests relating to operations crucial to learning, that hydrocephalic children will master higher level academic tasks less well than the basic educational skills. Even though hydrocephalic children's language does not appear to deteriorate in the course of development, they apparently acquire certain language skills at a progressively slower rate, with the result that they are increasingly less able to match their age peers in learning material that involves a high degree of language competence or that relies heavily on language-related operations.

Some medical variables were predictive of later language functioning, while others were not. Extraventricular hydrocephalus and spinal dysraphism, both preserved higher order language functions but disrupted fluent speech reproduction, suggesting that subtentorial areas might be functionally important for verbal fluency. In contrast, hydrocephalus occurring as the result of intraventricular obstruction preserved fluency while impairing word finding and the understanding of grammar. Impairments in producing speech in the correct serial order (the tendency to make speech perseverations, anticipations, or incorrect sequencing) occurred in those individuals with intraventricular shunt procedures as compared with those whose shunts were extraventricular (lumboperitoneal). As a group, hydrocephalic children and adolescents improved with age less than the controls in their ability to understand grammar used in the context of sentences and to monitor their language for errors and anomalies. It was concluded that language is not a unitary function any more than hydrocephalus is a disease entity or a homogeneous condition. The results reflect the diversity of both language and brain. Not only was language separable from intelligence after early hydrocephalus, but it was composed of internally dissociable domains that bore a complex, but identifiable, relationship to the set of variables coding the aetiology, signs, symptoms, pathologies and treatments associated with early hydrocephalus. The use of terms like 'Cocktail Party Syndrome' do not address such basic questions as how well and how rapidly language develops after early hydrocephalus, or whether a particular hydrocephalic child has a medical history that would indicate a significant risk of compromised language and social development. Throughout the literature concerned with the intelligence and functioning of hydrocephalic children, the frequency and number of shunt procedures was not a significant variable. A medical history of recurrent infections involving the ventricular system, with or without shunt infection, appeared to play a significant role in the reduction of existing intelligence or reduction in the ability to develop further intelligence or linguistic abilities.

Sexual activity, marriage, and pregnancy

In the author's experience, sexual activity in the treated hydrocephalic patient, in the absence of other anomalies, has been normal. These patients are fully capable of marriage and successful parenthood. The difficulties arise when the hydrocephalus is associated with myelomeningocele. The problems are, for the most part, confined to the male patient, with lack of sexual function related to lower sacral nerve involvement. Young women with myelomeningoceles have had no problem with marriage and subsequent pregnancy, although success depends upon an understanding partner. Interestingly, it has come to the author's attention recently, that pregnancy in the hydrocephalic patient with a ventri-culoperitoneal shunt, may produce temporary obstruction of the intraperitoneal portion of the shunt during the last 4–6 weeks of pregnancy, resulting in intermittent blockage and the occurrence of symptoms of increased intracranial pressure. The obstruction resolved spontaneously following delivery. As time goes on, and experience with treated hydrocephalic patients extends over a longer period, there will be more information on problems related to sexual activity, marriage, and pregnancy. At the present time, however, the number of studies of adult hydrocephalics, treated in infancy, are so few that most of the experiences have not been published and exist only in anecdotal form.

Life expectancy

The mortality rate in hydrocephalic patients is more related to associated anomalies or disease than to the direct effects of hydrocephalus. It is difficult to obtain information concerning mortality because of the broad spectrum of associated problems, such as congenital anomalies and infection. Keucher and Mealey[25] reviewed a series of 228 children with non-neoplastic hydrocephalus with a follow-up of at least 7 years. They found that there was a mortality rate of 19 per cent for those treated with vascular shunts and 11 per cent for those treated with peritoneal shunts. Amacher and Wellington[53] reviewed the 5-year survival in children with infantile hydrocephalus and children with myelomeningocele associated with hydrocephalus. The 5-year survival rate in infantile hydro-cephalus was 98.3 per cent as compared to 71 per cent in patients with myelomeningocele. In those patients whose hydrocephalus was post-traumatic their survival was 100 per cent.

It is acknowledged that there have been no adequate studies comparing the short- or long term outcome of surgical and medical treatment. The natural course of untreated hydrocephalus is well documented.[54–56] It is suggested that approximately 50 per cent of untreated patients die as a direct result of hydrocephalus. Of the surviving 50 per cent, with arrested hydrocephalus, only 11–18 per cent had normal cognitive and neurological findings when examined at follow up. The remaining 82–89 per cent had varying degrees of cognitive delay and neurological abnormalities, which may not become apparent until years after the presumed arrest of hydrocephalus.[57] The irreversible ultrastruc-tural and chemical changes produced by hydrocephalus on the cerebral white matter, and to some extent on the grey matter, have been well documented. There is a general consensus of feeling, that treatment of all hydrocephalic patients should be undertaken early in order to prevent such changes.

Treated hydrocephalics, with a functional intelligence and without other gross anomalies, have the potential for a normal existence and life expectancy. In the author's 36 year experience, the majority of patients who have been successfully shunted early in life and who have avoided infections during the course of their shunt revisions, have done very well, going on to higher education and successful careers in the professions and industry. The limitations of the enjoyment of life are related most often to the physical side-effects of the shunting procedures, such as the restriction of back movement due to scoliosis and facet fusion as the result of laminectomy, and the tethering effect of shunts extending from the head into the pleura or peritoneal cavity. With newer shunt materials and surgical techniques, the quality of life for hydrocephalic patients has dramatically improved over the past 36 years.

REFERENCES

1. McLaurin, R.L. Ventricular shunts: complications and results. In *Pediatric neurosurgery*, (ed. McLaurin, R.L., Schut, L., Venes, J.L., and Epstein, F.), pp. 219–29. W.B. Saunders, Philadelphia (1989).
2. Ruge, J.R., Cerullo, L.J., and McClone, O.G. Pneumocephalus in patients with CSF shunts. *Journal of Neurosurgery*, **63**, 532–6 (1985).
3. Collman, H., Mauersberg, W., and Mohr, G. Clinical observations and CSF absorp-tion studies in the slit ventricle syndrome. *Advances in Neurosurgery*, **8**, 183–6 (1980).
4. Engel, M., Carmel, P.W., and Chutorian, A.M. Increased intraventricular pressure without ventriculomegaly in children with shunts. 'Normal Volume' hydrocephalus. *Neurosurgery*, **5**, 549–52 (1979).

5. Epstein, F., Marlin, A., and Wald, A. Chronic headaches in the shunt-dependent adolescent with nearly normal ventricular volume: Diagnosis and treatment. *Neurosurgery*, **3**, 351–5 (1979).

6. Hyde-Rowan, M.O., Rekate, H.L., and Nulsen, F.E. Re-expansion of previously collapsed ventricles: The slit ventricle syndrome. *Journal of Neurosurgery*, **55**, 536–9 (1982).

7. Epstein, F. Increased intracranial pressure in hydrocephalic children with functioning shunts: A complication of shunt dependency. *Concepts in Pediatric Neurosurgery*, **4**, 119–30 (1983).

8. Kierken, R., Mortier, W., Pothman, R., Bock, W.J., and Seibert, H. The slit ventricle syndrome after shunting in hydrocephalic children. *Neuropediatrics*, **13**, 190–4 (1982).

9. Wisoff, J. and Epstein, F.J. Diagnosis and treatment of the slit ventricle syndrome. In *Concepts in neurosurgery. Hydrocephalus*, (ed. Scott, R.M.), Chapter 7, pp. 79–85. Williams and Wilkins, Baltimore (1990).

10. Epstein, F., Lapras, C., and Wisoff, J.H. 'Slit Ventricle Syndrome': Etiology and treatment. *Pediatric Neuroscience*, **14**, 5–10 (1988).

11. Holness, R.O., Hoffman, H.J., and Hendrick, E.B. Subtemporal decompression for the slit ventricle syndrome after shunting in hydrocephalic children. *Child's Brain*, **5**, 137–44 (1979).

12. George, R., Lelbrock, L., and Epstein, M. Long term analysis of CSF shunt infection. *Journal of Neurosurgery*, **51**, 804–11 (1979).

13. Walters, B.C., Hoffman, H.J., Hendrick, E.B., Humphreys, R.P. *et al.* CSF shunt infections. *Journal of Neurosurgery*, **60**, 1014–21 (1984).

14. McClone, D.G., Czyzewski, D. Raimondi, A.S., and Sommers, R.E. Central nervous system infections as a limiting factor in the intelligence of children with myelomeningocele. *Pediatrics*, **70**, 338–42 (1982).

15. Raimondi, A.S. and Soare, P. Intellectual development in shunted hydrocephalic children. *American Journal of Diseases of Children*, **127**, 664–71 (1974).

16. Luthardt, T. Bacterial infections in ventriculo–auricular shunt systems. *Developmental Medicine and Child Neurology*, **12** (Suppl. 22), 105–9 (1970).

17. Ammirati, M. and Raimondi, A.J. CSF shunt infections in children. *Child's Nervous System*, **3**, 106–9 (1987).

18. Klein, D.M. Comparison of antibiotic methods in the prophylaxis of operative shunt infections. *Concepts in Pediatric Neurosurgery*, **4**, 131–41 (1983).

19. McCullough, Q.C., Kane, J.G., Presper, J.H. *et al.* Antibiotic prophylaxis in ventricular shunt surgery. 1. Reduction of operative infection rates with methicillin. *Child's Brain*, **7**, 182–9 (1980).

20. Shapiro, S., Bosz, J., Kleiman, M. *et al.* Origin of organisms infecting ventricular shunts. *Neurosurgery*, **22**, 868–72 (1988).

21. Shurtleff, O.B., Stuntz, J.T., and Hayden, P.Y. Experience with 1201 CSF shunts. *Pediatric Neuroscience*, **12**, 49–57 (1985–86).

22. Haines, S.J. Antibiotic prophylaxis in neurosurgery. *Clinical Neurosurgery*, **33**, 633–42 (1985).

23. Ignelzi, R.J. and Kirsch, W.M. Follow-up analysis of ventriculoperitoneal and ventriculoatrial shunts for hydrocephalus. *Journal of Neurosurgery*, **42**, 679–82 (1975).

24. Odio, C., McCracken, G.H. Jr, and Nelsen, J.D. CSF shunt infections in pediatrics. A seven year experience. *American Journal of Diseases of Children*, **138**, 103–8 (1984).

25. Keucher, T.R. and Mealey, J. Jr. Long-term results after ventriculoatrial and ventriculoperitoneal shunting for infantile hydrocephalus. *Journal of Neurosurgery*, **50**, 179–86 (1979).

26. Salmon, J.H. Adult hydrocephalus. Evaluation of shunt therapy in 80 patients. *Journal of Neurosurgery*, **37**, 423–8 (1972).

27. Remer, P., Lacombe, J., Pierre-Kahn, A. *et al.* Factors causing acute shunt infection. Computer analysis of 1174 operations. *Journal of Neurosurgery*, **61**, 1072–8 (1984).

28. Ajir, F., Levin, A.V., and Duff, F.A. The effect of prophylactic methicillin in CSF shunt infections in children. *Neurosurgery*, **9**, 6–8 (1981).

29. Bayston, R. and Lari, J. A study of the sources of infection in colonized shunts. *Developmental Medicine and Child Neurology*, **16** (Suppl. 32), 16–22 (1974).

30. Schimke, R., Black, P.H., Mark, V.H., and Swartz, M.N. Indolent *Staphylococcus albus* or *aureus* bacteremia after ventriculoatriostomy: Role of foreign body in its initiation and perpetuation. *New England Journal of Medicine*, **264**, 264–70 (1961).

31. Guevara, J.A., LaTorre, J., Denoya, C., and Zuccaro, G. Microscopic studies in shunts for hydrocephalus. *Child's Brain*, **8**, 284–3 (1980).

32. Bayston, R. and Penny, S.P. Excessive production of mucoid substance in Staphylococcus SIIA: a possible factor in colonization of Holter shunts. *Developmental Medicine and Child Neurology*, **14** (Suppl. 27), 25–8 (1972).

33. Borges, L.F. Cerebrospinal fluid shunts interfere with host defenses. *Neurosurgery*, **10**, 55–69 (1982).

34. Finney, H.L. and Roberts, T.S. Nephritis secondary to chronic cerebrospinal fluid–vascular shunt infection, 'shunt nephritis'. *Child's Brain*, **6**, 189–93 (1980).

35. Schoenbaum, S.C., Gardner, P., and Shillito, J. Infections in cerebrospinal fluid shunts: Epidemiology, clinical manifestations and therapy. *Journal of Infectious Diseases*, **131**, 543–52 (1975).

36. Shurtleff, O.B., Foltz, E.L., Weeks, R.D. *et al.* Therapy of *Staphylococcus epidermis* infections associated with CSF shunts. *Pediatrics*, **53**, 55–62 (1974).

37. Haines, S.J. Systemic antibiotic prophylaxis in neurological surgery. *Neurosurgery*, **6**, 355–61 (1980).

38. Young, R.F. and Lawner, P.M. Perioperative antibiotic prophylaxis for the prevention of postoperative neurosurgical infections. *Journal of Neurosurgery*, **66**, 701–5 (1987).

39. Tenney, J.H., Vlahov, P., Salcman, M. *et al.* Wide variation in risk of wound infection following clean neurosurgery. *Journal of Neurosurgery*, **62**, 243–7 (1985).

40. Burke, J.F. The effective period of preventive antibiotic action in experimental incisions and dermal lesions. *Surgery*, **50**, 161–8 (1961).

41. Young, H.F., Nulsen, F.E., Weiss, M.H. *et al.* The relationship of intelligence and cerebral mantle in treated infantile hydrocephalus (IQ potential) in hydrocephalic children. *Pediatrics*, **52**, 38–44 (1972).

42. Nulsen, F.E. and Rekate, H.L. Results of treatment of hydrocephalus as a guide to future management. In *Pediatric neurosurgery*, (ed. section of Pediatric Neurosurgery of the American Association of Neurological Surgeons), pp. 229–41. Grune and Stratton, New York (1982).

43. Oberbauer, R.W. The significance of morphological details for developmental outcome in infantile hydrocephalus. *Child's Nervous System*, **1**, 329 (1985).

44. Dennis, M., Fitz, C.R., Netley, C.T. *et al.* The intelligence of hydrocephalic children. *Archives of Neurology*, **38**, 607–15 (1981).

45. Dennis, M., Hendrick, E.B., Hoffman, H.J., and Humphreys, R.P. Language of hydrocephalic children and adolescents. *Journal of Clinical and Experimental Neuropsychology*, **9**, 593–621 (1987).

46. Fletcher, J.M. and Levine, H.S. Neurobehavioural effects of brain injury in children. In *Handbook of pediatric psychology*, (ed. Routh, D.), pp. 258–95. Guilford, New York (1987).

47. Parsons, J.G. Short term verbal memory in hydrocephalic children. *Developmental Medicine and Child Neurology,* **11** (Suppl. 20), 1–9 (1969).

48. Ingram, T.T.S. and Naughton, J.A. Paediatric and psychological aspects of cerebral palsy associated with hydrocephalus. *Developmental Medicine and Child Neurology*, **4**, 287–92 (1962).

49. Swisher, L.P. and Pinsker, E.J. The language characteristics of hyperverbal hydrocephalic children. *Developmental Medicine and Child Neurology*, **13**, 746–55 (1971).

50. MacNab, G.H. The development of the knowledge and treatment of hydrocephalus. *Developmental Medicine and Child Neurology*, **8** (Suppl. 11), 1–9 (1969).

51. Spain, B. Verbal and performance ability in pre-school children with spina bifida. *Developmental Medicine and Child Neurology*, **16**, 773–80 (1974).

52. Tew, B.J. and Laurence, K.M. The clinical and psychological characteristics of children with 'cocktail party' syndrome. *Zeitschrift für Kinderchirurgie*, **28**, 360–7 (1979).

53. Amacher, A. L. and Wellington J. Infantile hydrocephalus. Long term results of surgical therapy. *Child's Brain*, **11**, 217–29 (1984).

54. Foltz, E.L. and Shurtleff, B. Five year comparative study of hydrocephalus in children, with and without operation, in 113 cases. *Journal of Neurosurgery*, **20**, 164–8 (1963).

55. Laurence, K.M. The natural history of hydrocephalus. *Lancet*, **ii**, 1152–4 (1958).

56. Yashon, D. Prognosis in infantile hydrocephalus. Past and present. *Journal of Neurosurgery*, **20**, 105–11 (1979).

57. James, H.E. and Schut, L. Pitfalls in the diagnosis of arrested hydrocephalus. *Acta Neurochirgugica*, **43**, 13–17 (1978).

8 Investigation and management of hydrocephalus in adults

R. V. Jeffreys

INTRODUCTION

It is essential to define hydrocephalus occurring in any age group accurately, but nowhere more so than in the adult; since atrophy occurs with increasing frequency in the older age groups. Cerebral atrophy leads to increasing accumulations of CSF as space replacement in a skull cavity that cannot change its size — hydrocephalus *ex vacuo*. In so far as hydrocephalus results from an imbalance of CSF formation and absorption, the term should be reserved for these and defined as 'an excessive accumulation of CSF within the head due to a disturbance of formation, flow, and absorption'.

There are various classifications of hydrocephalus which are based on clinical findings, morbid anatomy, or time of onset; none are perfect. Dandy and Blackfan[1] subdivided hydrocephalus into two major groups: communicating and non-communicating. In the former there is a full communication between the ventricles and subarachnoid spaces and in the latter CSF cannot not escape fully from the ventricles. This classification has found most favour particularly since it can be modified by aetiological description.[2]

Many of the causes of hydrocephalus occur both in children and adults, though with varying age dependency; for example in hydrocephalus due to neoplasms of the posterior fossa, medulloblastoma is more common in children and acoustic neuromas more common in the adult. Other causes, such as aqueduct stenosis, can present in childhood but can also manifest themselves slowly, such that it is only as an adult that the patient develops overt problems even though the primary pathological process was present in childhood. Others are uniquely problems of the adult, such as hydrocephalus secondary to basilar invagination due to Paget's disease or the so-called normal pressure hydrocephalus.

There are two main unique differences between children and adults — the skull and the brain. The adult skull cannot expand and, therefore, any increase in a tumour and/or CSF must be at the expense of the brain, which may well undergo secondary pressure atrophy. The skull of the child, at least until 10 years of age, can expand by suture diastasis if the volume increase of the pathological process is relatively slow; it cannot expand rapidly as, for example, with an acute extradural haematoma.

The adult brain is fully developed, and, in the vast majority of cases, any deterioration of cerebral function occurs against an already established background of intellect and behaviour; whereas a child is only on the threshold of intellectual activity and of environmental problems demanding abstract thought, as such it may be very difficult to assess and apportion blame to hydrocephalus, the aetiological cause, or to some other factor.

HYDRODYNAMICS OF HYDROCEPHALUS

It is easier to understand the hydrodynamics of hydrocephalus in the adult with an intact non-expandable skull by considering chronic hydrocephalus first. In such cases the lateral ventricles may be dilated to a capacity of several hundred millilitres, compared to the capacity of the normal human lateral and third ventricles of about 20 ml (Last and Tompsett[3] give 22.4 ml; Bull[4] gives 20 ml for all ventricles). The normal production of CSF in man has been estimated to be 0.35–40 ml/min or about 500 ml/24 hours (Davson and Segal[5]). Assuming that three-quarters of CSF production is within the lateral and third ventricles, then one can expect production of 0.30 ml/min, hence the contents of these ventricles will be replaced in just over one hour. If an obstruction of the aqueduct occurs then hydrocephalus, of the order of 300 ml in the ventricles, ensues; this is a volume which normally would take 15 hours to produce. From the experiments of Bering and Sato[6] it can be calculated that in the normal dog the contents of the lateral and third ventricles would be replaced every 2 hours; in the hydrocephalic dog, in which the aqueduct was blocked, replacement takes just over 7 hours. These figures can only be approximate, but they clearly beg the question: what happens to the CSF which is apparently being produced in chronic hydrocephalus and which cannot drain through the aqueduct? It has been assumed by clinicians that secretion of CSF diminishes in chronic hydrocephalus, as a failure to secrete against a high pressure, and there is some experimental evidence to support this hypothesis (Børgesen and Gjerris).[7] However, the reduction in the hydrocephalic cat was only of the order of 30 per cent (Bering and Sato[6]). There are other possible compensatory mechanisms that have to be considered; all of which might serve to dissipate the pressure gradient between the ventricles and the brain, and might, if the CSF obstruction is incomplete (as it usually is in man), reduce the pathological process of CSF accumulation.[2] These mechanisms include reduction in the cerebrovascular volume, enlargement of the ventricular system, and absorption of CSF by the brain across the ventricular lining; all may serve to slow down the evolution of hydrocephalus. Later cerebral atrophy may also serve to slow the process.

In an attempt to rationalize the problems of CSF accumulation in hydrocephalus, Hakim[8] suggested that one of the laws of mechanics might be applied:

$$\text{pressure} = \text{force/area}.$$

What this in fact means is that a normal CSF pressure will apply greater force upon an expanded ventricle than upon one of normal size, and that although the intraventricular pressure may be only slightly raised the ventricles will continue to expand. Whereas this principle may well have some validity in developing hydrocephalus, it must also be stressed that there are other factors to be considered in such a complex environment as the brain and surrounding skull. One such factor is the compensatory mechanism of transventricular absorption of CSF; this suggestion was made by Bering and Sato[6] and has been supported by other workers. The sites of transventricular absorption have not been fully identified, though the two most likely are transchoroidal and transependymal, and there is some experimental evidence to support both of these hypotheses.[2]

The resistance to outflow of CSF is a major determinant of intracranial pressure (ICP) and by measuring outflow resistance (see below) in communicating hydrocephalus it appears that there is a continuing spectrum from those patients with unequivocally raised ICP, through those with intermediate ICP, to those with normal ICP and resistance.[9] Another intriguing condition is when the CSF acquires an increased viscosity with a high protein content (for example due to neurofibromas within the vertebral canal) which in turn leads to an increased outflow resistance and thence to hydrocephalus even though the primary problem is within the vertebral canal.

The situation is quite different in acute hydrocephalus, for example that occurring in a posterior fossa abscess or a shunt blockage in a patient successfully treated and whose ventricles have shrunk back to normal. Clinical experience shows that coma and even death occur rapidly if relief is not rapidly forthcoming. It is presumed that this happens because there is insufficient space reserve within the skull and insufficient time for pressure atrophy to occur.

CLINICAL FEATURES

The clinical features may be due to hydrocephalus, or the underlying aetiological factor, or to combinations of the two. Since there are many aetiological factors, each with their own locality and producing specific focal neurological deficits, one can only give an outline of those symptoms which appear to be specific to hydrocephalus. At the same time consideration must be given to the rapidity or otherwise of evolution of the hydrocephalic state.

When the hydrocephalus is relatively acute, over days, weeks, or a few months, symptoms of raised intracranial pressure predominate. These include recurring and increasingly unremittent headache often exacerbated by coughing, sneezing, and straining at stool, together with nausea and occasionally vomiting. (Headache is of course an extremely common symptom in the population at large, but if two or more of the features listed above occur in the same patient then one should assume a high index of suspicion for an elevated ICP). In raised intracranial pressure papilloedema is frequently, though not invariably, found on fundoscopy. There may also be disturbances of gaze, most commonly sixth nerve pareses. Occasionally these features may be overlooked, with the patient developing a confusional state often misdiagnosed as a psychosis from which he may rapidly pass into coma. This pattern may be seen well in some patients after the successful clipping of an intracerebral aneurysm or treatment of bacterial meningitis.

If the hydrocephalus evolves more slowly over months, or even years, the features are those of diffuse organic brain damage. These events may be preceded by symptoms of raised intracranial pressure, but these may have been so insidious that they have been ignored. The predominant feature is one of a dementia in which there is a progressive deterioration of intellect and behaviour. The patient may lose insight into himself and be unaware of his decline, but often colleagues and relatives will have noticed it. There will a falling off of short-term memory together with an inability to acquire new information, coupled with a reduction in deductive reasoning. There will be a slowing of thought and speech processes, and physical activities leading to apathy in both intellectual and personal activities and in relationships with others. Pride in personal appearance and hygiene will decline, and may culminate in urinary incontinence similar to that seen with frontal lobe problems in which the patient lacks concern and may even be unaware that he is incontinent. Ultimately the patient will decline to total apathy, both in thought and physical processes, and may progress to stupor.

Although the clinician can perform simple mental and memory testing and gain a suspicion of an oncoming dementia, clinical neuropsychometry can provide a useful service in assessing higher cerebral function in a more detailed fashion; the testing is best performed by neuropsychologists. This may aid diagnosis as well as providing a useful baseline against which the effects of treatment can be assessed. For example, psychiatrists will often comment on how difficult it is to distinguish between an early dementia and a severe depression, though neuropsychologists may be able to distinguish between them.

Neurological symptoms develop gradually, the most important of which is ataxia of gait. Initially, the gait disturbance appears as a lack of co-ordination particularly over uneven ground such that the patient can easily trip, fall, and fracture bones since the righting mechanisms are slow to accommodate to sudden changes in posture. Thereafter, gait deteriorates further to become slow and broad-based, the patient lurches off balance in any direction, even on flat surfaces, and eventually the patient becomes chair- and even bed-bound. These gait disturbances are thought to be due to stretching of the pyramidal fibres from the motor cortex as they pass around the ventricle.[10] Incoordination of the upper limbs is less obvious, though observers will often comment that the patient is clumsy at feeding and dressing, and that handwriting has deteriorated. However, it must be pointed out that some of these features may simply be the result of the dementia and lack of care by the patient.

All the symptoms listed above can occur with the various types of cerebral atrophic processes. However, over the years it has become apparent that in hydrocephalus the dementia and gait disturbance occur together, whilst in atrophic processes it is more common for dementia to occur early and gait disturbance to occur later or not at all. Urinary incontinence is a late symptoms in both hydrocephalus and atrophy.

Many other symptoms can develop but the vast majority occur as a result of the primary cause (for example hearing loss and facial weakness in large acoustic neuromas) rather than as a result of the hydrocephalus alone.

NORMAL PRESSURE HYDROCEPHALUS

History

In 1964 Adams *et al.*[11] reported three cases with what they called occult hydrocephalus. The three cases consisted of two with a subarachnoid block to CSF and one of a paraphyseal third ventricular cyst. A clinical picture was described of psychomotor retardation together with imbalance of gait and urinary incontinence. The term occult was later replaced by the term normal pressure, based on the fact that at lumbar puncture the pressure was normal even in the presence of hydrocephalus. Such clinical findings as described above are common particularly in cerebral atrophy due to a variety of causes, most of which are untreatable. Not surprisingly, since some of the original cases were considerably improved by CSF diversion operations, there rapidly emerged a situation in which many demented patients with enlarged ventricles on lumbar air encephalography also underwent CSF diversion. Not surprisingly very few of these cases were helped and some were even made worse. As a result, matters seemed to be deteriorating to such a degree that the whole concept and the value of CSF diversion was called into question.

Fortunately at about this time Lundberg[12] evolved a method for continuous intracranial pressure monitoring by the ventricular route. This technique was then applied to these cases and what emerged was what had been anticipated by some, namely that in the midst of all these large numbers of dementing patients was a smaller cohort who had genuine CSF handling problems rather than atrophy. Continuous ICP monitoring showed that some patients, although having normal CSF pressures during large parts of the 24 hours, also at times developed periods of raised ICP in the form of short or long plateau waves.[13,14] These were the cases that responded well, often dramatically to CSF diversion. It was therefore thought that a better name for the condition would be either intermittently raised pressure hydrocephalus or adult non-tumorous hydrocephalus; however, the term normal pressure hydrocephalus continues to find most favour, but this must be reserved for those cases of communicating hydrocephalus in which there is no very obvious antecedent space occupying factor.

Pathophysiology

The pathological findings are disappointing from the standpoint of providing an explanation of the syndrome. Incomplete leptomeningeal fibrosis with or without changes in the arachnoid granulations are the most common findings; how-ever, some patients with Alzheimer's disease have similar findings.[15] Further-more, ventricular ependymal disruption, subependymal glial reaction, and periventricular loss of myelin have all been found; however, these are the findings in other forms of chronic hydrocephalus.

Clearly there must first be some factor which initiates the obstruction to flow or malabsorption of CSF, so that a damming-back pressure gradient occurs which causes the ventricles to progressively dilate. Thereafter, it is possible to postulate that the expanding ventricles compress the cortical subarachnoid spaces, compounding the problem by further reducing the flow of CSF.

Continuous intracranial pressure monitoring has established that although the pressure may be normal for long periods there are times when the pressure exhibits beta waves either spontaneously (usually during sleep) or in response to a rise in intrathoracic pressure as occurs during coughing or sneezing.[13,14,16] Challenge tests have been developed which either involve a single bolus intraventricular injection of a small volume of saline[14] or a continuous infusion of saline into the lumbar subarachnoid space at about twice the normal rate of CSF production (0.7 ml/min).[17] In the former test the intraventricular pressure rises quickly in a hydrocephalic patient and may even provoke beta waves, but, it barely rises in a patient with cerebral atrophy. In the latter test the pressure normally reaches a plateau below 22 mm Hg, but does not do so in hydro-cephalus where the pressure may continue to rise. These tests have produced much interesting data and they are justified in the clinical situation when trying to distinguish hydrocephalus, that might benefit from CSF diversion, from atrophy which will not.[18] However, they must be applied cautiously and only used when it is felt that the evidence from ICP monitoring might significantly aid management policy when other non-invasive tests have proved inconclusive.

METHODS OF INVESTIGATION

First-line investigation

In the vast majority of cases it is not possible, on clinical grounds alone, to diagnose hydrocephalus, but rather one is investigating a patient for either presumptive evidence of a space-occupying lesion and/or a dementia. It is CT scanning which will demonstrate the hydrocephalus together with any under-lying causative lesion and it usually with this radiological investigation that one starts. Some purists would insist that plain skull X-rays still have a place in diagnosis. In truth, one has to admit there is some validity to this argument in that altered configuration of the skull base which can lead to hydrocephalus (for example basilar invagination) and pre-existing skull changes from a hydro-cephalus of childhood will be demonstrated; however, CT scanning can show all these and so much more. Currently if a CT scanner is available it is probably better to use this method first and to obtain skull X-rays later if required; however, if a CT scanner is not easily available then skull X-rays should be performed. The role of Magnetic Resonance Imaging (MRI) will clearly become more established with its wider availability. Recently the intriguing possibility of using MRI for the measurement of intracranial CSF volume[19] has been propounded and more may well be heard of this technique in the foreseeable future.

Apart from identifying the presence or absence of any aetiological agent, what are the cardinal CT features to look for? Enlargement of the lateral ventricles clearly comes first, and rounding of the anterior horns is a clear feature. Of further import is the presence of periventricular lucencies around the anterior horns which clearly sets hydrocephalus apart from atrophy where this sign does not occur (Fig. 8.1). The presence of enlarged sulci over the cerebral hemispheres is contentious since this can either represent availability of intracranial spare space, meaning that the hydrocephalus is not under tension, or that the CSF is accumulating due to reduced absorption by the arachnoid granulations and the hydrocephalus is under tension (Fig. 8.2(a), (b)). When in doubt in the presence of this sign it is wise to turn to other methods of investigation, such as ICP monitoring. For those without the facilities for ICP monitoring, draining CSF several times daily by lumbar puncture and assessing any clinical improvement can sometimes be of help in establishing whether or not permanent CSF drainage is required. However, one must state that this is rather second-best management for new cases (and in whom it is dangerous if a space-occupying

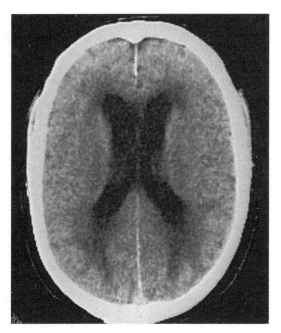

Fig. 8.1 CT scan showing hydrocephalus with periventricular lucencies in a 55-year-old man with normal pressure hydrocephalus.

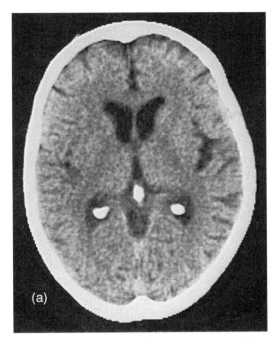

Fig. 8.2(a) CT scan showing large ventricles in a 60-year-old woman. Note also dilated cortical subarachnoid spaces. This was a case of cerebral atrophy.

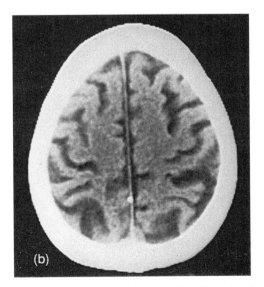

Fig. 8.2(b) Same patient as in Fig. 8.2(a). Note the dilated subarachnoid spaces over the top of the cerebral hemispheres.

lesion is present), though it can be adequate for the assessment of hydrocephalus continuing after other treatments, such as clipping of an intracranial aneurysm. Most of the other CT signs relate to the aetiological agents as well and will be dealt with as appropriate below.

It may be easier to follow the convention of communicating and non-communicating hydrocephalus in discussing the aetiological lesions and further possible investigations that may be necessary.

Non-communicating hydrocephalus

Any space-occupying lesion in or close to the 'narrows' of the ventricular system of aqueduct of Sylvius can lead to hydrocephalus, fortunately most of these are apparent on iodine-enhanced CT scans. A list of all possible causative lesions would be very long and for present purposes only common lesions will be mentioned.

In the case of the third ventricle one can see lesions within it, such as colloid cysts (Fig. 8.3), craniopharyngiomas, and gliomas (Fig. 8.4) which produce hydrocephalus usually by obstructing one or both of the foramina of Monro. Lesions external to the ventricle, such as large pituitary adenomas (Figs 8.5(a), (b)), giant aneurysms of the basilar and anterior communicating arteries, and craniopharyngiomas will indent and distort the third ventricle from without.

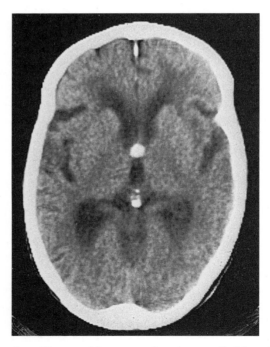

Fig. 8.3 CT scan in a 40-year-old woman showing a colloid cyst of the third ventricle.

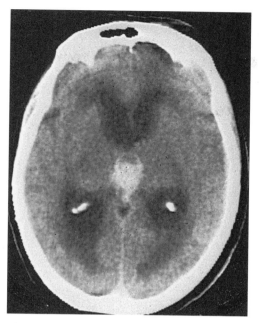

Fig. 8.4 CT scan of 20 year old woman showing hydrocephalus due to an astrocytoma of the thalamus bulging into the third ventricle.

Lesions which further narrow the aqueduct of Sylvius include some cases of congenital stenosis whose presentation is delayed until adulthood. Lesions without the aqueduct include pineal neoplasms (Fig. 8.6) and some intrinsic brainstem gliomas. If lesions do not obviously enhance with contrast they may still be suspected by a discrepancy in size between the enlarged supratentorial ventricles and normal sized fourth ventricle. The diagnosis of pure aqueduct stenosis must be made cautiously, and only after compression from space-occupying lesions (particularly peri-aqueductal gliomas) has been excluded by MRI or contrast ventriculography.

Nearly every space-occupying lesion of the posterior fossa once it reaches a certain size will, given time, lead to distortion of the entrance of the aqueduct into the fourth ventricle or of the fourth ventricle itself. The lesions may be extra-axial or intra-axial. Cerebellopontine angle neoplasms such as acoustic neuromas (Figs 8.7(a), (b), (c)) or meningiomas (Fig. 8.8), once they exceed 2 cm in diameter, nearly always cause hydrocephalus. Other extra-axial lesions to be considered include glomus jugulare tumours and epidermoids. Intra-axial lesions such as cerebellar gliomas, haemangioblastomas (Figs 8.9(a), (b)), and metastases will cause hydrocephalus chronically, but one must not forget abscesses of the cerebellum or large infarcts and haematomas of the cerebellum which may cause an acute hydrocephalus very quickly in a matter of a few days. Distortions from the skull base such as Paget's disease and basilar invagination

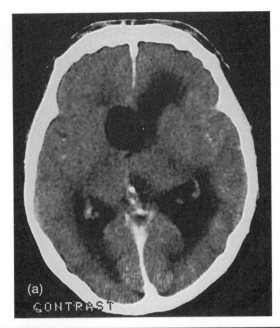

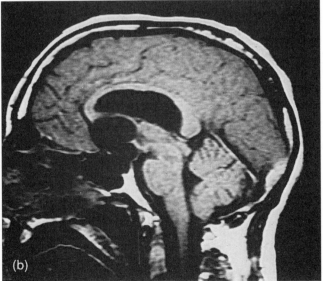

Fig. 8.5(a) CT scan of a 45-year-old man with chiasmal compression and hydrocephalus due to a large cyst arising from the pituitary fossa and which has indented the third ventricle. **(b)** Same case as Fig. 8.5(a) an MRI scan showing the anatomy more easily than in the CT scan of Fig. 8.5(a).

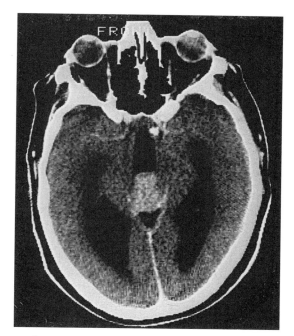

Fig. 8.6 CT scan of 53-year-old man showing hydrocephalus due to a pinealoma.

(Fig. 8.10) will also cause hydrocephalus by kinking the brainstem, as will lesions of the foramen magnum such as meningiomas. A small number of adults have Arnold–Chiari type 1 malformation and these cases may develop hydrocephalus;[20] in type 1, cerebellar tissue lies below the level of the foramen magnum and the medulla oblongata may or may not also be displaced caudally. The theories for the development of hydrocephalus in this condition are many and varied.[21]

Communicating hydrocephalus

This results from obstruction to the flow of CSF in the subarachnoid spaces or some obstruction to the re-absorption of CSF into the venous system. In the adult the most common cause is that of subarachnoid haemorrhage from ruptured intracranial aneurysms, where it has been shown that 63 per cent cases have hydrocephalus in the early stages after haemorrhage,[22] though in the majority CSF pathways return to normal within a few days or weeks following aneurysmal surgery.[23] Another cause of blood in the CSF is trauma, and although hydrocephalus can occur subsequently (Figs 8.11(a), (b)) it is surprising how infrequently this happens when one considers the frequency of major craniocerebral trauma.

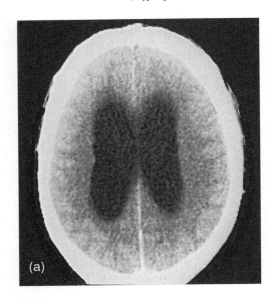

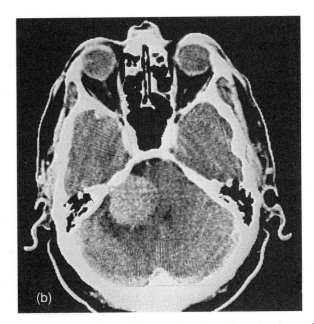

Fig. 8.7(a) CT scan in a 50-year-old man showing a large hydrocephalus due to a large acoustic neuroma. **(b)** Same case as Fig. 8.7(a) showing large acoustic neuroma.

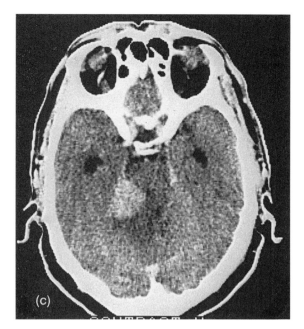

Fig. 8.7(c) Same case as Figs 8.7(a) and (b) showing the large acoustic neuroma extending through the tentorial hiatus.

Any arachnoiditis can lead to hydrocephalus; and the causes range from infective meningitis (due to bacteria or other micro-organisms), aseptic meningitis after posterior fossa surgery, and granulomatous meningitis (for example sarcoid). Hydrocephalus may occur acutely or chronically even after the agent has been successfully treated, and presumably this is due to chronic scar tissue within the meninges.

The case of adult non-tumorous intermittent raised pressure hydrocephalus (normal pressure hydrocephalus) is a curious one and has been dealt with separately (see above). Finally, mention must be made of those patients who after excision of a posterior fossa mass lesion develop a pseudomeningocele. When such patients are CT scanned the ventricles are often small, since the extra volume of CSF is being accommodated within the pseudomeningocele sac. Such cases are either simply mechanical or some are due to the curious condition of aseptic meningitis that can occur after posterior fossa surgery. If the sac does not remain flat after a few lumbar punctures and drainage of CSF then these patients will require CSF diversion.

Second-line investigation

After the CT scan what does one do next? In the case of non-communicating hydrocephalus with an obvious cause it is the latter that may require further

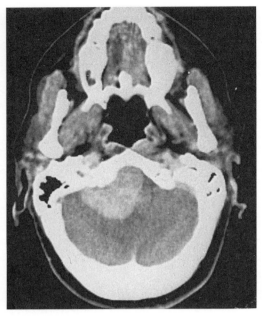

Fig. 8.8 CT scan in a 40-year-old woman with hydrocephalus ataxia, and a bulbar palsy; the causative agent is a large meningioma arising from the skull base and extending down to the foramen magnum.

investigation. For example, an enhancing lesion in the third ventricle may require cerebral angiography to confirm or refute a vascular pathology such as an aneurysm. Magnetic resonance imaging (MRI) may yield further information, particularly if gadolinium enhancement is used. Contrast ventriculography still has a place for lesions in/around the third ventricle and around the aqueduct of Sylvius if MRI is unavailable. But basically the decision needs to be taken whether or not to explore and excise the offending lesion. If surgery is carried out the hydrocephalus may or may not settle and if not subsequent CSF diversion will be needed. If excision surgery is not attempted then CT-guided biopsy may be attempted followed by CSF diversion and other appropriate treatments such as radiotherapy.

At this stage one should mention the role of burr-hole ventricular drainage of CSF to temporarily improve the condition of a patient drowsy or stuporose from hydrocephalus, thus allowing reduction of the mass effect of neoplasm and surrounding oedema by dexamethasone, and better fluid and electrolyte balance. This can be a few days well bought before other investigations can be performed or before undertaking what can often be major surgery. However, one should stress that this should not be a routine procedure since it will be unnecessary in a large number of cases, and furthermore it is probably better to operate on alert

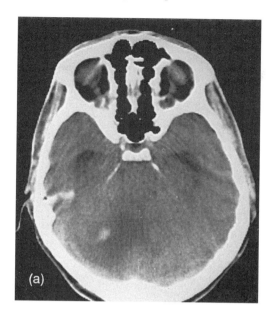

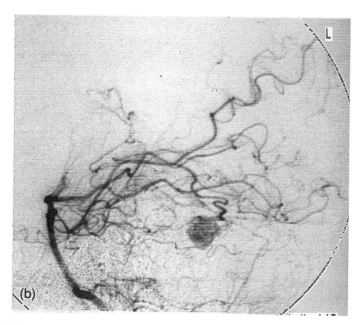

Fig. 8.9(a) CT scan of a 31-year-old man showing a left cerebellar cyst and an enhancing nodule. **(b)** Same case as Fig. 8.9(a) with a vertebral angiogram showing the enhancing nodule which was a haemangioblastoma.

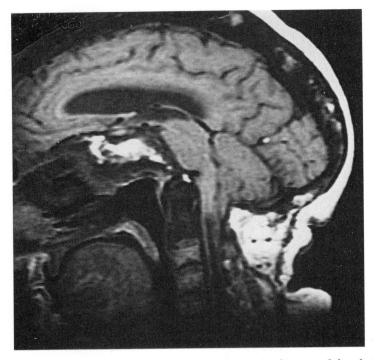

Fig. 8.10 MRI scan in 60-year-old woman with Paget's disease of the skull. The scan shows hydrocephalus due to basilar invagination, such that the tip of the odontoid process is well within the skull and is causing upward kinking of the brainstem.

patients with a virgin CSF uncontaminated by bacteria or other agents. Additionally, with large posterior fossa space-occupying lesions there is the risk of the potentially lethal complication of upward coning of the cerebellum into the tentorial hiatus.

If there is a hydrocephalus without a causative space-occupying lesion one has to look for a possible cause. Stenosis of the aqueduct of Sylvius is suspected if there is a significant disproportion in the size of the supratentorial ventricles compared to the fourth ventricle. This can be shown on MRI, but if this technique is unavailable then contrast ventriculography is required. Distortions of the skull base, such as basilar invagination can be easily seen both on CT scan and plain skull X-rays. A meningitis can often be surmised clinically but will need examination of the CSF by lumbar puncture. Blood in the CSF is easily identified, either on CT scan or lumbar puncture, and usually the clinical findings will have already suggested a subarachnoid haemorrhage from a ruptured aneurysm or arteriovenous malformation. Bacterial meningitis is

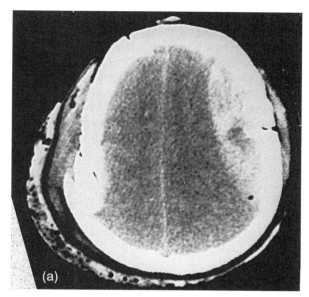

Fig. 8.11(a) CT scan of 50-year-old man a few hours after he had fallen over a cliff. Note the right extradural haematoma and the left subdural haematoma. These were evacuated by bilateral craniotomies.

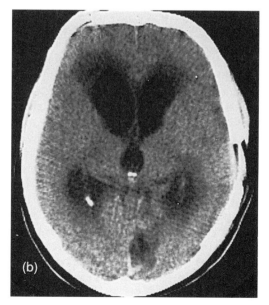

Fig. 8.11(b) CT scan of same patient 6 weeks later showing gross hydrocephalus which required CSF shunting.

likewise clinically suspected and confirmed by CSF examination and enlisting the aid of the microbiological department. The more difficult forms of chronic leptomeningitis are suggested by changes in the CSF of protein content, cell count, and the presence or absence of other micro-organisms such as fungi or cryptococci, and close co-operation with a microbiologist is essential. Cytocentrifugation of the CSF may be of help both for infective arachnoiditis as well as for carcinomatous meningitis which can occasionally present as hydrocephalus before the original primary malignancy becomes manifest.

INTRACRANIAL PRESSURE MONITORING

Much of the original work on ICP monitoring was done at a time when the only radiological assessment of the CSF pathways was by contrast ventriculography (usually with air). Such a test was unpleasant and could not be frequently repeated. The advent of CT scanning allowed repetitive monitoring of the size of the CSF pathways by a non-invasive technique to be undertaken. This can be used to follow the size of the CSF pathways, particularly after treatment, and any increase in size is usually an indication that pressure is developing and a CSF diversion is required. This particularly applies to the majority of cases of non-communicating hydrocephalus management even after treatment of the causative lesion; if the hydrocephalus does not resolve on CT scanning then it can be reasonably assumed that CSF diversion is required, though if there is doubt then ICP monitoring can be carried out. CT scanning also has a very useful role in monitoring the success or otherwise of CSF diversion operations by sequential scanning at a frequency dictated by the clinical state of the patient.

Intracranial pressure (ICP) monitoring still has a place in distinguishing those cases of communicating hydrocephalus which will respond to CSF diversion and those which might well be due cerebral atrophy and made worse. It is unnecessary for aqueduct stenosis since the mere presence of enlarged ventricles is sufficient evidence that there is both an anatomical and physiological block in the CSF pathways which requires treatment.

Although ICP can be measured from within the ventricle or on the surface of the brain in the case of hydrocephalus it is best monitored from within the ventricle, since it is this component of the intracranial contents which is particularly under test; access is also gained to the CSF for examination of CSF. A frontal burr-hole is fashioned through which a fluid-filled catheter is placed into the frontal horn; a technique first described by Lundberg.[12] The catheter runs to an external pressure-transducer. The result is either displayed real-time on a monitor or for a more permanent record on to a chart recorder. Both methods can be subjected to computer analysis. The record should continue for at least 24 hours. Those with intermittently raised ICP will exhibit some rises of ICP during this time, most commonly during sleep. The pressure may be continuously raised, or paroxysmally with pressure waves lasting either 30 minutes or more (alpha waves) or over periods of 2–10 minutes (beta waves). If alpha waves appear this is a sign of severely raised ICP and it would be wise to terminate the recording by opening the catheter to drain the excess CSF. If the baseline pressure has been more than 10 mm Hg, and more particularly if beta or alpha waves have occurred, then it is clear that CSF diversion is required. If no pressure waves have occurred and the baseline pressure has been normal or only marginally raised during 24 hours then the CSF pathways can be challenged, either abruptly by a bolus injection of normal saline into the ventricles[14,24] or by a continuous slow infusion of normal saline over a few hours.[17,25] An atrophic brain will cope with these challenges by exhibiting no or only a very small rise in ICP; such a patient does not require CSF diversion and might well be made worse. A brain whose CSF pathways are beginning to decompensate will show rises in ICP and even beta waves may be provoked; such a patient requires CSF diversion. If such changes occur during the test then it is wise to aspirate some CSF to return the ventricular pressure to normal levels whilst arrangements are made for operation.

CEREBRAL BLOOD FLOW (CBF)

In 1969 Greitz et al.[26] reported reduced CBF correlated with both ventricular enlargement and neurological deficits in patients with non-tumorous hydrocephalus. Using a CT scan ^{133}Xe method Meyer et al.[27] found that white matter CBF was particularly reduced in periventricular white matter, they suggested that this might well be due to CSF passing from the ventricles into the white matter. Furthermore, cortical grey matter blood flow was also reduced and these changes were different from those occurring in Alzheimer's dementia and multi-infarct dementia. Vorstrup et al.[28] also found a decrease in blood flow in central areas which improved after shunting. But Kushner et al.[29] found that CBF was unaltered by shunting, and this would seem to indicate that autoregulation is unaltered in non-tumorous hydrocephalus. Their findings would also suggest that in some patients, at least, irreversible changes have taken place. Whereas CBF estimations have increased to some extent our knowledge of non-tumorous hydrocephalus, it is doubtful whether they will contribute much in the way of differentiating between non-tumorous hydrocephalus and cerebral atrophy. It would not be unreasonable for those with access to CBF estimations to use this method in further studies, but for those without the facility the other methods mentioned above will be quite adequate.

TREATMENT

There is nothing intrinsically different in the methods of treatment for adults compared to those for children or adolescents. The indications are similar. For non-communicating hydrocephalus this means removal, if possible, of the aetiological lesion first and then CSF diversion if there is continuing persistent hydrocephalus. For communicating hydrocephalus CSF diversion will be required once the CSF is sterile and free from material which can block shunts (for example blood). The range of operations and types of CSF diversions have been discussed in Chapter 6. The vast majority of patients can be adequately treated by either a ventriculoatrial shunt or a ventriculoperitoneal shunt. Due to the fact that body length will not change in an adult, shunt revisions for alterations of the length of shunt tubing are unnecessary in a properly inserted shunt system, unlike the situation that pertains in children. Either the atrial or peritoneal route can be used and both have their protagonists, though it is probably true to state that the majority of neurosurgeons now favour the peritoneal route. Although antisyphon shunt systems are being introduced probably what is more important in preventing over-drainage of CSF is the opening pressure of the valve; in the rigid skull of the adult an opening pressure of between 70–90 mm H_2O will prove satisfactory for the vast majority of patients. For all cases, other than third ventricular masses (see below), in the first instance the burr-hole is placed just above and behind the ear in order to insert the catheter into the body of the lateral ventricle. If ventricular blockages occur then the ventricular catheters can be transposed to the frontal horn.

Occasionally these routes are unsuitable and the lumbarperitoneal route can be used for communicating hydrocephalus, as for example in cases with normal sized ventricles and a pseudomeningocele after posterior fossa surgery (see above), or in cases with persistently malfunctioning shunts. Some neurosurgeons still favour Torkildsen's operation (drainage of CSF by a simple conduit tube from the lateral ventricle to the cisterna magna) for cases of non-communicating hydrocephalus, such as stenosis of the aqueduct of Sylvius. However, it must be pointed out that there are no valves controlling the drainage of CSF is such a system and overdrainage can present problems.

In cases with third ventricular masses, with blockage to the foramina of Monro, bilateral ventricular tubes into the frontal horns are necessary though they may be attached to a common lower end through a T- or Y-connector.

There is a disturbing trend for shunt operations to be thought of as minor procedures, the performance of which may be delegated to inexperienced surgeons. A shunt will dramatically change the intracranial pressure dynamics and have a wide ranging effect on all its components parts. Scrupulous attention to detail is necessary to minimize potential complications and to maximize the efficacy of the shunt.

If CSF diversion is performed for the right reasons in the right patients then recovery can begin immediately, but rehabilitation, in the form of physiotherapy, occupational therapy, and psychological therapy will help maximize such recovery. In addition to arranging rehabilitation, it is mandatory for the neurosurgeon to explain to the immediate relatives the concepts of CSF diversion and to warn them about complications and what symptoms to expect in the advent of a shunt complication so that they will report back early rather be transferred in *extremis*.

Complications

These fall into six main categories:

(1) obstruction

(2) infection

(3) intracranial haematoma

(4) over-drainage

(5) mechanical failure

(6) thromboembolism.

Obstruction

Obstruction of an external ventricular shunt may be insidious, intermittent, or sudden in onset, and the clinical effect corresponds. Where the hydrocephalus was initially of the non-communicating type failure of the shunt produces severe and rapidly progressive symptoms of raised intracranial pressure, often worse than those preceding the operation. If the hydrocephalus was initially communicating the relapse evolves more slowly, probably because the basal cisterns and spinal theca can accommodate some of the CSF which is not passing through the shunt. However, caution must be exercised since it is possible for shunting to convert a communicating into a non-communicating hydrocephalus. The obliteration of the perimesencephalic cistern on CT scanning can be a useful sign of life threatening shunt failure.[30]

Obstructions that are slow in evolution may be suspected by the recurrence of symptoms that occurred initially.

Palpation of either the valve (in the Holter system) or the reservoir (in the Pudenz system) may suggest that:

1. The ventricular catheter is blocked, for the contents can be compressed but the valve/reservoir refills very slowly or not at all.

2. The block lies in the valve or distal catheter, because the valve/reservoir is incompressible.

3. The shunt is apparently working normally.

A normally working shunt should empty easily without resistance and refill within a short time, i.e. 5–30 seconds. The refilling rate will lengthen as the ventricles become smaller and some allowance must be made for this phenomenon. Some shunt systems do not have a palpable reservoir or valve to feel.

The clinical details are paramount and should override any conclusions reached on shunt patency from palpation of the valve/reservoir. If there is any suspicion of a shunt obstruction then it is wiser to evaluate the shunt by a repeat CT scan (looking at the size of the CSF pathways) and to measure the intracranial pressure either through the valve/reservoir or by ventricular tap in the case of non-communicating hydrocephalus or by lumbar puncture for communicating hydrocephalus. The patency of the shunt system can be tested by injecting water-soluble iodine contrast materials into the valve/reservoir (shuntogram); this technique not only outlines the shunt (which can also be seen on plain X-ray since most shunt tubing is impregnated with radio-opaque barium) but, by taking serial X-rays over 30 minutes, also gives an indication of the rate at which the dye is cleared through the system. Recently Graham et al.[31] have advocated using radioactive [99mTc] DTPA (diethylenetriamine pentacetic acid) as a method of performing a shuntogram.

The ventricular catheter may be obstructed by debris or coagulum, by contact with the choroid plexus, or brain as a result of diminution of the size of the ventricle. It is rare for the distal atrial catheter to block in adults once it has been accurately placed.[32] In the case of V–P shunts the distal catheter may become occluded by omentum or peritoneal adhesions as commonly in adults as in children.

The management of a shunt blockage is clear; it must be explored and all aspects of the shunt rechecked at surgery. In the case of recurrent blockages to the ventricular catheter it is often wiser to reposition it in the frontal horn, in the hope that in this position it will be less likely to come into contact with choroid plexus. If the current shunt system cannot be made to work then it will be necessary to change the system i.e. V–A to V–P or vice versa. Caution must also be exercised in attempting to withdraw the ventricular catheter; if it will not come out easily it is unwise to tug hard since it is possible that a ventricular or cerebral haemorrhage may be produced due to the adherence of the catheter to choroid plexus or brain. If the catheter will not come easily it is wiser to amputate it at the brain surface and leave the deeper portion in situ and place a fresh catheter at a different site, usually frontal.

The frequency of shunt blockage seems to depend on the age at which the first shunt was inserted; in neonates and children the incidence is 25–40 per cent within 2 years of operation, and 40–100 per cent at 5 years or longer;[2] in adults the rate is lower, ranging from 7 per cent[32] to 21 per cent.[33] The most important reason for this discrepancy between children and adults relates to the growth of the child and the inability of the shunt system to accommodate, thus children require more operations for the insertion of longer shunt catheters; and generally the adage is that the greater the number of shunt operations the more the likelihood of shunt infection.

Infection

This is more common in children.[34] Renier et al.[35] reported a commendably low rate of 10.5 per cent. The rate in adults should be less than 5 per cent.[32] The reasons for this are two-fold; first, many of the children are infants in whom the level of IgM antibodies, which are required to fight off Gram-negative bacteria, are low;[35] and secondly, series of children contain within their midst those with open myelomeningocele with all the attendant problems of introducing bacteria into the shunt system from an already contaminated CSF. The effects of infection tend to be more numerous and more serious in patients with V–A shunts than those with V–P shunts; the reason being that infection of a V–A shunt may lead to bacteraemia.

Shunt infection is encountered in three main forms:

1. Wound infection from imperfect healing or from faulty technique. The skin over the valve/reservoir may necrose, and this complication can be minimized by ensuring pericranial cover in addition to skin cover. In adults this should be a rare complication and only occur in debilitated patients.

2. Ventriculitis and meningitis may occur from a spread of skin infection, from an open myelomeningocele, or from contamination of the shunt system during operation.

3. Infection of the shunt system may lead to infection within the blood system in the case of V–A shunts; bacterial endocarditis, infected pulmonary embolism, bacteraemia and septicaemia, and proliferating glomerulonephritis have all been described.[2] In the case of V–P shunts peritoneal infections may occur, though usually these are not as devastating as is the case for V–A shunts.

The majority of shunt infections occur immediately or within a few months of insertion; in which case it is difficult to refute the opinion that bacterial contamination occurred during operation. However, in some patients a V–A shunt can work well for many months or even years, seemingly without any evidence of infection, only for a shunt infection to become apparent a short while after a systemic infection (such as pneumonia or urinary tract infection); in such cases it is less easy to incriminate intra-operative contamination.

The most common bacteria is *Staphylococcus epidermidis* (*S. albus*) which is coagulase-negative and is a common skin contaminant. Less commonly *S. aureus, Pseudomonas aeruginosa*, and *Escherichia coli* are found.

The treatment of shunt infections must be aggressive so that the coincidental effects mentioned above are prevented or eliminated. Initially, a course of intravenous antibiotic can be tried, but if the infection has not been eliminated within 7–10 days the shunt system must be removed in its entirety, the hydrocephalus controlled by continuous external ventricular drainage, and again the appropriate antibiotic administered intravenously. A new shunt system can only be inserted after all infection has been eliminated, particularly assessed by a normal cell count in the CSF.

The question of whether or not prophylactic antibiotics should be used at the time of shunt insertion is difficult to answer. The antibiotics can either be given systemically and/or into the shunt at the time of insertion. Again, although there is no proof as to the efficacy, it is probably wise to use prophylactic antibiotics in patients with shunts who are to undergo surgery in other potentially infected areas of the body, such as infected teeth.

Intracranial haematoma

After a hydrocephalus has been drained by the insertion of a shunt system a variable period of time will elapse before the brain can expand and occupy the skull fully. During this period there exists a considerable potential for the formation of subdural haematoma from a ruptured cortical vein leaking into the potential space that exists; this possibility is enhanced by trauma to the head, albeit of a minor nature; this particularly applies if the skull is enlarged. Furthermore, shunts produce a syphon effect when the patient is in the erect or sitting position, whereby the intracranial pressure may be subatmospheric,[36] and for this reason some shunt systems incorporate an antisyphon device; recently a new type of three-stage valve system has been introduced which seeks to mimic the physiological flow of CSF.[37] The incidence of intracranial haematoma was 4 per cent in the series of Illingworth *et al.*[33] and 2 per cent in Jeffreys' series,[32] who felt that the incidence might be lessened by avoiding excessive drainage of CSF during the insertion of the shunt, and by keeping the patient supine for the first 3–4 post-operative days.

Once the complication occurs it can be very difficult to treat. Burr-hole drainage of the haematoma should be attempted first and this may be all that is required. Unfortunately, in some patients the haematoma may recur, and in this event it may be necessary to temporarily clamp off the shunt system for a few days in order to allow the brain to expand and occlude the subdural space.

Over-drainage of CSF

In some patients over-drainage of CSF can occur without necessarily producing an intracranial haematoma. Symptoms such as headache, nausea and vomiting, lethargy, and minimal strabismi can occur typically when in the upright posture and relieved when lying down.[38] To check for this the ICP needs to be tested in different postures. If confirmed, by the finding of low ICP on standing and normal ICP on lying down, the shunt system requires revision and substitution by a new system, either with some form of antisyphon device or a shunt with a higher opening pressure.

Mechanical failure

The modern shunt system is well manufactured and faulty systems are rare. However, it is prudent to check the opening pressure of the system prior to insertion by connecting it to a column of fluid in order that the opening hydrostatic pressure can be verified. Most shunt systems are impregnated with agents which are opaque to X-rays and as a consequence saline cannot easily be seen through the walls; this problem is easily overcome by using a coloured solution (such as methylene blue) which can later be flushed out of the shunt with saline.

Those shunt systems that are not supplied as one piece can come apart at connectors. Careful technique at insertion should prevent this happening spontaneously. However, blows to the head can cause the connectors to come adrift or even fracture the silastic tubing. Such a complication can be suspected by the accumulation of subgaleal CSF; plain X-rays may indicate a gap in the system. Re-exploration of the shunt is necessary.

Thromboembolism

In the earlier days of V–A shunting thromboembolism was a common complication such that Anderson[39] mentioned the presence of pulmonary embolism in 2 out of 12 post-mortem examinations in a series of 36 operations and Friedman *et al.*[40] found pulmonary vascular lesions in 57 per cent of cases reaching autopsy. Since the introduction of modern plastics (silastic) the incidence of this complication appears to have fallen dramatically and little mention is made in more recent series.

Results

The results of non-communicating hydrocephalus relate more to the results of treatment of the aetiological lesion than to the hydrocephalus *per se.* Many treatments can successfully remove the lesion and allow natural healing to re-institute normal CSF pathways. Careful clinical follow-up of such patients together with follow-up CT scanning will ensure that patients make the best possible recovery. It is wise to perform a post-operative CT scan a few weeks after primary treatment of a lesion that causes a non-communicating hydro-cephalus, to check that the CSF pathways are returning to normal. If they are not then CSF diversion must be considered. Moreover, hydrocephalus can develop very insidiously and the possibility must be kept in mind, and if long-term follow-up of patients is not carried out by the surgeon then the general medical practitioner must be warned of this possibility.

In the case of adult non-tumorous hydrocephalus, complete recovery can occur in 35 per cent of patients and useful improvement to social acceptability in another 30 per cent.[18] In some patients the recovery can be quite dramatic with recovery from dementia, incontinence, and a chair-bound existence to the state of being capable of earning a living, and the Wechsler Adult Intelligence Scale (WAIS) can improve by up to 20 points from the pre-operative state. Although the neurological physical deficits can improve very early post-operatively, improvement in intellectual processes is slower and is usually maximal at 3–6 months.[14] The slower recovery of the latter is probably due to the fact that the patient has to re-educate his brain with new learning and retention of data, and thus cross correlate.

It is interesting to speculate why patients improve. One of the more imme-diate effects of CSF diversion is the improvement in cerebral blood flow (CBF) which is diminished beforehand and which quickly improves.[26] The pre-operative CBF is associated with decreased cerebral oxidative, glucose and amino acid metabolism and it is not unreasonable to hypothesize that neurones that are viable, but working at suboptimal efficiency, can improve efficiency with a better blood supply. In the longer term prevention of raised ICP and stretching of the cerebral mantle must also improve the situation, but there is no consistent relationship between increases in CBF and reduction in ventricular size.[27] The improvement in gait may relate to relief of the stretching on the long fibres.[10]

REFERENCES

1. Dandy, W.E. and Blackfan, K.D. Internal hydrocephalus. An experimental, clinical and pathological study. *American Journal of Diseases in Children*, **8**, 406–20 (1914).

2. Milhorat, T.H. *Hydrocephalus and the cerebrospinal fluid*. Williams & Wilkins, Baltimore (1972).

3. Last, R.J. and Tompsett, D.H. Casts of the cerebral ventricles. *British Journal of Surgery*, **40**, 525–35 (1953).

4. Bull, J.W.D. Cerebrospinal fluid pathways. *Neurology*, **11**, 1–20 (1961).

5. Davson, H. and Segal, M.B. Secretion and drainage of the cerebrospinal fluid. *Acta Neurologica Latin America*, (Suppl. 1), **17**, 99–110 (1971).

6. Bering, E.A. and Sato, O. Hydrocephalus: changes in formation and absorption of cerebrospinal fluid within the cerebral ventricles. *Journal of Neurosurgery*, **20**, 1050–9 (1963).

7. Børgesen, S.E. and Gjerris, F. Relationship between intracranial pressure, ventricular size and resistance to outflow. *Journal of Neurosurgery*, **76**, 535–9 (1987).

8. Hakim, S. Algunas observaciones sobre la presion del L.C.R. hidrocefalico en el adulto con 'presion normal'. *Tesis de Grado Universidad Javeriana*, Bogota, Colombia (1964).

9. Kosteljanetz, M. CSF dynamics and pressure–volume relationships in communicating hydrocephalus. *Journal of Neurosurgery*, **64**, 45–52 (1986).

10. Yakovlev, P.I. Hydrocephalus. *American Journal of Mental Deficiency*, **51**, 561–70 (1947).

11. Adams, R.D., Fisher, C.M., Hakim, S., Ojemannn, R.G., and Sweet, W.H. Symptomatic occult hydrocephalus with 'normal' cerebrospinal fluid pressure. A treatable condition. *New England Journal of Medicine*, **273**, 117–30 (1964).

12. Lundberg, N. Continuous recording and control of ventricular fluid pressure in neurosurgical practice. *Acta Psychiatrica Neurologica Scandinavica*, **36** (Suppl. 149), 1–163 (1960).

13. Chawla, J.C., Hulme, A., and Cooper, R. Intracranial pressure in patients with dementia and communicating hydrocephalus. *Journal of Neurosurgery*, **40**, 37–9 (1974).

14. Jeffreys, R.V. and Wood, M.M. Adult non-tumourous dementia and hydrocephalus. *Acta Neurochirugica*, **45**, 103–14 (1978).

15. Di Rocco, C., Di Trapani, G., Maira, G., Bentivoglio, M., Macchi G., and Rossi, G.F. Pathological findings in presenile dementias. *Journal of Neurological Science*, **33**, 437–50 (1977).

16. Symon, L., Dorsch, N.W.C. and Stephens, R.J. Pressure waves in so called normal pressure hydrocephalus. *Lancet*, **iii**, 1291–2 (1972).

17. Katzman, R. and Hussey, F. A simple constant-infusion manometric test for measurement of CSF absorption. II. Clinical studies. *Neurology*, **20**, 665–80 (1970).
18. Pickard, J.D. Adult communicating hydrocephalus. *British Journal of Hospital Medicine*, **7**, 35–44 (1982).
19. Condon, B., Wyper, D., Grant, R., Patterson, J., Hadley, D. and Teasdale, G. Use of magnetic resonance imaging to measure intracranial cerebrospinal fluid volume. *Lancet*, **i**, 1355–7 (1986).
20. Paul, K.S., Lye, R.H., Strang, F.A., and Dutton, J. Arnold–Chiari malformation. *Journal of Neurosurgery*, **58**, 183–7 (1983).
21. Jeffreys, R.V. Hydrocephalus. In *Northfield's textbook of neurosurgery*, (2nd edn), (ed. J.D. Miller, 543–73). Blackwell, London (1987).
22. Wenig, C., Huber, G., and Emde, H. Hydrocephalus after subarachnoid bleeding. *European Neurology* **18**, 1–7 (1979).
23. Jeffreys, R.V. Early complications and results of surgery for ruptured intracranial aneurysms. *Acta Neurochirugica*, **56**, 39–52 (1981).
24. Marmorou, A., Shulman, K., and Rosende, R.M. A non-linear analysis of the cerebrospinal fluid system and intracranial pressure dynamics. *Journal of Neurosurgery*, **48**, 332–44 (1978).
25. Lorenzo, A.V., Bresnan, M.J., and Barlow, C.F. Cerebrospinal fluid absorption deficit in normal pressure hydrocephalus. *Archives of Neurology*, **30**, 387–93 (1974).
26. Greitz, T.V.B., Grepe, A.O.L. and Kalmer, M.S.F. Pre- and post-operative evaluation of cerebral blood flow in low pressure hydrocephalus. *Journal of Neurosurgery*, **31**, 644–51 (1969).
27. Meyer, J.S., Kitagawa, Y., Tanahashi, N., Tachibana, H., Kandula, P., Cech, D.A., Clifton, G.L., and Rose, J.E. Evaluation of treatment of normal pressure hydrocephalus. *Journal of Neurosurgery*, **62**, 513–21 (1985).
28. Vorstrup, S., Christensen, J., Gjerris, F., Sørensen, P.S., Thomsen, A., and Paulson, O.B. Cerebral blood flow in patients with normal pressure hydrocephalus before and after shunting. *Journal of Neurosurgery*, **6**, 379–87 (1987).
29. Kushner, M., Younkin, D., and Weinberger, J. Cerebral haemodynamics in the diagnosis of normal pressure hydrocephalus. *Neurology*, **34**, 96–9 (1984).
30. Johnson, D.L., Fitz, C., McCullough, D.C., and Schwarz, S. Perimesencephalic cistern obliteration: a CT sign of life-threatening shunt failure. *Journal of Neurosurgery*, **64**, 386–9 (1986).
31. Graham, P., Howman-Giles, R., Johnston, I., and Besser, M. Evaluation of CSF shunt patency by means of technetium-99m DPTA. *Journal of Neurosurgery*, **57**, 262–6 (1982).
32. Jeffreys, R.V. The complications of ventriculo–atrial shunting in hydrocephalus. In *Advances in neurosurgery, No. 6* (ed. R. Wullenweber, H. Weker, M. Brock, and M. Klinger) pp. 17–22. Springer, Berlin (1978).
33. Illingworth, R.D., Logue, V., and Symon, L. The ventriculocaval shunt in the treatment of adult hydrocephalus: results and complications in 107 patients. *Journal of Neurosurgery*, **35**, 681–5 (1971).
34. Schoenbaum, D.C., Gardner, P., and Shillito, J. Infections of cerebrospinal shunts: epidemiology, clinical manifestations and therapy. *Journal of Infectious Diseases*, **131**, 543–52 (1975).

35. Renier, D., Lacombe, J., Pierre-Kahn, A., Sainte-Rose, C., and Hirsch, J. Factors causing acute shunt infection. *Journal of Neurosurgery*, **61**, 1072–8 (1984).

36. McCullough, D.C. and Fox, J.L. Negative intracranial pressure. Hydrocephalus in adults and its relationship to the production of subdural hematoma. *Journal of Neurosurgery*, **40**, 272–5 (1974).

37. Sainte-Rose, C., Hooven, M.D., and Hirsch, J. A new approach in the treatment of hydrocephalus. *Journal of Neurosurgery*, **66**, 213–26 (1987).

38. Foltz, E.L. and Blanks, J.P. Symptomatic low intracranial pressure in shunted hydrocephalus. *Journal of Neurosurgery*, **68**, 401–8 (1988).

39. Anderson, F.M. Ventriculo–auriculostomy in treatment of hydrocephalus. *Journal of Neurosurgery*, **16**, 551–9 (1959).

40. Friedman, S., Zita-Gozum, C., and Chatten, J. Pulmonary vascular changes complicating ventriculovascular shunting for hydrocephalus. *Journal of Paediatrics*, **64**, 305–14 (1964).

9 Psychiatric disorders in patients with hydrocephalus

J. Corbett, S. Cumella, B. Chipchase

INTRODUCTION

The emotional and behavioural problems associated with hydrocephalus arise from an interaction between a number of factors:

(1) the stage at which the hydrocephalus occurs, together with the extent, site, and nature of brain damage or dysfunction;

(2) the presence of spina bifida;

(3) the presence of associated physical impairment, such as paraplegia, epilepsy, or incontinence;

(4) the extent and degree of any specific or generalized psychological impairment;

(5) the disability of the individual patient, and his caring network arising from these impairments.

It follows that the psychiatric complications of hydrocephalus will vary considerably depending upon whether it is associated with spina bifida, whether shunting has been performed, or if the hydrocephalus has been arrested spontaneously. The changing pattern of psychiatric morbidity is reflected in the literature of the past 30 years, following the introduction of the Spitz–Holter valve. These early developments are recorded largely in the *Proceedings of the Society for Research into Hydrocephalus and Spina Bifida.* Prior to this period, prognosis was particularly poor for children with progressive hydrocephalus, and survival into adult life was unusual. The sight of untreated hydrocephalic in infants nursed with loving care in institutions will be engraved on the memories of visitors.

The introduction of the Spitz–Holter valve led to increased interest in the intellectual functioning of children who were shunted and those who had arrested spontaneously. Initially there was most concern with global cognitive performance, but an interest in the 'Cocktail Party Syndrome' has persisted, with an increasing delineation of specific cognitive defects. During the past decade there have been a number of reports of the impact on families on learning of the diagnosis of spina bifida. To this must be added the stress of coping with disabilities which could be multiple and severe where non-selective surgery was practised. Recently there have been reports of the social adjustment and psychiatric morbidity in survivors of this early treatment who have reached adolescence and early adult life.

The literature on the psychiatric aspects of arrested and normal pressure hydrocephalus in adult life has been relatively sparse and anecdotal, but the introduction of non-invasive brain imaging has unveiled a potential for research which has yet to be fully realized. Because the pattern of disability has changed radically, it is difficult to assess psychiatric disorder, or give prevalence rates for it. But a number of factors may be identified which could guide management. In this chapter, studies of intellectual functioning, psychiatric morbidity and disability, impact on families of the diagnosis, and social adjustment of older children and adolescents will be considered.

COGNITIVE FUNCTIONING

Hagberg[1] in 1962 reviewing 'The sequelae of spontaneously arrested infantile hydrocephalus' pointed out that it constitutes a syndrome in which relatively slow, mild, and transient adverse influences have been influencing the brain. The consequences of what was then termed 'minimal brain dysfunction' were studied in 26 children selected from a larger Swedish series of untreated cases of hydrocephalus. Many of the children were late in their mental development and five had suffered convulsions. Signs of ataxia were common, occurring in six cases, but cerebral palsy was only occasionally seen. Intelligence tests using the Terman–Merrill Scale showed variations in intellectual capacity larger than would be expected in a healthy population, and behavioural difficulties occurred particularly in those in the lower IQ groups and with neurological abnormalities.[1]

In a study of 16 children selected from 700 seen in a cerebral palsy clinic, who had a head circumference above the 97th percentile, Ingram and Naughton[2] found that intelligence was in the normal range and they also identified the behavioural symptoms which they called the 'chatterbox' syndrome. The term 'Cocktail Party' Syndrome[3] has, however, continued to win favour and perhaps best encapsulates the particular behavioural characteristics which are seen in a proportion of cases. Subsequently a number of reports appeared confirming that some children with hydrocephalus talk excessively and that their speech is lacking in content. Taylor[4] pointed out that these children do well in repeating stories from memory but were unable to explain their content. The limits of their language abilities were reflected in their responses to intelligence tests so that they did well on some verbal tasks, such as picture vocabulary tests, but failed on other tasks which required reasoning and comprehension. Parsons[5] found no difference in vocabulary learning scores between controls and children with spina bifida and hydrocephalus, although the full scale IQ in the control group was higher. Swisher and Pinsker,[6] examining 11 severely affected children with spina bifida and hydrocephalus, recorded ten minutes conversation on magnetic tape and analysed these conversations using the Illinois Test for Psycholinguistic Abilities (ITPA). They found more bizarre speech and poorer language function in the affected children when compared with controls, and they also found delay in speech development until two years of age followed by a rapid increase in production.

Further investigation of a group of 14 hydrocephalic children by Miller and Sethi[7] suggested that the children also had a severe deficit in the perception of visuospatial relationships. Studies of 145 children aged three years with spina bifida and cranium bifidum by Spain,[8] Anderson,[9,10] Anderson and Spain,[11] and Anderson and Plewis[12] showed that the 96 children who required a shunt to control their hydrocephalus had lower mean scores on all tests compared with children without shunts, particularly in the non-verbal tests. Only one-third of the children with shunts seemed to be developing normally, and many of these children had moderate or severe physical handicap. Children with shunts and with below average scores on performance tests also tended to show poor verbal ability scores and 40 per cent of this group were rated as 'hyperverbal'. These children showed a characteristic pattern of scores on the verbal scales with good syntax but poor comprehension and inability to use language creatively. Tew and Laurence[13] reporting on the findings in a cohort of spina bifida cases born in South Wales between 1964 and 1966, the majority of whom had hydrocephalus, showed that the scores of the children with spina bifida alone were closer to those of normal children but still below average. Of the 59 children who were compared with a group of matched controls, eight with a spontaneously 'arrested' hydrocephalus were in the dull backward range of abilities (mean IQ 83.8) and 31 with shunt treated hydrocephalus had a lower mean score of 70 with half functioning within the retarded range. Abnormal visuoperceptual function closely correlated with defects in intelligence and the results of school attainment tests paralleled the distribution of intelligence, although many children were found to be functioning below expectation for both age and measured ability. Richardson,[14] describing two cases of spontaneously arrested hydrocephalus whose educational progress appeared normal, found that on examination they had a reduced performance IQ but normal verbal IQ. They showed a significant impairment in immediate free recall when their memory was tested and they suggested that impairment of verbal memory might be an important underlying defect. Cull and Wyke[15] investigating memory in ten children with spina bifida compared with ten matched for IQ but without physical impairment and ten controls found a difficulty in learning unrelated verbal material in those with hydrocephalus.

Boccher and colleagues,[16] found no significant relationship between ventricular size (as estimated by ventriculography prior to surgery) and subsequent intellectual development in 13 shunted children who were leading normal social lives for their age group. Tew[17] reviewed the subject of the 'Cocktail Party Syndrome' in the 59 surviving children of the South Wales cohort of children with spina bifida and hydrocephalus born between 1964 and 1966 and studied at the age of five. Those children with the 'Cocktail Party Syndrome' differed from the other children in having significantly lower scores on the Wechsler Scales and very retarded social skills. They confirmed the finding that visuoperceptual abilities were also significantly worse. They reported that the verbal fluency of children with the 'Cocktail Party Syndrome' did not, however, lead to superior scores on the Reynell Expressive Language Scales, for these children found difficulty in using language creatively in spite of good syntax. Further studies of these children at the age of seven showed them to be significantly worse than other cases of spina bifida, in reading, spelling and arithmetic, and they all had a shorter concentration span and slightly more behavioural problems in school according to their teachers. There was evidence that the 'Cocktail Party Syndrome' declines with age and its presence at the age of ten is indicative of a lower level of intelligence. The children with this syndrome were more likely to be female and to be less intelligent than the boys, and it was suggested that this was because they had more severe physical handicaps. The condition was much commoner among shunted children than those with spontaneously arrested hydrocephalus and this may be also related to their lower level of ability.

Billard and colleagues[18] and Dennis and colleagues,[19] reviewing the previous studies of intelligence in hydrocephalic children, concluded that it was related to the type of hydrocephalus,[13,20–22] the thickness of the cortical mantle before and after treatment,[23,24] the brain mass,[25] and the need for a shunt, as has been previously described. No significant relationship was found in reported studies between the level of intelligence and the rate of increase of head size,[23,26] critical cortical thickness before shunt treatment,[22] the severity of hydrocephalus prior to surgery, 'head circumference', the degree of paralytic defect, or the number of shunt revisions. In their own study of 78 children with hydrocephalus Billard and colleagues[18] found that the common outcome of early hydrocephalus is an uneven development of intelligence during childhood. Non-verbal intelligence developed less well than verbal intelligence. This selective cognitive defect did not have its origin in the hydrocephalic condition itself, or in the treatment, but rather in the developmental brain anomalies and associated disabilities to which the hydrocephalic child is prone. These include (in children with aqueduct stenosis and other non-communicating hydrocephalus) a selectively thin cortex, ocular abnormalities, motor deficits, and seizures.

The specific cognitive impairments seen in children with hydrocephalus include perceptual–motor abnormalities, and these are not readily explicable on the basis of gross neuropathology and enlarged ventricular size. It was suggested by Miller and Sethi[7] that the phenomena might be due to stretching of the fibres of the corpus callosum resulting in partial callosum dysfunction, but this was not supported by the studies of Zeiner and Prigatano.[27] Neither of these studies consider the possibility that generalized stretching of association fibres might be implicated, as suggested by MacNab,[28] and the striking finding of superior cognitive achievement in some subjects with considerable hydrocephalus, but presumably normal brain mass, is not fully explained.[29] Lonton,[30] examining the

CT scan appearances of 261 children with meningomyelocele and 98 children with hydrocephalus alone, found a significant relationship between the CT appearances and the performance IQ but not verbal IQ.

Horn and colleagues[31] tested the hypothesis that children with spina bifida and hydrocephalus are more distractible than normal children and that the distractibility partially accounts for the language deficits. Fifteen primary school children with spina bifida and hydrocephalus were compared with controls matched for mental age on a non-verbal task. It was found that hydrocephalic children were more easily distracted and showed more vocabulary deficits when irrelevant items were present. Dennis and colleagues[19] also found that language development was not uniform in their study of the intelligence of hydrocephalic children.

Summarizing the effect of hydrocephalus on cognitive functioning, specific abnormalities, including the 'Cocktail Party Syndrome', are found in which there is good vocabulary and syntax but poor comprehension. Motor difficulties, visuospatial abnormalities, and memory defects which are also seen may relate to underlying distractibility, but the neuropathological basis for these disabilities remains a topic for future study.

PSYCHIATRIC DISORDER

Although many of the studies mentioned previously described behavioural difficulties, there have been few systematic studies of the prevalence of psychiatric disorder in children with spina bifida and hydrocephalus. Connell and McConnel[32] studied 45 children of school age who had been treated surgically for hydrocephalus in the early months of life; there were 25 boys and 20 girls. They administered a standardized rating scale completed by parents and teachers together with semi-structured interviews of parents and children. By the middle years of childhood, a baby born with hydrocephalus was at least four times as likely as his normal peers to develop psychiatric disorder. This was related to the degree of brain damage, associated physical handicaps, shunt malfunction requiring periods in hospital, and to other psychosocial factors. Psychiatric disorder was more common in boys and was associated with low intelligence, perceptual and dyspraxia problems, together with hyperkinesia. The coping mechanisms of the child were closely related to parental attitudes towards him and their management of the child's disabilities. It was concluded that the predominance of emotional disorder suggested that early intervention, through family counselling and efforts to strengthen the child's defences for coping with his multifarious problems, could improve the quality of life.

IMPACT ON THE FAMILY

A number of studies have examined the effect on the family of the birth of a handicapped child. Murdoch[33–35] examined the way in which the parents of 109 children with spina bifida, born in Scotland over the previous ten years, were told about the diagnosis and compared these with the families of 123 children with Down syndrome. One-third of the mothers of children with Down syndrome, and half of the mothers of children with the spina bifida, realized that something was different before they were told of the diagnosis.

Murdoch concluded that the way in which the parents were told about their baby's abnormality could be of crucial importance for the future development of the child. It was found that over one-third of the mothers of children with Down syndrome and half of the mothers of spina bifida sufferers were given little opportunity to discuss their feelings and anxieties about the baby. Only a minority were referred to social workers whilst in hospital, and their separation from the child shortly after birth was a significant factor, so that 61 per cent of the mothers of spina bifida children never saw their child during the stay in hospital, and subsequently received little emotional support.

Bearing in mind that nearly all children with spina bifida aperta subsequently develop hydrocephalus, the following studies are relevant. Charney[36] interviewed parents of 50 children with spina bifida born in Philadelphia between 1978 and 1982. Of the 47 mothers and 29 fathers interviewed, only 26 were satisfied with the information which they received after the delivery, although 61 felt that the information given at the tertiary care hospital was adequate. Satisfaction was significantly more common when parents had been involved in decisions about the management of their new-born infant. Most felt that they should have the final decision about the medical management of their child. Although decisions about surgical closure of the lesion in spina bifida have to be made rapidly, Charney found that there was usually sufficient time for comprehensive discussion, counselling, and emotional support for parents before requiring them to decide whether or not to consent to proceed with surgical management. Hare and colleagues,[37,38] studying the South Wales cohort of 120 families, concluded that there was a need for care, skill, and sympathy in telling parents about the malformation. Parents associations and specialized social workers, together with the referral of a child to a specialized centre, must be regarded as acceptable service provision.

Although initial feelings may be of shocked disbelief and denial, the common immediate reaction is one of guilt and feelings of responsibility mixed with grief and confusion and a sense of personal inadequacy. An understanding of the genetic background and of the chances of recurrence in future pregnancies does little at this stage to assuage this sense of responsibility. Any process of selection produces particular emotional reactions whether it follows uniform early closure of the back or not.[39,40] Although parents of children not selected for active treatment may suffer a distorted grief reaction, this may be less traumatic than that following surgery with its promise of survival.

The death of any child should not be seen as the end of the episode, and social case work needs to continue over a period of several months until mourning is over and emotional equilibrium restored. Richardson and Goodall[41] and Delight and Goodall[42,43] have reported in detail on the experiences of families of 98 untreated children born between 1971 and 1981 at one centre, giving valuable guidance on management emphasizing that even a short life can be of great value, both to that child's family and to a wider society.

It is tempting to suggest that the counselling and support which families need could be provided by the domiciliary team of the general practitioner, health visitor, and social worker. The evidence from most studies is that it is uncommon in community practice for comprehensive support to be forthcoming, and a specialist team is desirable consulting closely with the primary care and district handicap services.

Query and colleagues,[44] carried out a retrospective study of patients shunted for hydrocephalus and their families, studying the impact of living with chronic illness. In doing this they followed 36 patients previously studied 20 years earlier. The small size of the sample is compensated for by the detailed interviews with the subjects and their families. Despite reports by parents and siblings of severe financial and emotional stress, most judged the quality of their family relationships and lives to be good. The poorest social outcomes were in those with an unfavourable medical outlook and/or questionable prospects for future independence, or both.

Attention has already been paid to specific disabilities, and Scott *et al.*[45] examined the psychosexual problems of 26 patients with spina bifida aged between 12–16 years. They interviewed the subjects and their parents using a structured questionnaire. Particular attention was paid to problems related to urinary diversion and those wearing penile appliances. Very few of the children knew much about the nature of their disability or the reasons for having had surgery. Their ignorance was thought to reflect their parents' lack of knowledge resulting in repression of feelings and denial of problems by the families.

It was recommended that the full implication of urinary diversion be clearly explained to the parents and to the children as they grow older, and that support and counselling be made more readily available to deal with psychosexual problems.

Dorner[46] interviewed 40 adolescents with spina bifida at home to find out how they felt about their situation. Some degree of misery was very common, but this was more likely to be severe in the girls than in the boys. About half the girls had, on some occasion in the past year, felt that life was not worth living. It was concluded that these feelings were related to their social isolation outside school and that they might be alleviated by improved opportunity for contact with peers.

As with many of the studies of the psychosocial impact of hydrocephalus and spina bifida on individuals and their families there was no control group in this study and it must be remembered that nearly half of normal adolescents report similar feelings of adolescent turmoil.[47] It is reasonable to conclude, however, that such feelings are likely to be more severe in children with multiple disability.

In Dorner's study[46] half of those who had left school were either unemployed or very dissatisfied with their job, and in addition to worries about work they reported preoccupations concerning sexual relationships, sexual function, and marriage. About two-thirds of the teenagers hoped to get married and half of these thought they could have children, but girls were particularly worried about their capacity to conceive and boys had understandable concerns about potency. Very few had consulted anyone about this, and Dorner pointed out a clear need for adequate counselling of adolescents to enable them to distinguish between real and imagined fears about the consequences of their condition.

In a more recent study, Cromer et al.[48] studied the level of knowledge, attitudes, and activity related to sexuality in a group of 21 adolescents and young adults with meningomyelocele, a group of control relatives, and a group of adolescents with cystic fibrosis matched for age and sex. Slightly more than half of the sample were female; the mean age was 17.2 years and their backgrounds were mainly middle class. Twenty eight per cent of the myelodysplastic group reported previous sexual activity compared with 60 per cent of the controls and 43 per cent of those with cystic fibrosis. As in Dorner's study[46] most of the disabled adolescents expressed a desire to marry and have children, but fewer than 20 per cent had sought information about their sexual or reproductive function from their physician, while only 16 per cent of those with myelo-dysplasia who reported sexual activity had used contraception, emphasizing the need for sex education and contraceptive advice.

Lord and colleagues[49] from California examined the social and academic implications of mainstream, mainstream and special class combined, or segregated special school for 31 adolescents with spina bifida. This elegant study is particularly relevant to the move towards integrated education for disabled pupils in other parts of the world.

They administered the Peabody Picture Vocabulary Test and UCLA Loneliness Scale (Adolescents) as well as the Personality Inventory for Children (Caretakers). Adolescents in mainstream classes had the most normal scores for academic and social skills. Those in combined classes had intermediate scores, while those in specialized classes had the lowest scores. Paradoxically adolescents in combined classes reported the least loneliness, and this study suggested that even in young people with relatively good social skills mainstream placement was associated with a greater subjective experience of loneliness than combined placement.

Lord and colleagues[49] also found from interviewing parents and carers that there was difficulty not only in acknowledging their child's problems, but also their own psychological discomfort and the stress placed on families as a result of the disability. Parents of students in the combined educational placements seemed to have most difficulty and the reason for this was unclear.

Much has been written about the denial, sadness, guilt, and stress that can chronically affect the parents of disabled children with spina bifida,[50–52] but parents' discomfort may also arise from uncertainty about their child's true status and potential. This is particularly likely to occur in the case of hydrocephalus, where the child's superficial verbal facility may lead to an overestimate of their academic and social potential. Inappropriate expectations, which may not be realized because of the child's more severe performance difficulties, may lead to role failure and secondary emotional and behavioural reactions which can affect the whole family.

Lord and colleagues[49] point out that professionals often refuse to provide a specific functional prognosis for an individual child, and parents often find themselves bewildered and anxious. In that context, ill-judged attempts at integration through combined placements could be interpreted as yet another confusing message about the child's potential, thus generating more anxiety than mainstream or full-time special school placements, which leave less room for doubt.

The poor prognosis of children undergoing unselective early treatment is emphasized by the findings of follow-up studies carried out by Lorber[53] and more recently by Hunt.[54] The latter study reviewed the outcome in 117 cases treated unselectively from birth, between 1963 and 1971 in Cambridge, who were followed up for between 16–20 years. Forty eight had died before their sixteenth birthday and of the survivors 60 had had a shunt inserted. Two were blind following shunt malfunction; 22 were mentally retarded with an IQ of less than 80; 35 were wheelchair dependent; 52 were incontinent, and 32 of these need help to manage their incontinence; 9 weighed more than 75 kg, and one-third of both sexes had undergone precocious puberty; three had insulin-dependent diabetes, while 12 continued to need anticonvulsant drugs for the treatment of epilepsy; 32 had suffered from pressure sores, and only 33 were unable to live without help or supervision, whilst only 17 were capable of open employment.

Both these studies emphasized the high degree of multiple disability in cohorts of children born and first treated during the era of unselective surgery who are now surviving into adult life. The degree of long-term disability following selective surgical management will undoubtedly be much less,[55–57] but the longer term outcome remains to be documented, and the studies of children subjected to unselective surgery remain a salutary reminder of the complexity and severity of disability in the worst situation.

It will be noted that most of the literature on the psychiatric aspects of hydrocephalus concerns the complex pattern of disability in those with spina bifida. While it is possible that uncomplicated arrested hydrocephalus is not usually complicated by psychiatric disorder it seems more likely that it has not been subject to systematic study or that, as in the case of spina bifida, psychiatric disorder is related more to the underlying cause of brain damage, for example meningitis or cerebral malformation, or to associated disability such as epilepsy, than to the hydrocephalus itself.

'NORMAL PRESSURE' HYDROCEPHALUS

Rice and Gendelman[58] reported on the psychiatric symptomatology of five patients with normal pressure hydrocephalus, originally described by Adams,[59,60] these patients aged 61–77 years presented with organic brain syndromes, including dementia. Rice and Gendelman[58] pointed out that in all the cases the symptomatology was non-specific and the presenting complaint was often related to pre-existing emotional or personality difficulties, but that an abrupt change in personality should lead to the possibility of such a diagnosis.

Price and Tucker[61] and Lying-Tunell[62] report cases presenting with both clear cut depressive symptomatology and periodic psychosis, with paranoid delusional ideation and auditory hallucinosis occurring before the onset of clear-cut dementia or gait disturbance. These patients had received prolonged psychiatric treatment including ECT before a diagnosis of normal pressure hydrocephalus was made and ventriculoatrial shunting carried out.

A prospective study of 25 adult patients with normal pressure hydrocephalus was reported by Jeffreys and Wood[63] emphasizing the clinical picture of disabling dementia associated with psychomotor retardation, imbalance of gait, and urinary incontinence. They preferred the term non-tumorous dementia to normal pressure or normotensive hydrocephalus, as they found, from intracranial pressure monitoring over 24-hour periods, that there were cases with intermittently raised pressure. They felt that their description would exclude not only tumours but also conditions causing internal hydrocephalus, such as third ventricular cysts and aqueduct stenosis, and recommended that any patient under the age of 70 years suffering from dementia, in the absence of any clear-cut neurological causes for it, should be suspected of hydrocephalus and investigated. They also felt that care should be taken only to embark on ventricular shunting when psychometric assessment, intracranial pressure monitoring, and the appearance of the lateral ventricles indicate a good prognosis.

This is not to deny that functional psychosis may occur in patients with arrested hydrocephalus and this may respond to psychiatric treatment, including ECT.[64]

Finally the possibility of 'occult' hydrocephalus leading to dementia should not be dismissed. Corbett *et al.*[65] described the case of a 36-year-old woman with XO mosaicism (Turner syndrome) and marked webbing of the neck who developed a poorly controlled seizure disorder at the age of nine. Her intellectual deterioration and gait imbalance developing later in life was initially diagnosed as due to anticonvulsant intoxication and 'epileptic dementia', until she was found to be suffering from obstructive hydrocephalus. It is this sort of case which illustrates the importance of the accurate differential diagnosis of progressive hydrocephalus as the most important single cause of dementia spanning birth to senility.

CONCLUSION

The psychopathological associations of hydrocephalus provide a window on the mind which merits close attention and investigation. The psychological complications of arrested hydrocephalus and the complex of disabilities associated with spina bifida illustrate the impact of neurological impairment not only on the developing individual but on the family and wider caring network. The onset of hydrocephalus in adult life is an important and potentially treatable condition which, therefore, should always be suspected in appropriate circumstances and which requires close collaboration between the psychiatrist, psychologist, and neurosurgeon.

REFERENCES

1. Hagberg, B. The sequelae of spontaneously arrested infantile hydrocephalus. *Developmental Medicine and Child Neurology*, **4**, 583–7 (1962).
2. Ingram, T.T.S. and Naughton, J.A. Paediatric and psychological aspects of cerebral palsy associated with hydrocephalus. *Developmental Medicine and Child Neurology*, **4**, 287–92 (1962).
3. Hagberg, B. and Sjorgen, I. The chronic brain syndrome in infantile hydrocephalus. *American Journal of Diseases in Children*, **112**, 189–96 (1966).
4. Taylor, E.M. *Psychological appraisal of children with cerebral defects*. Harvard University Press, Cambridge, Mass. (1961).
5. Parsons, J.G. An investigation into the verbal facility of hydrocephalus children with special reference to vocabulary, morphology and fluency. *Developmental Medicine and Child Neurology*, Supplement 16, 109–10 (1968).
6. Swisher, L.P. and Pinsker, E.J. The language characteristics of hyperverbal, hydrocephalic children. *Developmental Medicine and Child Neurology*, **13**, 746–55 (1971).
7. Miller, E. and Sethi, L. The effect of hydrocephalus perception. *Developmental Medicine and Child Neurology*, **13** (Suppl. 25), 77–81 (1971).
8. Spain, B. Verbal and performance ability in preschool children with spina bifida. *Developmental Medicine and Child Neurology*, **16**, 773–80 (1974).
9. Anderson, E.M. Cognitive deficits in children with spina bifida and hydrocephalus: a review of the literature. *British Journal of Educational Psychology*, **45**, 257–68 (1975).
10. Anderson, E.M. The psychological and social adjustment of adolescents with cerebral palsy or spina bifida and hydrocephalus. *International Journal of Rehabilitation Research*, **2**, 245–7 (1979).
11. Anderson, E.M. and Spain, B. *The child with spina bifida*, p. 34. Methuen & Co. Ltd., London (1977).
12. Anderson, E.M. and Plewis, I. Impairment of a motor skill in children with spina bifida cystica and hydrocephalus: an exploratory study. *British Journal of Psychology*, **68**, 61–70 (1977).

13. Tew, B. and Laurence, K.M. The effects of hydrocephalus on intelligence, visual perception and school attainment. *Developmental Medicine and Child Neurology*, **17** (Suppl. 35), 129–34 (1975).

14. Richardson, J.T.E. Memory and intelligence following spontaneously arrested congenital hydrocephalus. *British Journal of Social and Clinical Psychology*, **17**, 261–7 (1978).

15. Cull, C. and Wyke, M.A. Memory function of children with spina bifida and shunted hydrocephalus. *Developmental Medicine and Child Neurology*, **26**, 177–83 (1984).

16. Boccher, J., Jacobsen, S., Gyldensted, C., Harmsen, A., and Gloerfelt-Tarp, B. Intellectual development and brain size in 13 shunted hydrocephalic children. *Neuropadiatrie*, **9**, 369–77 (1978).

17. Tew, B. The 'Cocktail Party Syndrome' in children with hydrocephalus and spina bifida. *British Journal of Disorders of Communication*, **14**, 89–101 (1979).

18. Billard, C., Santini, J.J., Gillet, P., Nargeot, M.C., and Adrien, J.L. Long-term intellectual prognosis of hydrocephalus with reference to 77 children. *Paediatric Neuroscience*, **12**, 219–25 (1985).

19. Dennis, M., Fitz, L.R., Netley, C.T., Sugar, J., Harwood-Nash, D.C.F., Hendrick, E.B., Hoffman, H.J., and Humphreys, R.P. The intelligence of hydrocephalic children. *Archives of Neurology*, **38**, 607–15 (1981).

20. Badell-Ribera, A., Schulman, K., and Paddock, N. The relationship non-progressive hydrocephalus to intellectual functioning in children. *Pediatrics*, **37**, 787–93 (1966).

21. Soare, P. and Raimondi, A.J. Intellectual and perceptual motor characteristics of treated myelomeningocele children. *American Journal of Diseases of Children*, **131**, 199–204 (1977).

22. Tromp, C.N., Van den Burg, W., and Jansen, A. Nature and severity of hydrocephalus and its relation to later intellectual function. *Zeitschrift für Kinderchirurgie*, **28**, 354–60 (1979).

23. Hunt, G.M. and Holmes, A.E. Some factors relating to intelligence in treated children with spina bifida cystica. *Developmental Medicine and Child Neurology*, **35**, 65–70 (1975).

24. Young, H.F., Nulsen, F.E., and Weiss, M.H. The relationship of intelligence and cerebral mantle in treated infantile hydrocephalus. *Paediatrics*, **52**, 54–60 (1973).

25. Shurtleff, A.B., Foltz, E.L., and Loeser, J.B. Hydrocephalus: A definition of its progression and relationship to intellectual function, diagnosis and complications. *American Journal of Diseases of Children*, **125**, 688–93 (1973).

26. Hunt, G.M. and Holmes, A.E. Factors relating to intelligence in treated cases of spina bifida cystica. *American Journal of Diseases of Children*, **130**, 823–7 (1976).

27. Zeiner, H.K. and Prigatano, G.P. Information processing deficits in hydrocephalus and letter reversal children. *Neuropsychologia*, **20**, 483–92 (1982).

28. MacNab, G.H. The development of the knowledge and treatment of hydrocephalus. *Developmental Medicine and Child Neurology*, **8** (Suppl. 11), 1–9 (1969).

29. Lorber, J. Is your brain really necessary? *Science*, **210**, 1232–4 (1980).

30. Lonton, A.P. The relationship between intellectual skills and the computerised axial tomograms of children with spina bifida and hydrocephalus. *Kinderchirurgie und Grenzgebiete*, **28**, 368–74 (1979).

31. Horn, D.G., Pugzleslorch, E., Lorch, R.F. Jr, and Culatta, B. Distractibility and vocabulary deficits in children with spina bifida and hydrocephalus. *Developmental Medicine and Child Neurology*, **27**, 713–20 (1985).

32. Connell, H.M. and McConnel, T.S. Psychiatric sequelae in children treated operatively for hydrocephalus in infancy. *Developmental Medicine and Child Neurology*, **23**, 505–17 (1981).

33. Murdoch, J.C. Communication of the diagnosis of Down's Syndrome and spina bifida in Scotland 1971–1981. *Journal of Mental Deficiency Research*, **27**, 247–53 (1983).

34. Murdoch, J.C. Immediate post-natal management of the mothers of Down's syndrome and spina bifida children in Scotland 1971–1981. *Journal of Mental Deficiency Research*, **28**, 67–72 (1984).

35. Murdoch, J.C. Experience of the mothers of Down's syndrome and spina bifida children on going home from hospital in Scotland 1971–1981. *Journal of Mental Deficiency Research*, **28**, 123–7 (1984).

36. Charney, E.B. Parental attitudes toward management of newborns with myelomeningocoele. *Developmental Medicine and Child Neurology*, **32**, 14–9 (1990).

37. Hare, E.H., Laurence, K.M., Paynes, H., and Rawnsley, K. Spina bifida cystica and family stress. *British Medical Journal*, **2**, 757–60 (1966).

38. Hare, E.H., Laurence, K.M., Payne, H., and Rawnsley, K. *Spina bifida and family stress. Research into Hydrocephalus and Spina Bifida, Spastics Society*, pp. 28–32. Wm. Heinemann, London (1967).

39. Matson, D.D. *Neurosurgery of infancy and childhood*. Charles C. Thomas, Springfield, Ill. (1969).

40. Tew, B. and Laurence, K.M. The ability and attainments of spina bifida patients born in South Wales between 1956–1962. *Developmental Medicine and Child Neurology*, **14** (Suppl. 27), 124 (1972).

41. Richardson, S.A. and Goodall, J. Trends in the management of spina bifida babies, 1971–81: home care for non-surgical group. *Maternal and Child Health*, **9** (8), 252–7 (1984).

42. Delight, E. and Goodall, J. Babies with spina bifida treated without surgery: parents' views on home versus hospital care. *British Medical Journal*, **297**, 1230–3 (1988).

43. Delight, E. and Goodall, J. Love and loss: Conversations with parents of babies with spina bifida managed without surgery 1971–1978. *Developmental Medicine and Child Neurology*, **32** (Suppl. 61), 1–58 (1990).

44. Query, J.M., Reichelt, C., and Christoferson, L.A. Living with a chronic illness: a retrospective study of patients shunted for hydrocephalus and their families. *Developmental Medicine and Child Neurology*, **32**, 119–28 (1990).

45. Scott, M., Roberts, E.G.G., and Tew, B. Psychosexual problems of adolescent spina bifida patients. *Developmental Medicine and Child Neurology*, **17** (Suppl. 35), 158–9 (1975).

46. Dorner, S. Adolescents with spina bifida — How they see their situation. *Archives of Disease in Childhood*, **51**, 439 (1976).

47. Rutter, M., Graham, P., Chadwick, O., and Yule, W. Adolescent turmoil: fact or fiction? *Journal of Child Psychology and Psychiatry*, **17**, 35–6 (1976).

48. Cromer, B.A., Enrille, B., McCoy, B., Gerhardstein, M.J., Fitzpatrick, M., and Judis, J. Knowledge, attitudes and behaviour related to sexuality in adolescents with chronic disability. *Developmental Medicine and Child Neurology*, **32**, 602–10 (1990).

49. Lord, J., Varzos, N., Behrman, B., Wicks, J., and Wicks D. Implications of mainstream classrooms for adolescents with spina bifida. *Developmental Medicine and Child Neurology*, **32**, 20–9 (1990).

50. Freeston, B. An enquiry into the effect of a spina bifida child upon family life. *Developmental Medicine and Child Neurology*, **13**, 456–61 (1971).

51. Walker, J.H., Thomas, M., and Russell, I.T. Spina bifida and the parents. *Developmental Medicine and Child Neurology*, **13**, 462–76 (1971).

52. Martin, P. Marital breakdown in families of patients with spina bifida cystica. *Developmental Medicine and Child Neurology*, **17**, 757–64 (1975).

53. Lorber, J. Results of treatment of myelomeningocoele. *Developmental Medicine and Child Neurology*, **13**, 279–303 (1971).

54. Hunt, G.M. Open spina bifida: outcome for a complete cohort treated unselectively and followed into adulthood. *Developmental Medicine and Child Neurology*, **32**, 108–18 (1990).

55. Stark, G.D. and Drummond, M. Results of early selective operation in meningomyelocoele. *Archives of Disease in Childhood*, **48**, 476–83 (1973).

56. Gross, R.H. Newborns with myelodysplasia: the rest of the story. *New England Journal of Medicine*, **312**, 1632–4 (1985).

57. Evans, R.C., Tew, B., Thomas, M.D., and Ford J. Selective surgical management of neural tube malformations. *Archives of Disease in Childhood*, **60**, 415–19 (1985).

58. Rice, E.M. and Gendelman, S. Psychiatric aspects of normal pressure hydrocephalus. *Journal of the American Medical Association*, **223**, 409–12 (1973).

59. Hakin, S. and Adams, R.D. The special clinical problem of symptomatic hydrocephalus with normal cerebrospinal fluid pressure. *Journal of Neurological Science*, **2**, 307–27 (1965).

60. Adams, R. D., Fisher, C. M., Hakin, S., Ojemann, R. D., and Sweet W. H. Symptomatic occult hydrocephalus with 'normal' cerebrospinal fluid pressure. *New England Journal of Medicine*, **273**, 117–26 (1965).

61. Price, T.R.P. and Tucker, G.J. Psychiatric and behavioural manifestations of normal pressure hydrocephalus. *Journal of Nervous and Mental Disease*, **164**, 51–5 (1977).

62. Lying-Tunell, U. Psychotic symptoms in normal pressure hydrocephalus. *Acta Psychiatrica Scandinavica*, **59**, 415–19 (1979).

63. Jeffreys, R.V. and Wood, M.M. Adult non-tumourous dementia and hydrocephalus. *Acta Neurochirurgica*, **45**, 103–14 (1978).

64. Mansheim, P. ECT in the treatment of a depressed adolescent with meningo-myelocoele, hydrocephalus and seizures. *Journal of Clinical Psychiatry*, **44**, 385–6 (1983).

65. Corbett, J.A., Krishnan, V., and Roy, M. Hydrocephalus associated with XO mosaicism (Turner's Syndrome). (In preparation.) (1992).

10 Social aspects of hydrocephalus

D. Simpson and R. Hemmer

INTRODUCTION

Hydrocephalus becomes a social problem when it impairs cerebral function to such an extent that the patient is handicapped in school, employment, or family life. The physical and intellectual disabilities caused by hydrocephalus have been discussed (Chapters 7 and 9); they are often increased, or even dominated, by the disabilities resulting from associated conditions such as cerebral palsy or myelomeningocele. In varying degrees or combinations, many cases of hydrocephalus suffer from intellectual retardation, leg weakness, faecal and/or urinary incontinence, epilepsy and impaired vision: these disabilities can all be major social handicaps. By no means all hydrocephalus patients are disabled: in many, successful surgical treatment or spontaneous arrest will preserve normal neurological function. Indeed, appropriate treatment by shunt placement will sometimes reverse functional impairments, especially mental impairment and disorders of gait. But the treatment of hydrocephalus has its own social costs and problems, and in some communities the economic costs of treatment are prohibitive. Macias[1] has noted that this is so, for example, in Mexico, where very many families live in poverty without real social security; the same is true in many parts of Africa and Asia. Even in richer communities, the treatment and upbringing of a child with hydrocephalus, especially with an associated myelomeningocele, represent a considerable financial burden, as well as an enormous emotional load on the child's family. In the longer term, maintenance of a shunt may have social and psychosocial costs: sudden shunt blockage can disrupt the patient's life, and the fear of blockage can in itself cause emotional stresses. Seemingly arrested hydrocephalus may also suddenly decompensate, with similar effects.[2,3]

PREVENTIVE CONSIDERATIONS

Since the surgical treatment of hydrocephalus is neither cheap nor invariably successful, it is important to consider whether this serious pathophysiological disorder can be prevented. Primary prophylaxis, in the sense of preventive treatment of the causative condition, is sometimes possible in cases due to causes operating after birth. Intraventricular haemorrhage due to prematurity, and neonatal meningitis, are important causes of acquired infantile hydrocephalus;

obstetrical trauma may also result in hydrocephalus presenting in infancy and even later. These causes of hydrocephalus are to a considerable degree amenable to preventive measures. Better obstetrical management has greatly reduced the incidence of trauma during delivery, and more effective antibiotics are reducing the severity of neonatal meningitis and (presumably) the likelihood of post-meningitic hydrocephalus. There is hope that some causes of prematurity will become preventable. Intrauterine microbial infection has been incriminated as a cause of preterm labour, and appropriate chemotherapy may increase the likelihood of delivery at full term[4] (Chapters 5 and 6). Most causes of congenital hydrocephalus are not at present amenable to primary preventive measures, but early antenatal diagnosis is often possible, and this does offer the possibility of secondary prevention, by abortion.

The antenatal diagnosis of hydrocephalus has been discussed in Chapter 5. The presence of an open neural tube defect (myelomeningocele or anencephaly) may be suspected if there is an elevated maternal serum level of alpha-feto-protein (AFP). Brock,[5] who pioneered this important screening procedure, found that some 80 per cent of all neural tube defects may be detected in this way. Elevated alpha-feto-protein in the amniotic fluid is found in an even higher percentage of cases. An elevated alpha-feto-protein level, whether in the serum or in the amniotic fluid, is not pathognomonic of a neural tube defect, and ultrasonic visualization of the lesion is always desirable. Serum screening for alpha-feto-protein can be offered routinely, and is usually done at the sixteenth week of gestation.

Amniocentesis may be done as the investigation of first choice if there is a family history of neural tube defect; Carter and Evans[6] found that a neural tube defect in an older sibling increased the risk to about 1 in 25, in a British population with an overall neural tube defect incidence of about 1 in 300. The risks are similar in Australia, a country with a lower incidence.[7]

Antenatal ultrasonography can visualize most cases of myelomeningocele and almost all cases of anencephaly. Ultrasound may also demonstrate significant ventricular enlargement as early as the seventeenth week (Fig. 10.1). However, the examination needs skill and patience: in our experience, routine obstetrical ultrasonography may not diagnose hydrocephalus or myelodysplasia during the first 20 weeks. Bernard et al.,[8] from the UK, have emphasized that ultrasound is not at present a substitute for maternal serum AFP screening: the procedures are complementary.

The combined procedures of maternal serum screening, amniocentesis in selected cases, and ultrasonography will detect most cases of neural tube defect, with or without hydrocephalus, at a gestational age when the fetus is not viable. This allows termination of pregnancy. For many communities and many parents, this is an acceptable choice, given that the life of a severely disabled child may be very unhappy, and a heavy burden on the parents and on the community, a burden which can be costed for the community,[9,10] but which is incalculable for

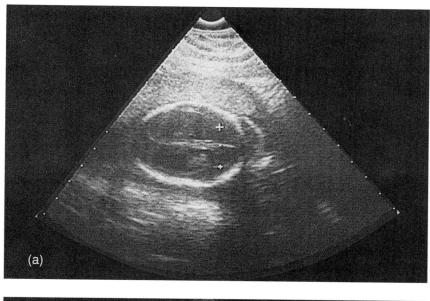

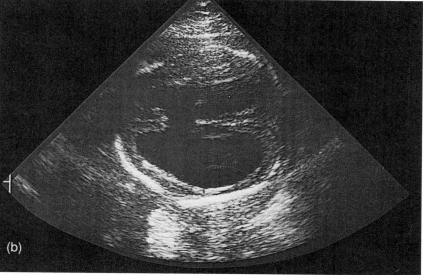

Fig. 10.1 Diagnosis of hydrocephalus in utero by ultrasound: the ventricular dilatation is clearly seen (a) at 17 weeks' and (b) at 24 weeks' gestation. The parents were initially reluctant to consider termination; however, the progress of the disease convinced them of the severity of the hydrocephalus, and pregnancy was terminated soon after the second sonogram.

the parents. Nevertheless, there are parents for whom abortion is not an acceptable procedure, and it is important to ensure that screening procedures are not done without explanation of the implications. Twin pregnancies, with one unaffected fetus, are an agonizing challenge even for parents who would wish a singleton pregnancy to be terminated. Selective feticide of the affected twin can be considered, but in two recent cases treated by one of us, the parents could not accept the risk to the normal fetuses, and in consequence two normal infants and two infants with paraplegia and very gross hydrocephalus have been born. It must however be emphasized that in the world today there are great variations in attitudes, both religious and legal, to 'prevention' by abortion. The Roman Catholic Church explicitly condemns termination of pregnancy if the malformation is compatible with life.[11] Many Protestant Christian theologians condone termination, explicitly or tacitly. This is also the case among exponents of the Jewish faith: in Israel today, secular law permits termination of pregnancy when there is a gross fetal malformation, and we are informed that some rabbis, even those of Orthodox convictions, have found this theologically acceptable. There is also diversity of opinion among the adherents of other great religions; a distinguished Hindu friend has told us that in his faith such a decision is left to the individual conscience, but in his country abortion is illegal under civil laws that are a legacy of a previous imperial administration. The problems become still more agonizing when the parents are adherents of different faiths, or have different views on the acceptability of life with severe disabilities.

Cases of hydrocephalus without myelomeningocele are also being diagnosed by ultrasound.[12] The presence of an associated gross cerebral anomaly may justify abortion. Examples of such gross anomalies include cephaloceles,[13] hydranencephaly, and holoprosencephaly. When a cephalocele contains a large mass of brain tissue extruded from the skull, then the outlook for mental normality is bad; the same is true when ultrasound shows virtual absence of the cerebral cortex (hydranencephaly) or fusion of the cerebral ventricles into a single cavity (holoprosencephaly). If it is decided to allow the pregnancy to go to term, serial monitoring of ventricular size will guide the obstetrician in deciding when and how to deliver the infant (see Chapter 5).

Antenatal diagnosis of a major fetal abnormality usually has important psychological repercussions: the parents may reject the diagnosis, or they may disagree on the best choice to make. They must be given the most exact possible ultrasonic diagnosis of the probable severity of the anomaly; thus, they may be helped if they can be told of the level of a myelomeningocele, and the severity of associated hydrocephalus. If they choose to allow the pregnancy to go on, or if the pregnancy is already advanced, then emotional support will be needed. If the pregnancy is terminated, grief and guilt may be helped by sensitive counselling.[14] In these varied situations, the obstetrician, the paediatric neurosurgeon, the social worker, the psychologist, and the minister of religion may all be involved; help may also come from the parent of a child with a similar abnormality, or from a victim of the condition. We stress especially the role of the neurosurgeon, who is usually best qualified to explain the probable significance of hydrocephalus and any associated malformation in terms of lifelong disability.

DISABILITIES AND HANDICAPS

The physical and intellectual disabilities suffered by people with hydrocephalus can be related to the pathology of the cerebral lesions, and to any associated spinal lesions. These disabilities can be measured objectively with reasonable accuracy, and many authors have published large series of cases of hydrocephalus with and without spina bifida. In the period before the advent of effective shunt treatment, Laurence[15,16] reported on 182 paediatric cases referred to a single neurosurgeon and not treated actively. For the present purpose, it is relevant that in 81 of these, the hydrocephalus appeared to have arrested and of these, 41 per cent had normal intelligence; moreover, 33 per cent had little or no physical disability. This careful study, and a similar Swedish study of untreated cases,[17] should not be taken too seriously today: these series were selected both by death, which eliminated many severe cases, and by the referral process, which doubtless excluded many less severe cases. But these early studies do remind us of what can still be seen in many developing countries: that untreated hydrocephalus is sometimes compatible with normal abilities. It is also true that untreated hydrocephalus can progress to total disability, with a vegetative level of function and an enormous, immobile head (Fig. 10.2). Surviving cases of this type can be seen often enough in all parts of the world, though they are happily becoming rare in developed countries. Modern treatment by shunting undoubtedly increases not only the chances of survival but also the quality of survival. This is most evident in cases of hydrocephalus without the complicating effects of spinal malformations or prematurity.[18]

Our own experience of the disabilities due to hydrocephalus is based on cases referred for paediatric neurosurgical management in two countries with quite similar socio-economic and medical characteristics, Freiburg-im-Breisgau (Germany) and Adelaide(Australia) (Table 10.1). The Freiburg experience with cases treated surgically between 1961–8 has been published in detail.[2,19–21] The Adelaide experience has been published briefly and incompletely reported.[22–24] One of us also has some experience of treating hydrocephalus in less fortunate countries, derived from brief periods of work as a visiting specialist in various medical centres in south-east Asia and elsewhere.

Intellectual disabilities

By the very simplistic measure of the Wechsler IQ scale, many cases of hydrocephalus function in the normal range (IQ score > 80): indeed, this was so in about half the patients in both the Freiburg (57 per cent) and the Adelaide (47 per cent) series. In both series there were a few of above average intelligence. Some aetiological types of hydrocephalus show, on average, better preservation of intelligence. Hemmer[21] found an average IQ of 92 ± 20.75 SD in cases of

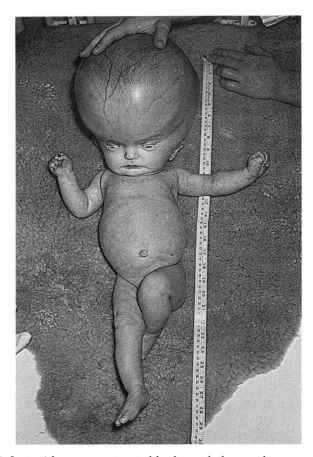

Fig. 10.2 Infant with severe untreated hydrocephalus: such cases are rarely seen in developed countries today, but are not rare in communities unable to afford surgical treatment.

hydrocephalus with spina bifida, higher than in other categories; in the Adelaide series, however, best results were seen in cases of aqueduct stenosis. Hydrocephalus due to obstruction of the aqueduct of Sylvius is of course not a disease entity: blockages of the aqueduct can result from many causes. In some cases, onset is in childhood rather than infancy, or even in adult life; late onset cases are likely to do well if treated properly. Most authors have noted that the worst outcomes are seen in cases of hydrocephalus secondary to meningitis or to severe closed head injury; such cases have often suffered severe brain damage from the infection or the head injury, rather than from the hydrocephalus.

Normality on the Wechsler scale does not necessarily mean normal intellect. As has been indicated (Chapters 7 and 9) many cases of hydrocephalus scoring

Table 10.1 Mobility in cases of myelodysplasia: reduced mobility is primarily due to the spinal impairment, but hydrocephalus was a contributory factor in some severely disabled cases. The Adelaide series was followed for 12–22 years, the Freiburg series for 3–15 years: this may explain the higher Adelaide incidence of wheelchair users, as this series includes some examples of delayed worsening.

Mobility	Adelaide series[24]		Freiburg series[21]	
	No. cases	% series	No. cases	% series
Normal	28	33.3	35	35
With crutches or appliances	23	27.4	40	40
In wheelchair	29	34.5	18	18
Virtually immobile (severe mental or physical disabilities)	1	1.2	7	7
Uncertain	3	3.6	—	—
Total	84	100	100	100

normally on the IQ scale have disabling impairments of concentration and memory. Nevertheless, it can be said that a substantial number of cases of surgically-treated hydrocephalus have no overt intellectual disabilities, and no consequent handicaps in school or employment. A somewhat larger number do have varying degrees of intellectual disability, but in the majority these disabilities do not prevent integration in normal school. Gross mental impairment does occur in a few cases, and may require education in a special school, or even institutional care in later life.

Uncomplicated hydrocephalus is less often associated with locomotor disabilities, though many cases do suffer from some degree of spastic leg weakness, especially in cases of hydrocephalus secondary to prematurity.[25] Lack of facility in fine finger movements is often also seen, and may be handicapping in competitive employment.

Incontinence

Most cases of myelomeningocele are incontinent of urine: this was so in 90 per cent of the Freiburg series and 86 per cent of the Adelaide series. Children who smell of urine are likely to be rejected by their peers, and faecal incontinence is also a great social handicap. Self-catheterization or an artificial urinary stoma will, however, usually achieve social continence, given proper training and accessible toilets; faecal incontinence is also as a rule manageable. The struggle to achieve social continence is most burdensome in the first few years of school life. In cases of hydrocephalus without myelomeningocele, sphincteric control is almost always normal.

Sexuality

In most cases of myelomeningocele, impairment of sacral cord function causes impotence in the male, though there are occasional well-attested exceptions. Chronic bladder infection may result in sterility. Females, on the other hand, can conceive and bear children: as early as 1969 Salmon[26] reported the memorable case of Jojo, a Marseillaise who achieved five magnificent infants (*sic*) despite sphincteric paralysis and bilateral leg amputations. This record of enterprise and fecundity is unequalled in the Freiburg and Adelaide series, but in both there have been fertile marriages. Hydrocephalus *per se* should not interfere with pregnancy; we have seen one case of serious malfunction of a ventriculoatrial shunt due to ascent of the diaphragm and passage of the atrial catheter into the cardiac ventricle, but this does not occur if the initial catheter position is relatively high. This is the only major complication that we have seen in pregnant women with ventriculoatrial shunts. We have no personal experience of pregnancy in women with peritoneal shunts, but Frolich *et al.*,[27] reporting three cases and reviewing the literature, found no difficulties attributable to the presence of the catheter in the abdomen. In cases of hydrocephalus complicated by epilepsy, the possibility of drug-induced malformations of the fetus needs consideration: all the common anticonvulsants have been blamed, carbamazepine (Tegretol) being the least suspect as a teratogen.

Epilepsy

Many hydrocephalic children experience at least one epileptic fit: this was recorded in 33 per cent of cases both in the Adelaide and Freiburg series, and Blaauw[28] found a similar incidence in a Dutch series. The causes of epilepsy in hydrocephalus have been discussed (see Chapter 7). From the social viewpoint, epilepsy is sometimes a serious disability, but in the majority of cases fits are infrequent and respond well to medication. In cases that do suffer from serious epilepsy, there are other signs of cerebral damage and often mental retardation: in the Freiburg series of hydrocephalic children with epilepsy, the average IQ was 73 ± 23.1, well below the series mean. However, there are exceptions: the Adelaide series includes a very intelligent young woman with aqueduct stenosis who suffers frequent temporal lobe seizures and occasional major fits. She has worked as a scientific technician and has borne two normal infants, while receiving primidone and carbamazepine, but the epilepsy is a very real handicap, since it debars her from driving a car. Such cases are, however, unusual, and in general epilepsy is not prominent among the social handicaps of people with hydrocephalus.

Visual impairment

Acute or chronic raised intracranial hypertension can damage vision. In the era before the advent of treatment by effective shunts, blindness from hydrocephalus was not very rare: Fraser and Friedmann,[29] in a study of 776 blind children in England and Wales, concluded that optic atrophy secondary to hydrocephalus was the leading cause of blindness from congenital malformations. Study of their protocols suggests that hydrocephalus was present in at least 15 (1.9 per cent) cases: a small but not insignificant element in the large social problem of blindness. Early diagnosis and effective treatment should prevent many of these tragedies. Nevertheless, cases still occur. In the Freiburg series, visual impairment from optic atrophy was recorded in 18 cases (11 per cent). Loss of vision can be the penalty of delay in diagnosing shunt blockage: an infant in the Adelaide series suffered acute bilateral occipital infarction (Fig. 10.3) and is left with cortical blindness. Severe visual impairment is obviously a social handicap: in most developed countries, education and employment for the blind are well established and often generously funded, but

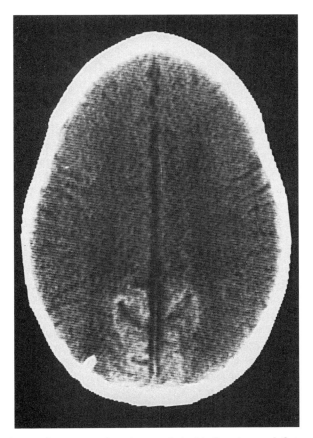

Fig. 10.3 Enhanced CT scan showing occipital infarction as bilateral hyperdense areas. This was a consequence of acute shunt blockage. The symptoms were not specific, and diagnosis was delayed.

hydrocephalics with visual loss often suffer from other disabilities and may have very limited educability. This was so in half the Freiburg cases of severe visual loss.

Deafness

This is a rare disability among hydrocephalics; there were four cases (2.5 per cent) in the Freiburg series. Interestingly, children with hydrocephalus often complain of increased sensitivity to noise (hyperacusis).

Psychosocial implications

Here, as elsewhere, it is necessary to distinguish between the effects of hydrocephalus and those of the associated impairments. The child with successfully treated hydrocephalus and no major disabilities can live a normal life: marriage, a career, and a full social life are all possible. In this group the chief psychosocial effect of the hydrocephalus lies in the possibility of shunt blockage. This can make residence distant from a neurosurgical unit very hazardous: in the Adelaide series, one very successfully treated girl died in coma during an air flight from her far distant home, with a blockage that was almost certainly remediable. It is very important to ensure that parents and family medical practitioners know the symptoms of shunt blockage; in most developed countries, air rescue services are well developed, and if the diagnosis is made, it should usually be possible to avoid a tragic outcome by flying the patient to a neurosurgical centre, dehydration by mannitol and/or frusemide being used to gain time.[23] There are, however, other adverse psychosocial effects of shunt malfunction. A fit, intelligent lad who has forgotten about his shunt for a decade or more suddenly has a blockage and an emergency operation. His confidence is abruptly shattered, and thereafter every headache is a threat to him. Such cases require very careful assessment and sensitive management. CT scanning, isotope shunt function tests, and even intracranial pressure manometry are often necessary to reassure the patient (and the physician); in occasional cases, psychiatric counselling may be required to assist such patients to regain their confidence and to live with the knowledge that blockages are unpredictable events in his or her life.

There are also a few physical restrictions on the life of a person with successfully treated hydrocephalus and no significant disabilities. Head injuries should be avoided: this is certainly so when there is ventricular dilatation, and probably also when the ventricles are small. Boxing should certainly be avoided, and probably also football: this is a social handicap for boys in communities that regard football highly, though in practice there are plenty of alternative winter sports that do not necessarily entail knocks on the head. Some employments are likely to be barred to someone with a shunt or with arrested hydrocephalus, such as the police or the armed forces.

The social problems are very different in those cases of hydrocephalus with major disabilities, whether from primary cerebral or cerebellar damage, from an associated spinal malformation, or from optic atrophy. There is an abundant literature setting out the impact of these disabilities in education, in employment, and in family life. Much of this literature relates only indirectly to hydrocephalus, since most writers are concerned with specific disabilities rather than with the causative disease process. An exception to this is spina bifida: the unique complexities of the hydrocephalus–myelomeningocele syndrome have attracted much attention, and much of what follows is based on our own experience in this field and on the publications of the Society for Research into Hydrocephalus and Spina Bifida. It has to be remembered that not every patient with spina bifida has significant hydrocephalus.

EDUCATIONAL NEEDS OF CHILDREN WITH HYDROCEPHALUS

In the past, and for very good reasons, disabled children were often segregated in special schools, usually with medical orientations; there were schools for the physically disabled, for children with intellectual retardation, for the blind, and even for such specialized problems as urinary incontinence. Such schools give protection, special teaching skills, and facilities for medical treatment where this is needed. But these advantages are offset by isolation from normal life, and often by a lack of the competitive spirit and the educational facilities to foster excellence. In most developed countries, educationists have rejected the philosophy of segregation in special schools, or even special classes. It has been argued that intellectual disabilities, unless very severe, can be accommodated in normal ('mainstream') classes, provided that teachers are numerous, sufficiently skilled, and not too busy to give one-to-one tuition. Locomotor disabilities can also be accommodated in normal schools, provided that classes are not inaccessible to pupils who move in wheelchairs or on crutches. Lifts and ramps are essential: any expedient which impairs independence, such as carrying a disabled child up a few steps, is to be condemned. Incontinence can also be accommodated, provided that timetables and toilets allow the disabled child opportunity and privacy to empty the bladder: younger children will need a carer (parent or visiting nurse) to help with this. Only the visually handicapped are likely to need a special school, at least initially, since the techniques of educating the blind are very specialized. When the Adelaide experience of spina bifida was first reviewed 20 years ago,[30] only 14 (27 per cent) of 52 children went to a school for the physically disabled, five (10 per cent) were ineducable, and the remainder (63 per cent) attended normal primary or secondary schools. With better school facilities, the percentage of children in special schools has fallen to 12 per cent. In the Freiburg series of 160 cases, special schools were used in 70 (43 per cent) of cases: interestingly, the proportion was much the same both for cases of myelomeningocele and for other types of hydrocephalus. In Germany also, the policy of placing disabled children in normal classes has further reduced the role of special schools.

Integration in a normal school has, theoretically, many advantages, and there are some objective studies showing that better educational achievements can be expected, as well as the social benefits of independence and association with able-bodied peers.[31,32] It is also optimistically believed that disabled children in a normal school do something to educate able-bodied children in humanity and breadth of mind.

Nevertheless, it seems likely that in most communities there is a place for the special school. Such schools can accommodate children needing continued medical treatment; they can also provide a refuge for those children who find a normal school too competitive or too cruel. Especially at the kindergarten level, the staff of a special school can prepare disabled children for the environment of the normal school, and can later assist schoolteachers in dealing with special educational problems. In Adelaide, the Regency Park Centre for Young Disabled, once only a residential school for crippled children, has found a new role in preparing children with disabilities for normal school and as a resource centre for children and schoolteachers alike. Such schools can also promote sports, games, and recreational hobbies for disabled children and adolescents.

Mainstream integration is an educational ideal that some individuals, and some communities, cannot always achieve. For the individual, a special school may offer a necessary sense of security and a comprehending, less competitive environment; for the community, a special school may be an easier option than providing schools with sufficiently well-trained teachers in sufficient numbers. We believe that in relatively affluent countries, comprehensive mainstream education is preferable and achievable in most cases; however, there should be flexibility in educational placing, and a readiness to use special schools or special classes when necessary. Such flexibility is best achieved if there is close liaison between teachers and medical practitioners; in practice, this means letters, visits, and case conferences.

Sport is also important for most children, and there are great difficulties in providing rewarding opportunities for sport in many cases of hydrocephalus. Quite apart from the limitations imposed by spinal or cerebral leg weakness, the impaired eye–hand coordination often seen in hydrocephalus can be a tremendous handicap. Non-competitive sports such as swimming and riding may be favoured, but competitive sports for the disabled have great value in many cases; wheelchair games and sports for the blind have been organized in most parts of the world, and the achievements of many disabled athletes have been spectacular (Fig. 10.4). Special schools, and adult organizations for disabled sport, can and do combine to give disabled children the excitements and the physical benefits of sports in competition against children with comparable disabilities.

Regional and inter-regional contests have been held for many years, and in August 1981, the first International Games for Disabled Children (aged 13–16 years) were held in Newcastle-on-Tyne, UK. International contests of this type enlarge the social experience of the participants enormously: they travel under

(a)

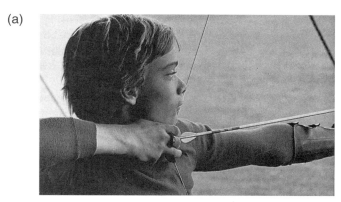

(b)

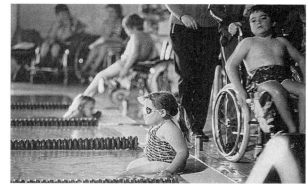

(c)

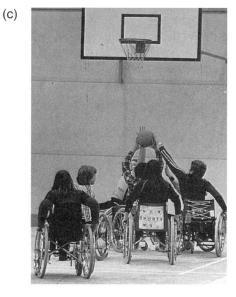

Fig. 10.4 Disabled child athletes, members of a team competing in (a) archery, (b) swimming, and (c) wheelchair basketball. In this team, all the children had spinal impairments; many also had hydrocephalus.

ideal conditions, they can make friendships with their peers in other countries, and they can gain maturity in an environment free from medical and parental supervision. Children and adults with hydrocephalus who enter into competitive games are usually categorized on the severity of associated impairments, for example paraplegia from myelodysplasia or blindness from optic atrophy. Wheelchair athletes are graded according to the level of the motor loss, on the basis of the experience of games for adults with acquired spinal injuries. This system of categorization may be somewhat unfair for the victim of congenital hydrocephalus, if there is an associated impairment of upper limb coordination. However, many people with hydrocephalus have overcome this additional handicap; at the Newcastle-on-Tyne games, 8 of the 22 Australian disabled athletes had hydrocephalus severe enough to need a shunt, and nevertheless received international acclaim in wheelchair racing, basketball, swimming, and archery.

HYDROCEPHALUS AND THE FAMILY

It has been said that a disabled child means a disabled family. The impact of disabilities often becomes evident very early. When hydrocephalus is congenital, the parents have to cope immediately with the emotional shock of a deformed or sickly infant, with the added dread of mental retardation: intelligent and ambitious parents are often especially shocked by these considerations, and may reject the infant. Less demanding parents may accept the hydrocephalic infant, but find the need for surgical treatment harder to comprehend. When hydrocephalus is diagnosed later in infancy, parental bonding is as a rule already established, and rejection is unlikely. However, a contrary problem of excessive concern may arise, and this can go on to an attitude of overprotection later in life. This is evident in some 50 per cent of the autobiographies of Freiburg patients.[21] Thus a 21-year-old girl with impaired vision but high intelligence (IQ 115) felt that her parents did not understand her ambitions and her hobbies.

I have left home because I had a difficult relationship with my parents, especially my mother, who clung to me from overanxiety. It was she who always made me aware that I was a problem child for her, and this role was again reinforced in my adolescence. She admitted to me that I had no future in independence, because I would need immediate help in the event of a shunt blockage, and seemingly only my family could do this. My father expressed his concern in narrow ideas about my career decision. He admitted to me that I had neither the ability nor the need for a higher school education or training for a career qualification. This came chiefly from his own job situation, he is an unskilled labourer. To this was added his experience with my sister, who married after the end of her education, which was therefore seemingly superfluous. I had a different relationship with my siblings. My brother (19-years-old) was always closer to me than my sister (26-years-old). She saw me as the most privileged one of us three children.

This bleak parental relationship was softened when the girl became the intimate friend of an older man, formed a circle of friends and found herself accepted.

When hydrocephalus is associated with myelomeningocele, the parents must often carry the burden of frequent illnesses, such as urinary infections and pathological fractures, and frequent operations. However, with good planning and conservative policies, the need for repeated orthopaedic and urological procedures can be reduced. Hospital out-patient attendances are always numerous for cases of hydrocephalus complicating spina bifida, and they are also numerous when the hydrocephalus is associated with cerebral palsy needing physiotherapy and other forms of habilitation. Even in cases of uncomplicated hydrocephalus, there is usually a need for out-patient attendances and occasional hospital admissions for shunt malfunctions: in the Adelaide series, the rate of shunt blockage was one per 5.6 years of life with a shunt, but only one case in five was entirely free from blockages.[23] Blockages are especially frequent in infancy: the parents must always be on guard for these major problems. They must also deal with mundane problems like clothes and shoes that wear out because of splints and orthoses, or frequent needs for laundry because of soiling: minor problems, but demanding in time and cumulatively costly.

The mother usually carries the chief burden: bringing up a disabled child is often a full-time job, and in the Freiburg series 69 per cent of all mothers were wholly committed to the home. This is an important deprivation, especially in societies in which housework has low prestige and women commonly hold jobs outside the house. The burden is less heavy in societies that involve grandparents and other family members in child-rearing, as in many parts of Asia. In societies such as Australia, where one in eight children now grows up in a single-parent family, the mother's burden is often increased by the absence of an effective father.

The father of a disabled child also carries substantial though less obvious burdens. In most marriages, he will be the provider of finances, and in no country known to us are the government benefits given for child disability likely to cover the costs and loss of maternal earnings. More subtly, he may find his disabled child engrossing his wife's time and emotional interests. He may well feel isolated, even neglected. Evans *et al.*[33] studied a cohort of fathers of children with spina bifida in Wales after 18 years: the divorce rate was not significantly elevated, but there was a very significant increase in illnesses, supposedly psychosomatic.

The siblings of a disabled child may also feel neglected, and indeed the pressures on their parents often make this really the case; a London study by Carr *et al.*[34] found that family social activities were restricted. Holidays, especially among working class families, usually had to include the disabled child; perhaps this is no bad thing in a united family, but it is of more concern that parents' outings by day and by night were markedly less frequent when the disabled child had a locomotor difficulty. Nearly half the mothers interviewed reported that they felt depressed and/or run-down. Nevertheless, the same study showed that the incidence of serious behavioural problems among siblings was actually lower than in a control population, and maternal stress was not measurably related either to the severity of the disability or to the degree of dependency.

It is a tribute to human spirit that very many families carry all these burdens successfully, and some appear to have been strengthened by the endeavour. The parents of one delightful, but severely disabled, girl with hydrocephalus have told us that the challenge had made them, and their other children, less egoistic and more loving; such families are not rare. Moilanen *et al.*[35] compared the family attitudes towards 55 Finnish children with uncomplicated hydrocephalus with those of controls: the families of hydrocephalic children were found to be significantly more cohesive and also more democratic, in that decisions and responsibilities were shared, and not dictated by traditional concepts of parental autocracy and its counterpart, rebellion by children and adolescents.

HYDROCEPHALUS IN ADULT LIFE

Many adults with hydrocephalus have achieved full employment and rewarding personal relationships, either because their disabilities were insignificant, or because their abilities outweighed their disabilities (Fig. 10.5). The Adelaide

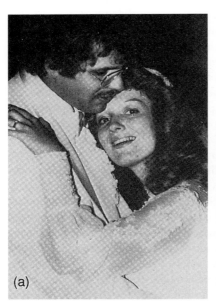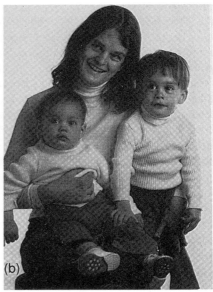

(a)   (b)

Fig. 10.5 Hydrocephalus in the family: (a) marriage of a 24-year-old secretary and (b) housewife, aged 24, with her two healthy children. Both women have surgically treated hydrocephalus. (Reproduced with permission from R. Hemmer, Der fruehkindliche Hydrozephalus.[21])

series includes examples of shunt-dependent hydrocephalics who have done well in university courses, banking, underground mining, and laboratory work. The Freiburg series has data on 102 adults who had left school by the end of 1984, 23 with myelomeningocele and 79 with other forms of hydrocephalus. Of these, 24 per cent had completed vocational training and were employed or ready for employment in a wide range of jobs, chiefly low-level positions in the service sector. Another 32 per cent were in training positions, mostly for better-paid employment of similar type; 27 per cent were in sheltered workshops. Both series record a substantial number of stable marriages or other partnerships. Psychiatric illness has not been prominent: cases of depression and social isolation have been encountered, but in a Freiburg series of 43 older cases, a standard personality questionnaire did not show a high incidence of such tendencies.

Even in developed countries, many hydrocephalic adults fail to obtain regular employment. In a recent study from Sheffield, there was a distressingly high (81 per cent) incidence of unemployment among adults with myelodysplasia, most of whom also had hydrocephalus.[36] Employment problems are greatest when there are significant intellectual disabilities. Locomotor disabilities can be over-come by making transport and workplace accessible to wheelchair users. In most developed countries, there are legislative measures enforcing wheelchair acces-sibility in public buildings; these are sometimes disregarded, especially by the more shameless public authorities, but consumer organizations for the disabled are increasingly able to demand their rights in this respect. Transport may be by private car or by appropriately modified public vehicles. Brief autobiographies of 20 young adults in the Freiburg series show how vital it is for the disabled person to have a driver's licence. In Germany, this is given only after a special assessment, and a speed limitation may be imposed: it is argued with some reason that a road crash would be especially detrimental to a hydrocephalic. In Australia, and in the United Kingdom, hydrocephalus receives no special consideration from licensing authorities: epilepsy, poor vision, and impaired manual motor control, however, may debar some people with hydrocephalus from driving. In Australia, persons with epilepsy are allowed to drive only if seizure-free for at least two years; some latitude is allowed when seizures are purely nocturnal. In other countries, more restrictive regulations are in force.

Does the adult with hydrocephalus face a shorter life span, with an earlier onset of old age? There are at present few if any data to answer this alarming question. Cases of spontaneously arrested hydrocephalus do sometimes show neurological worsening in middle life, but at present there is nothing to suggest that this is an inevitable event. Jansen[37] reviewed a cohort of 231 Danish cases diagnosed in the period 1946–1955 and found that most of the survivors were employed (57 per cent) or at least able to care for themselves (9 per cent): this does not suggest a high incidence of delayed cerebral failure, even in untreated cases, though the time base (21–35 years) may be considered too short. It is nevertheless true that adults with arrested hydrocephalus do sometimes show delayed neurological deterioration, sometimes from the hydrocephalus and sometimes from associated hydromyelia: one case in the Adelaide series slowly worsened from hydromyelia despite surgical treatment, and died at the age of 63.[38]

Efficient shunts have been in use in many parts of the world for some 30 years; in both Freiburg and Adelaide, many cases so treated have remained well for 25 years or more, and we see no reason for pessimism. Nevertheless, insurance companies are reluctant to insure the lives of persons known to be shunt-dependent.

Brackenridge,[39] in an authoritative work on medical aspects of life risks, concludes that 'only a very few carefully selected applicants having a history of hydrocephalus treated by a shunt procedure would be suitable candidates for life insurance.' No applicant is accepted during the first year, and a record of more than one blockage is taken as grounds for rejection. We believe that this view is unduly cautious, but there is a need for long-term actuarial studies to provide a firm basis for decision, both with respect to life insurance and in relation to eligibility for health insurance if this is conditional on a record of previous good health.

HYDROCEPHALUS AND THE COMMUNITY

A hydrocephalic infant makes moral and material demands on the community in which it is to live. In developed countries, infantile hydrocephalus is accepted as a treatable condition, and the necessary surgical and hospital treatments are made available at charges affordable by the parents, or in many countries under no direct charge at all: the community accepts the financial obligation and expenses are met from general revenue or by some kind of health insurance levy. The costs are obviously greatest when hydrocephalus is associated with myelomeningocele. In 1981, the in-patient and out-patient costs of a live-born infant with myelomeningocele treated in South Australia averaged about A$12 000; in 1989 this would amount to about US$9500. This was a tolerable cost in a community which then had a per capita annual gross national product of about US$12 000, given that only ten such infants were then surviving annually in South Australia; given also that euthanasia was not acceptable in this community, it is evident that refusal to treat would often be very expensive. It is true to say that in wealthy communities, surgical treatment of hydrocephalus is usually less costly than long-term institutional care. O'Brien and McLanahan[40] in 1981 alleged that the government of the US State of Georgia had issued the remarkable ruling that no infant with hydrocephalus and myelodysplasia could be admitted to any state medical facility unless a shunt was performed, and presumably this was on fiscal rather than humanitarian grounds, since these authors do not record any official objection to sending untreated infants to die in their homes.

Hydrocephalus not associated with myelodysplasia is usually a much less costly condition, since there are fewer long-term disabilities: even so, the standard operative treatment by a shunt may constitute a formidable expenditure in many developing countries.

We have tried to cost the treatment of hydrocephalus in different parts of the world by personal enquiries from neurosurgical colleagues in a number of centres in America, Africa, and Asia. It proved impossible to get meaningful estimates of the overall costs, but many prices for imported US-made shunts were received, and it is clear that these vary considerably from country to country. Thus, in Australia, the shunts bought in 1989 cost the equivalent of US$355–590 per three-piece unit; a comparable shunt sold in Malaysia at the equivalent of US$240–280.

These price variations represent many factors, such as governmental tax policies, retailers' profit margins, and the very real generosity of some suppliers. In an endeavour to make meaningful comparisons, we took the cost of a well-known one-piece shunt system, which in January 1990 sold in the USA at a retail price of about US$130, and considered this as a percentage of the per capita gross domestic product (GDP) of various countries with well-established neurosurgical services. (Figures for GDP were taken either from the *International Financial Statistics Yearbook*[41] or from a World Health Organization source[42]). In affluent countries such as the USA and western Germany, with per capita GDP around US$20 000, this price represented about 0.7 per cent of the per capita GDP. In Australia, a country then enjoying precarious prosperity, the same shunt sold at a somewhat higher retail price: even so, the cost was only about 1.8 per cent of the per capita GDP. South Africa, Mexico, and Malaysia are prosperous developing countries with GDP then in the range US$2000–2500: the quoted price would represent about 6 per cent of this, and it is understandable that neurosurgeons in these and similar countries see the cost of the shunt itself as a significant commitment. In the Socialist Republic of Vietnam, a country with long-established neurosurgical services, the per capita GDP in 1985 was reportedly[42] US$110: the cost of a shunt would, therefore, represent about 100 per cent of this figure, and it is not surprising that shunt procurement is difficult.

It is likely that such difficulties are as great, or even greater, in many parts of Africa and South America. In communities which are devastated by famine, war, AIDS, and other endemic diseases, hydrocephalus cannot be given a high priority by health economists, and few cases will undergo surgical treatment. Untreated cases often survive for years, and since parental love is not proportional to the wealth of the community, neurosurgical visitors to developing countries are often besought to treat hydrocephalic infants. The results of such treatment can be very saddening, since theatre asepsis may be poor, and even a successful operation may be only the prelude to later death from shunt blockage or infection. One approach to this situation is to devise cheaper shunts, and to improve local neurosurgical services. In India, the cost of the US-made one-piece shunt is about 50 per cent of the current per capita GDP. However, Upadhyaya[43] has devised an efficient shunt which in 1989 sold at about Rs130

(US$8.00), and which has given good results in a large series of cases. Upadhyaya (personal communication, 1989) indicates that some 80–90 000 shunts have been distributed. This very creditable achievement reminds us that in developed countries, the consumer of medical products may pay not only for a high standard of workmanship, but also for a high profit margin and for insurance against litigation. However, the provision of a cheap shunt does not end the commitment by a community: there must also be a surgical service to maintain the shunt at short notice, and medical practitioners alert to the symptoms of shunt blockage.

The community costs of hydrocephalus, and of the associated disabilities, go beyond the provision of medical services. Special education is expensive: Hagard *et al.*[9] found that the annual excess costs in primary schooling of a Scottish child with myelomeningocele represented 28 per cent of the medical costs incurred in the first year of life, secondary schooling being a smaller annual charge. In most developed countries, the costs of special schooling are largely met from public revenue, though private charity is important in many places. Other obvious community charges relate to the provision of public transport, access to buildings, and the funding of workshops and activity centres. National approaches vary in these areas according to ideology and resources. Even within nations and states, there are often very considerable local variations: local or municipal authorities may be richer or poorer, more or less responsible or shameless, disability pressure groups more or less eloquent. It is true to say that in the last 20 years there has been increasing worldwide concern over the welfare of the disabled; initially this was voiced chiefly by medical practitioners and social workers, but latterly organizations for the disabled have been able to present the consumer viewpoint, often with great eloquence.

However adequate the social services may be, a disabled child is a heavy financial drain on the family, and a disabled adult has financial needs that go beyond the requirements for life support. In many Western communities, disabilities due to accident are considered to deserve financial 'compensation', and such compensation payments can be enormous, especially if some person or institution can be held legally at fault. It is very rare for hydrocephalus to be a legally compensable condition, though occasionally legal ingenuity will find grounds for a suit for medical negligence. Recognizing this, many countries provide financial support for the parents of a disabled child and for the disabled adult, usually in the form of a periodic payment or pension, though special problems, such as distant residence or a need for an aid to mobility, are often funded in other ways. Thus, in Australia in 1990, the combined family and disability allowances for a severely disabled child amounted to A$1929 (US$1470) per annum, with additional refunds for travel on medical grounds and provision of aids to mobility, for example wheelchairs. A completely disabled adult received A$6947 (US$5280) per annum. These figures should be related to the national per capita GDP, then about US$12 000. Provisions in other countries vary and are often supplemented from private charity. In developing countries, the support of disabled children and adults is often provided, if at all, by street begging. Peter Rickham,[44] a great paediatric surgeon with a special interest in hydrocephalus, once quoted a professor of moral theology, to the effect that the moral calibre of a society can be judged by the care it gives to its sick, especially to those who have nothing to contribute directly to society. This yardstick is acceptable only if one remembers that the quality of care cannot be costed in financial terms alone: in many impoverished countries, one can see parental care of a quality that shames what is offered in many affluent societies. This is so in some Australian aboriginal tribes; several Adelaide cases of hydrocephalus treated by shunts have lived long and seemingly happy lives in remote tribal or partially tribal settings. Their lives are precarious, since their shunts may block, but they are nevertheless valued members of their families, despite their obvious disabilities.

CONCLUSIONS

Other authors in this book have shown that hydrocephalus can be treated effectively, though with an important incidence of complications. Shunt infection remains a troublesome problem, though good asepsis and antibiotic prophylaxis may reduce the incidence of this. Shunt blockage is even more troublesome; one hopes that better designed, flow-dependent valves may reduce the very real hazards of shunt-dependency. In this chapter, we have reviewed the social implications of current methods of treatment. Experience has shown that with proper management, hydrocephalus is compatible with virtually normal life; nevertheless, many cases of hydrocephalus are severely disabled, either because the condition was not treated until there was irreversible damage, or as a result of associated conditions like meningitis or myelodysplasia.

Neurological disabilities impose great burdens on the victims, and on their families; their disabilities also impose socio-economic burdens on the communities in which they live. In affluent communities, these burdens are tolerable, and with improved shunt technology will doubtless become still more so. In impoverished communities, there are other medical and social problems that have more immediate importance, and higher priority, than the requirements of hydrocephalic infants and children.

Research workers in the fields of hydrocephalus and of neurological disability should not neglect the importance of devising cost–effective management strategies that have wide applications throughout the world.

ACKNOWLEDGEMENTS

We thank Hippokrates Verlag, Stuttgart, for permission to reproduce Fig. 10.5 from *Der fruehkindliche Hydrozephalus,*[21] Dr M. Furness of the Adelaide Medical Centre for Women and Children for the sonograms in Fig. 10.1, and the Spina Bifida Society of South Australia for Fig. 10.4. We have received generous advice from colleagues and officials in many countries: we thank especially Dr F. Rueda-Franco (Mexico), Dr J. Maigrot (Mauritius), Dr V. Gunasekaran (Malaysia), Dr J.C. Peter (South Africa), Professor A. Sahar (Israel), Professor P. Upadhyaya (Saudi Arabia), and HE the High Commissioner of India in Australia. We are obliged to the Department of Medical Art, Adelaide Medical Centre for Women and Children, for preparation of illustrations. We thank Dr A. Carney and Miss A. Inglis for advice and help in the preparation of this chapter. And lastly, we thank the German, Australian, and Vietnamese patients, and their parents, who over the last 30 years have taught us the social significance of hydrocephalus.

REFERENCES

1. Macias, R. Surgical indications of myelomeningocele. *International Society for Pediatric Neurosurgery, Proceedings of 13th Annual Meeting*, p. 55 (1985).
2. Hemmer, R. and Boehm, B. Once a shunt, always a shunt? *Developmental Medicine and Child Neurology*, **18** (Suppl. 37), 69–73 (1976).
3. Vaishnav, A. and MacKinnon, A.E. Progressive hydrocephalus in teenage spina bifida patients. *Zeitschrift für Kinderchirurgie*, **41** (Suppl. 1), 36–7 (1986).
4. Romero, R. and Mazor, M. Infection and preterm labor. *Clinical Obstetrics and Gynecology*, **31**, 553–84 (1988).
5. Brock, D.J.H. Impact of maternal alpha-foeto-protein screening on antenatal diagnosis. *British Medical Journal*, **285**, 365–7 (1982).
6. Carter, C.O. and Evans, K. Spina bifida and anencephalus in Greater London. *Journal of Medical Genetics*, **10**, 209–34 (1973).
7. Field, B. Neural tube defects in New South Wales, Australia. *Journal of Medical Genetics*, **15**, 329–38 (1978).
8. Bernard, S.H., Walsworth-Bell, J.P., Super, M., Read, A.P., and Harris, R. A survey of neural tube defect pregnancies in North-West England. *Zeitschrift für Kinderchirurgie*, **43** (Suppl. 11), 15–16 (1988).
9. Hagard, S., Carter, F., and Milne, R.G. Screening for spina bifida cystica. A cost–benefit analysis. *British Journal of Preventive and Social Medicine*, **30**, 40–53 (1976).
10. Glass, N.J. and Cove, A.R. Cost effectiveness of screening for neural tube deformities. In *Towards the prevention of fetal malformations*, (ed. Scrymgeour, J.B), pp. 217–23. Edinburgh, University Press Edinburgh (1978).
11. Sacred Congregation for the Doctrine of the Faith. Declaration on procured abortion. In *Vatican II. More post conciliar documents*, (ed. Flannery, A.), Vol. 2, pp. 441–53. W.B. Eerdmans, Grand Rapids, Michigan (1982).
12. Drugan, A., Krause, B., Canady, A., Zador, I.F., Sacks, A.J., and Evans, M.I. The natural history of prenatally diagnosed cerebral ventriculomegaly. *Journal of the American Medical Association*, **261**, 1785–8 (1989).
13. Simpson, D.A., David, D.J., and White, J. Cephaloceles: Treatment, outcome and antenatal diagnosis. *Neurosurgery*, **15**, 14–21 (1984).
14. Lloyd, J. and Laurence, K.M. Response to termination of pregnancy for genetic reasons. *Zeitschrift für Kinderchirurgie*, **38** (Suppl. 11), 98–9 (1983).

15. Laurence, K.M. The natural history of hydrocephalus. *Lancet*, **ii**, 1152–4 (1958).
16. Laurence, K.M. and Coates, S. Further thoughts on the natural history of hydrocephalus. *Developmental Medicine and Child Neurology*, **4**, 263–7 (1962).
17. Hagberg, S. and Sjogren, I. The chronic brain syndrome of infantile hydrocephalus. A follow-up study of 63 spontaneously arrested cases. *American Journal of Diseases of Children*, **112**, 189–96 (1966).
18. Fernell, E., Hagberg, S., Hagberg, G., Hult, H., and von Wendt, L. Epidemiology of infantile hydrocephalus in Sweden: a clinical follow-up study in children born at term. *Neuropediatrics*, **19**, 135–42 (1988).
19. Hemmer, R. *Dringliche chirurgische Eingriffe an Gehirn, Rückenmark und Schädel im frühen Sauglingsalter*. Ferdinand Enke Verlag, Stuttgart (1969).
20. Hemmer, R. and Potthoff, P.C. Die Ventilinsuffizienz bei ventriculo–auriculaeren Drainage. *Zeitschrift für Kinderchirurgie*, **8**, 12–16 (1970).
21. Hemmer, R. *Der fruehkindliche Hydrozephalus*. Hippokrates Verlag, Stuttgart (1983).
22. Beal, S., Carney, A., Manson, J.I., and Simpson D.A. Hydrocephalus in childhood: survival and quality of survival. *Proceedings of the 15th International Congress of Pediatrics*, (ed Ghai, O.P and Taneja P.N), pp. 945–50. Indian Academy of Pediatrics, New Delhi (1977).
23. Simpson, D.A. Living with hydrocephalus. *British Medical Journal*, (Editorial), **288**, 813–14 (1984).
24. Simpson, D., Carney A., and Creswell, J. Myelomeningoceles: validity of early postnatal assessment. *Journal of Pediatric Neurosciences*, **1**, 187–202 (1985).
25. Fernell, E., Hagberg, B., Hagberg, G., Hult, G., and von Wendt, L. Current aspects of the outcome in preterm infants. *Neuropediatrics*, **19**, 143–5 (1988).
26. Salmon, M. Symposium sur les myelomeningoceles et leurs complications. *Annales de chirurgie infantile* **10**, 13–14 (1969).
27. Frolich, E.P., Russell, J.M., and van Gelderen, C.I. Pregnancy complicated by maternal hydrocephalus. A report of three cases. *South African Medical Journal*, **70**, 358–60 (1986).
28. Blaauw, G. Hydrocephalus and epilepsy. *Zeitschrift für Kinderchirurgie*, **25**, 341–5, (1978).
29. Fraser, G.R. and Friedmann, I.A. *The causes of blindness in childhood*. Johns Hopkins Press, Baltimore (1967).
30. Carney, A., Newbold, D.B., and Simpson, D.A. Spina bifida in South Australia. Problems in education. *Medical Journal of Australia*, **2**, 993–6 (1971).
31. Lonton, A.P., Cole, M.S.J., and Mercer, J. The integration of spina bifida children — are their needs being met? *Zeitschrift für Kinderchirurgie*, **41** (Suppl. 1), 45–7 (1986).
32. Tew, B.J. Spina bifida children in ordinary schools: handicap, attainment and behaviour. *Zeitschrift für Kinderchirurgie*, **43** (Suppl. 11), 46–8 (1988).
33. Evans, O., Tew, B., and Laurence, K.M. The fathers of children with spina bifida. *Zeitschrift für Kinderchirurgie*, **40** (Suppl. 1), 42–4 (1986).
34. Carr, J., Pearson, A., and Halliwell, M. The effect of disability on family life. *Zeitschrift für Kinderchirurgie*, **38** (Suppl. 11), 103–6 (1983).
35. Moilanen, I., Meira, L., Serlo, W., and von Wendt, L. Psychosocial adaptations of hydrocephalic children. *Zeitschrift für Kinderchirurgie*, **40** (Suppl. 1), 31–3 (1985).

36. Lonton, A.P., Laughlin, A.M., and O'Sullivan, A.M. The employment of adults with spina bifida. *Zeitschrift für Kinderchirurgie*, **39** (Suppl. 2), 132–4 (1984).
37. Jansen, J. A retrospective analysis 21 to 35 years after birth of hydrocephalic patients born from 1946 to 1955. An overall description of the material and the criteria used. *Acta Neurologica Scandinavica*, **71**, 436–47 (1985).
38. Hanieh, A. and Simpson, D.A. Cavitation of the spinal cord in association with spina bifida. *Zeitschrift für Kinderchirurgie*, **31**, 321–6 (1980).
39. Brackenridge, R.D.C. *Medical selection of life risks*, (2nd edn.), pp. 638–41. Nature Press, Basingstoke (1985).
40. O'Brien, M.S. and McLanahan, C.S. Review of the neurosurgical management of myelomeningocele at a regional pediatric medical center. *Concepts in Pediatric Neurosurgery*, **1**, 202–15 (1981).
41. *International financial statistics yearbook*. International Monetary Fund, Washington, DC (1989).
42. *Western Pacific Region Data Bank on Socioeconomic and Health Indicators*. World Health Organization, Manila (1987).
43. Upadhyaya, P., Bhargava, S., Dube, S., Sundaram, K.R., and Ochaney, M. Results of ventriculo–atrial shunt surgery for hydrocephalus using Indian shunt valve: evaluation of intellectual performance with particular reference to computerized axial tomography. *Progress in Pediatric Surgery*, **15**, 209–22 (1982).
44. Rickham, P. The swing of the pendulum: the indications for operating on myelomeningocele. *Medical Journal of Australia*, **2**, 743–6 (1976).

Appendix: growth charts

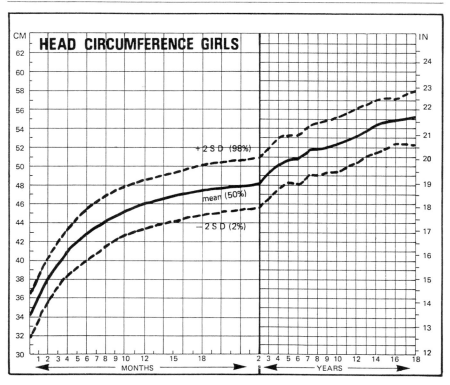

Fig. A.1 Head circumference chart for girls from birth to 18 years of age.

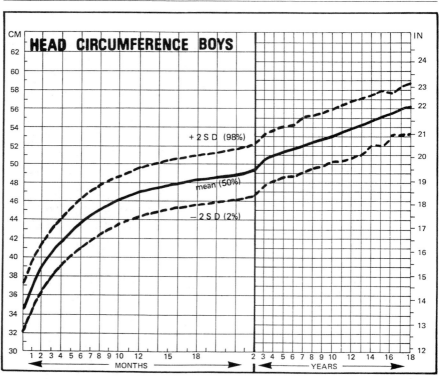

Fig. A.2 Head circumference chart for boys from birth to 18 years of age.

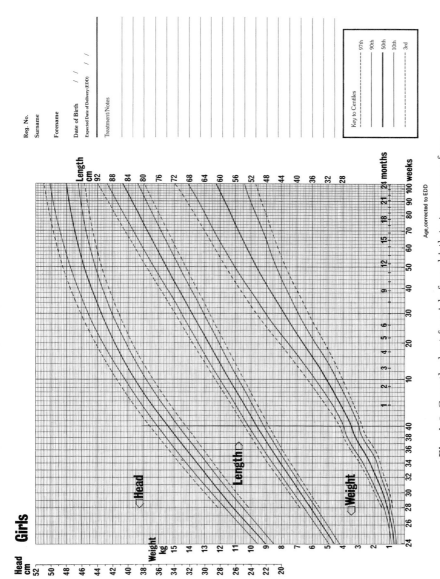

Fig. A.3 Growth chart for girls from birth to two years of age.

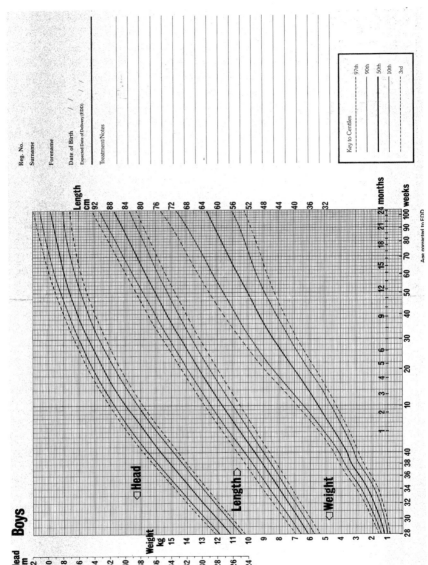

Fig. A.4 Growth chart for boys from birth to two years of age.

Index